Diploma Mill

Diploma Mill

The Rise and Fall of Dr. John Buchanan and the Eclectic Medical College of Pennsylvania

David Alan Johnson

The Kent State University Press ⬚ Kent, Ohio

Contents

Illustrations

Illustrations

Tables

Preface

I first encountered Dr. John Buchanan eight years ago while working on a history of medical regulation. At the time, I was researching a diploma scandal in 1923 involving several state medical boards. While reading various medical journals covering that scandal, I ran across references to Buchanan diplomas, along with assertions that the story I was researching constituted the worst diploma scandal since that of John Buchanan in 1880.

The phrasing in those stories piqued my interest. Their terse references to Buchanan seemed almost a form of insider shorthand, signaling their assumption that anyone familiar with medical licensing in the early 1920s would recognize immediately the allusion they were making, and that their readers would know not only who John Buchanan was but also what was implied by the phrase "Buchanan diploma." These writers were alluding to a man and a scandal in the history of American medical regulation that had occurred more than forty years earlier, yet they referenced Buchanan without offering any details of his misdeeds, confident that their readers would recognize the magnitude of the current scandal through their comparison of it with the scandal involving John Buchanan in 1880.

When I began investigating this subject in earnest several years later, even cursory research soon provided sufficient information to underscore the extent of Buchanan's diploma mill activities. I learned that John Buchanan and the Eclectic Medical College of Pennsylvania (EMC) represented the single biggest diploma mill of the nineteenth century and easily the best known. If that had been the extent of the story, however, I would have stopped digging at that point. Instead, a series of melodramatic incidents punctuating his career drew me ever deeper into Buchanan's story, notably his alleged suicide, his flight from justice, and the sensational events regarding his estate after his death. I became entangled in a story woven out of threads drawn from a variety of important mid- to late-nineteenth-century issues—the fitful steps toward modernizing medical education, the rebirth of medical licensing laws, the internecine conflicts

among the various schools of thought in American medicine, race relations in Philadelphia and America, and the rise of penny press newspapers
and investigative journalism—all of them fascinating.

I have structured *Diploma Mill* into three parts to reflect this tapestry
of events and help orient the reader. Part I describes the broad historical
context in which Buchanan implemented his criminal enterprise. This
section of *Diploma Mill* addresses not only the rise of eclectic medicine
as part of a reform movement in American medicine but the rise of the
Eclectic Medical College of Pennsylvania and John Buchanan specifically.
This portion of the book attempts to explain how and why Buchanan and
the EMC drifted into the sale of diplomas. Part II explores the critical
events of 1871–72 as a turning point in Buchanan's career, events including
his unsuccessful run for the Pennsylvania state legislature, a state senate
investigation of the school, the revocation of the EMC charter, and the
subsequent Pennsylvania Supreme Court decision that resurrected them
both. This section of the book also addresses the critical role played by
the reemergence of medical licensing laws in the United States at that
time. Part III relates the fall of Buchanan and the EMC triggered by the
melodramatic events that so captured my attention when I initially discovered them. In this section of the book, the narrative shifts to the events
of 1880–1881 (e.g., Buchanan's fake suicide, the manhunt for him, and
his criminal trial) and the cat-and-mouse game conducted between John
Buchanan and John Norris, editor of the *Philadelphia Record*, who almost
single-handedly brought down Buchanan and his school.

Every extended written work presents its own stylistic issues, requiring conscious decisions by the author. Several from this book warrant
mention. The first arises in Part I, regarding the use of contemporary
nineteenth-century labels applied to various philosophies of medicine and
their practitioners. Writers of the period, especially physicians, routinely
drew a line of demarcation dividing all physicians into two broad camps.
On one side stood the medical orthodoxy, with its physicians variously
identified as "regulars," "Old School" practitioners, and "allopaths."
These doctors were the intellectual descendants of Benjamin Rush and
others whose practices reflected the American medical norm in the late

eighteenth- and early nineteenth centuries. In modern parlance, these physicians represented the medical establishment.

On the other side stood all other physicians, categorized broadly as "irregulars." Under this umbrella we find physicians identifying themselves as botanics (later called physiomedicals), those naming themselves homeopaths, and the eclectics, who initially styled themselves as "Reformed" practitioners. Orthodox physicians, situated on the other side of this demarcation, scornfully referred to these irregulars by the derogatory epithet of "medical sects." Without question, the naming conventions (e.g., Old School, irregulars, sects) reflected the bias of the respective groups on either side of this divide. My use of these terms is intended solely to facilitate the readers' ease in following what may be unfamiliar players in an equally unfamiliar landscape. I intend no disparagement when using terms such as *irregulars* and *Old School*, although I am cognizant of the biases inherent in this terminology.

Another stylistic issue concerns the array of names for schools, organizations, and agencies inevitable in any written history in the field of medical education and medical regulation. Since constant use of the full titles of these institutions would be wearisome, I have opted to use established acronyms or shortened titles after the first use of the full name or have supplied one if none existed, referring to the Eclectic Medical College of Pennsylvania, for example, as the EMC.

Small portions of this book have been previously published, first appearing in my article "John Buchanan's Philadelphia Diploma Mill and the Rise of State Medical Boards," which was published in the *Bulletin of the History of Medicine* 89, no. 1 (Spring 2015): 25–58. All reference sources for this history appear in the endnotes.

Acknowledgments

Writing a book is a labor of love, but make no mistake: however dearly felt the subject matter, the labor involved is how authors pay their dues and for which they in turn have the privilege of formally acknowledging the contributions of others. I have been particularly fortunate, benefiting from the support of many individuals. I am deeply grateful to Professor James Mohr of the University of Oregon for his wise counsel on this book project and early reading of draft chapters. His guidance proved invaluable. Two of my colleagues at the Federation of State Medical Boards, Drew Carlson and Frances Cain, offered encouragement throughout this process, as well as keen eyes in proofreading the manuscript. Special thanks go to the Federation's president and CEO, Dr. Hank Chaudhry, who encouraged me to continue my efforts in historical research and publication.

Research can often be tedious and fruitless, as one chases down side paths that sometimes parallel and then rejoin the main trail but just as often lead nowhere. I am indebted to several people and institutions for their assistance in my research. My thanks go to staff in the newspaper reading room of the Philadelphia Free Library and to the library staff at the Historical Society of Pennsylvania. Special thanks go to Alex Herrlein and Devhra Bennett Jones at the Lloyd Library and Museum in Cincinnati, Ohio. Their kindness and prompt responses made it easy for me to remotely access several of the manuscripts housed at their institution. I would also like to thank Trish Weaver and Shelley Green at the National Board of Medical Examiners for tracking down a frustratingly elusive Pennsylvania Supreme Court case, *Allen v. Buchanan*. Connie King and Nicole Joniec, of the Library Company of Philadelphia, assisted me in finding several of Buchanan's publications and his political document "To my colored brothers of the Fourth Legislative District," as well as in digital image acquisition. Anne Brogan, Beth Lander, and their colleagues at the College of Physicians of Philadelphia proved most helpful, sharing manuscript materials on the Eclectic Medical College of Pennsylvania and on Drs. St. John Watkins Mintzer and William Paine, along with digital images of several items in their holdings. Kaitlyn Pettengill, archivist at the Historical Society of Pennsylvania, assisted with several digital image requests. I would also like to acknowledge the assistance of the Manuscript and Visual Collections Department of the William Henry Smith Memorial Library, associated with the Indiana Historical Society, in granting permission to print the photograph of Willis R. Revels. My thanks go to Katie Rudolph of the Denver Public Library for assistance with manuscript materials on EMC graduate Michael Beshoar, and to Christy Fic of the Ezra Lehman Memorial Library at Shippensburg University for helping me obtain copies of the *National Police Gazette*. My thanks as well go to Jaclyn Penny of the American Antiquarian Society for sharing the lyric broadsheet "Bogus Dr. John," to Thomas Lisanti of the New York Public Library for the image of John Buchanan, and to Arlene Shaner of the New York Academy of Medicine for an image of the Eclectic Medical College of Pennsylvania.

This book has benefited from the aid of these individuals and of others, whose contributions, great and small, have strengthened this story about a largely forgotten but consequential criminal episode in American medicine. The success of this book is attributable in part to these friends and colleagues. Any deficiencies, errors, or omissions rest with me.

Introduction

Despite the renown and infamy of John Buchanan and the Eclectic Medical College of Pennsylvania (EMC) at the height of their fame in 1880, very little of their story has survived in either the general or scholarly literature on the history of American medicine. On the one hand, this omission surprises because the story of Buchanan and the EMC resides at the intersection of three major developments in mid- to late-nineteenth-century American medicine: the aspirations of a fledgling medical profession, the advent of critical changes in medical education, and the rebirth of medical licensing laws throughout the United States. These intertwined threads from three distinct but complementary aspects of American medicine form the backdrop for the story of John Buchanan and the EMC.[1] The omission of this story also surprises because of the inherent fascination of such a dramatic and sensational tale. The descent of both Buchanan and his school into blatant criminal activities presented nineteenth-century readers with a riveting human-interest story that had the added benefit of a strong moral element in an era distinctly partial to instructive tales.

On the other hand, one could argue that the noticeable absence of John Buchanan and the EMC from the main stream of medical literature should come as no surprise at all, since Buchanan and the EMC were an acute embarrassment to the medical community, a front-page reminder of the failure of emerging medical professionalism and regulation. The twenty years of John Buchanan's medical practice and association with the EMC, from 1860 to 1880, coincided with profound developments in the medical profession as well as in medical education and licensing. The growing pains of these respective fields included the notable failure of physicians, educators, and regulators to work effectively and collaboratively with state legislators and leading professionals to eradicate an emerging, persistent problem—medical diploma mills. This failure allowed a dark corner of medical education to flourish even as physicians worked steadily to acquire the accoutrements of a genuine profession.

As several historians have noted, many mid-nineteenth-century physicians viewed themselves as professionals long before achieving recognition as such before the law. Despite the absence of the formal disciplines and mechanisms defining a profession, such as controlled entry into the field and oversight by fellow professionals, they regarded themselves as professionals. They believed that as physicians they were engaged in a distinct profession, as opposed to merely an occupation. Until later in the nineteenth century, this view of their status derived as much from their actual practice of medicine as from a shared body of knowledge with commonly accepted therapeutic regimens. And while physicians collectively sought greater social recognition and financial remuneration, they understood that only the enactment of legal constraints on the practice of medicine would ultimately consolidate the place of medicine as a true profession.[2]

To gain the desired legal recognition for the practice of medicine, physicians recognized that difficult questions would have to be addressed. For instance, what defined a physician? Was it mastery of a shared body of knowledge that reflected the physician as a professional? If so, who or what defined the parameters of this knowledge? Or was the role of physician defined by the possession of a credential (i.e., a medical degree)? If so, what educational standard should this credential reflect? Such questions were particularly problematic in the mid-nineteenth century, when the scientific underpinnings for much of medicine remained (from a modern perspective) relatively weak.

One result of these inherent definitional weaknesses was the flourishing of a variety of philosophical approaches to the practice of medicine. Some of these philosophical approaches, such as homeopathy or the botanically based eclectic practice of medicine, represented major challenges to the medical orthodoxy of the day. (Osteopathic medicine represented another challenger, but its growth and formalization in the 1890s fall outside the chronological focus of this narrative.) In this context, Buchanan's practice as a physician and role within the American reformed or eclectic school of medicine proved a bitter disappointment to the founders of the EMC and their dreams that the school would become the standard-bearer for eclectic medical education on the east coast, and ultimately an embarrassment to eclectics across the country.

In addition to its effect on the establishment of medicine as a profession, the story of John Buchanan and the Eclectic Medical College of Pennsylvania also resides in the world of nineteenth-century medical education. In many ways, the contentiousness, variability, and sometimes blurred boundaries among and between mid-nineteenth-century physicians and the profession as a whole were replicated within the medical schools of that era. One of the fundamental problems confronting many of these schools, including the EMC, stemmed from their governing and financial structures. Typical of the overwhelming majority of schools during this period, the EMC operated independently, rather than as part of a state-supported college or university, funding itself almost exclusively through student fees and tuition.[3] In essence, the EMC—like so many of the one hundred-plus medical schools listed in the United States' 1870 federal census—was a proprietary business established along the lines of a commercial venture undertaken by a group of investors, in this case a medical faculty and/or board of trustees. In addition, the clash of strong personalities that one might find within any small cadre of aspiring professionals in a start-up environment often plagued the small faculties of these schools. In the case of the EMC, these squabbles also mirrored the larger tensions arising among schools dedicated to differing philosophies of medicine.

Problems arising from the governing and financial structures of medical schools were aggravated by the fact that until 1890, these schools lacked both oversight by national accrediting bodies and an effective membership association supporting progressive improvements.[4] This meant that there were few constraints against financially driven decision making that may have been contrary to the best educational and pedagogical interests of the profession. The inherent financial instability characterizing the EMC and most other proprietary schools created a fundamental vulnerability at the core of their educational enterprise. The result was a temptation to cut corners while placing ever-greater pressure on school leaders like John Buchanan to maintain a steady stream of matriculants in order to continue to generate revenue for the school.

This characterization of the medical education landscape is not intended as an indictment of the proprietary model overall; for most American medical schools, this economic model represented the only option available. Some scholars have argued that this model worked reasonably well as a practical approach to medical education for much of the country, offering at least a modicum of didactic training for practice.[5] More importantly, relatively few legitimate schools appear to have succumbed to the temptation of selling diplomas outright, as did Buchanan and the

EMC. Nevertheless, the damage wrought by even a few rogue schools could be enormous, as we will see.

The story of John Buchanan and the EMC also resides in a third development in American medicine: the rebirth of medical licensing laws during the post–Civil War era. The push to reinstitute licensing laws arose to a great extent from pressures arising within the medical profession specific to medical education. Those practitioners representing the medical orthodoxy of the time, identified as allopathic physicians or medical "regulars," were the strongest advocates for licensing laws to regulate the practice of medicine. They demanded laws that would define what constituted the legal practice of medicine and set specific educational standards as minimum requirements for licensing physicians. In so doing, they hoped to stabilize what seemed to be an increasingly turbulent playing field with substandard schools churning out large numbers of physicians, some of whom were questionably educated and trained at best. For these medical regulars, professional and economic self-interest conveniently aligned with legitimate concern to protect the public against outright medical fakes, imposters, and charlatans.

Proponents of less orthodox medical philosophies, however, such as eclectic and homeopathic practitioners, were often leery of the push for medical licensing boards, although John Buchanan did call publicly (and disingenuously) for medical registration laws as one mechanism to combat medical charlatans. As challengers to the medical orthodoxy of the day, eclectic and homeopathic practitioners were understandably fearful that these laws would be used to exclude them from the legal practice of medicine. Ultimately, though, both of these groups of "irregular" practitioners chose to support such legislation, bowing to the seemingly irresistible wave of licensing laws arising in the last quarter of the nineteenth century and hoping that such laws might trigger a rising economic tide lifting all physicians. For John Buchanan and the EMC, licensing laws— even the rudimentary medical registration laws that predated most state medical boards—proved a boon to diploma sales by creating an added financial value to the medical degree as a gateway credential to licensed practice. Buchanan's diploma activities had found a market even before the introduction of licensing laws; the advent of these laws served to increase the potential market for his diplomas.

* * *

Having set the stage on which John Buchanan operated, it is time to explore his strange career, and the character that allowed him to pursue that career. It will soon become clear that Buchanan's personal and professional successes derived in large part from artifice and deception, from a keen understanding of human motivations, from influential contacts within the city and the state government, and from those personal qualities and attributes that combined to make him a savvy, if not always scrupulous, medical professional.

We see this in the language he used as editor of the *Eclectic Medical Journal of Pennsylvania (EMJP)*, the modest periodical serving as the voice of Buchanan and the EMC to the profession and the larger world. In its pages, he touted the virtues of the EMC to prospective students in language that vastly inflated the school's meager facilities and capacity to deliver quality education. Using the language of the classic "bait and switch" advertiser, Buchanan drew in not only unscrupulous individuals seeking a shortcut to a medical diploma but genuine students seeking legitimate instruction.

Buchanan's skills in deception and misdirection are also evident in the intellectual corner-cutting one finds in his many written works on medicine. His body of scholarly work—reaching ten volumes published between 1865 and 1890—seems impressive in its scale and in the breadth of its subject matter. A cursory look at his work conveys the impression of sustained intellectual labor over several decades. This positive perception fades, however, upon closer examination of his writing. Buchanan's reliance on repurposed text and multiple instances of outright plagiarism undermine the scholarly façade presented by the sheer volume of his published works.

Buchanan's self-interest and skill in manipulation are likewise demonstrated by his seemingly quixotic campaign for the Pennsylvania state legislature in 1871. As a candidate, he challenged an incumbent Republican and openly embraced Philadelphia's recently enfranchised black voters. But the realities behind his campaign reflected neither courage nor a politically progressive mind-set. Instead, Buchanan's candidacy showed an unexpected degree of political cunning and a willingness to exploit a newly enfranchised constituency using one of the major tools available to him—the actual diplomas issued by his legally chartered school.

We see this unscrupulousness, too, in his personal style and presence in front of audiences both large and small—an ability to dazzle students, confound critics, and give at least momentary pause to veteran journalists. His qualities combined those of the adept conversationalist, the knowledgeable man of medicine, and the successful salesman. Self-confidence and quick thinking characterized John Buchanan—as well as an unflappable demeanor under pressure and a sociopath's ability to persuade or convince himself and his audience of the truth of his assertions.

Given Buchanan's gift for self-serving flimflam, it seems fitting to open this narrative with a bit of self-created theater consistent with much that we now know of the man. Picture, then, John Buchanan standing at the rail of the ferryboat *Philadelphia* as it crossed the Delaware River from Philadelphia to Camden, ostensibly poised for a final leap designed to end his worldly legal and financial woes. The events of that night represented the single most audacious act of premeditated deception perpetrated by Buchanan during his tenure at the EMC, and only the sheer magnitude of the deception he attempted, not its nature, made his actions atypical. As will be seen, the arc of Buchanan's career spurred him to undertake an array of activities that would capture the attention of medical educators and regulators, fellow physicians, journalists, and ultimately the reading public, who followed his exploits through the daily press.

"The past is never dead. It's not even past."

—William Faulkner

Prologue

After midnight on Tuesday, August 17, 1880, the ferryboat *Philadelphia* prepared to launch from the Market Street landing in the city for which it was named for its final run across the Delaware River to New Jersey. The night was mild after a pleasant day topping out at just below 80 degrees.[1] A clear sky and the moonlight on the water provided ideal conditions for the ferry's routine ten-minute transit between Philadelphia and Camden. The boat slipped its mooring and headed for the channel between Smith and Windmill Islands in the middle of the Delaware, traversing these familiar landmarks before docking in Camden on the river's eastern bank. River traffic had slowed and the bustle of city activity had subsided as 1:00 A.M. approached. Apart from its crew, the boat carried only a handful of people on this last run.[2] Among the passengers that night was a short, heavyset Scotsman sporting the still-fashionable muttonchop whiskers. His name was John Buchanan, physician, educator, author, and for nearly a decade the dean of the Eclectic Medical College of Pennsylvania (EMC). In recent years, he had been one of Philadelphia's most controversial citizens.

The doctor had arrived at the boat landing accompanied by Thomas Vanduser, a friend of many years through the small artificial tooth facility he operated in New Jersey.[3] Once aboard the *Philadelphia*, the two men

approached a passenger, Louis Shober, as he leaned along the boat railing. The two men stood briefly before Shober and proffered their fare for
the trip across the river. Momentarily confused, Shober had demurred,
then pointed toward the crew member standing nearby collecting fares.
Shober later recalled the encounter as odd. Though the shorter of the two
men had stood before him for only a few seconds, something had seemed
amiss about his hair and side whiskers. Even in the dim lighting aboard
the ferry, Shober had thought the man looked "made up," like a stage ac-
tor in costume. The encounter had been so fleeting that Shober barely
had time to gain this impression before the two men stepped away to the
fare collector and Shober dismissed the incident from his mind.

Another passenger aboard the ferry that night was a local newspaper
reporter, W. R. Hamilton of the *Philadelphia Record*. Though Hamilton's
paper had doggedly pursued information on a criminal investigation into
John Buchanan and the EMC, this was not one of the stories Hamilton
worked on. He was initially unaware of the doctor's alleged presence on
the ferryboat that night. Similarly, two deckhands, William Wood and
William Rauch, and a passenger, William Gamble, later stated that while
they saw the man later identified as John Buchanan board the ferry, they
had not taken any particular notice of him at the time.

At least two crew members did know Buchanan. The *Philadelphia*'s
fireman, Joseph Middleton, knew the doctor by sight, though he had not
seen him for some time. Since Buchanan usually crossed at an earlier time
of day and Middleton worked a late shift on the ferry, his schedule no
longer brought him into regular contact with the doctor. The other crew
member familiar with Buchanan was the ship's engineer, John Holton. As
Buchanan had made his way past Holton on boarding the ferry, a brief
exchange took place. The usually "chatty and sociable" doctor offered
only a quick handshake and a simple "Good evening. . . . How do you
do?" as he moved along the deck, keeping his head bowed all the while
and hardly breaking stride. Later, Holton commented on the hoarse tenor
of Buchanan's voice and a certain "rough and hard" feel to his handshake.
This was odd, since professionals such as doctors, lawyers, or politicians
were notable for lacking rough calluses on their hands in a city where most
men earned their living through some kind of physical labor. Buchanan's
perfunctory greeting likewise struck Holton as odd, since the two men
were long-standing and cordial acquaintances. Holton claimed to have

known Buchanan since the 1860s, when the engineer sat for lectures at the EMC. They had always exchanged friendly greetings when they met over the ensuing years, and while the doctor's greeting that night had not been unfriendly, it had lacked the warmth Holton expected based upon their long acquaintance and many prior encounters. He ascribed it to illness or stress from the recent events covered so prominently in the local newspapers.

If John Buchanan seemed distant and distracted that night, he had good reason. In recent months, he had achieved notoriety throughout the country as the architect behind America's most notorious medical diploma mill. The prior week had proven particularly difficult, since a federal grand jury had indicted Buchanan for mail fraud. It had taken the doctor nearly two weeks and every friend, contact, and resource he knew to secure the necessary funds to meet his bail.[4] Arrest and indictment would understandably weigh heavily on any man, but it was not a new experience for John Buchanan. He had a long acquaintance with Philadelphia's legal system, as city authorities had arrested him many times between 1872 and 1876 on a range of offenses: medical malpractice, printing "obscene" circulars, and obtaining money under false pretenses. Two arrests on the last charge had stemmed from his thriving business in selling medical diplomas carrying the seal of the EMC.

A combination of good fortune, good connections, and perhaps even complicity by those in authority had saved Buchanan in each instance. None of the cases ever came to trial, as the legal charges were quietly dropped—an outcome infuriating to the doctor's critics within Philadelphia's medical and education communities. This time seemed different. Federal felony charges for mail fraud meant that Buchanan was no longer dealing with the local Philadelphia courts but was instead confronting a U.S. district court; the luck, pluck, and guile that had helped him out of trouble with state and local authorities for more than a decade was proving inadequate. This time, the probable outcome to the federal charges seemed clear: conviction, with a possible sentence of eighteen months in jail. These legal troubles were compounded by the financial repercussions arising from the charges. Even if Buchanan avoided a conviction, the costs of his legal defense and the monetary impact on the EMC were shaping up to be disastrous. For all intents and purposes, the EMC was a dying institution that threatened to drag Buchanan down with it.

In later statements to the police, Buchanan's friends and family talked of the profound changes they had observed in his behavior and demeanor, signaling depression. These signs first became evident in June, as he languished in Philadelphia's Moyamensing jail, struggling to raise bail funds. Friends visiting him were struck by his deflated spirit. His mood lifted briefly after his release on June 19, but as one legal setback followed upon another in the ensuing weeks, and as it became clear that the *Philadelphia Record* and its city editor, John Norris, were committed to destroying him professionally, Buchanan's intimates watched the cumulative effects of the legal ordeal begin to break him in body and spirit. In a later interview with the newspapers, his wife claimed that Buchanan had fallen into a suicidal despair, attempting to end his life with laudanum. Other unnamed sources claimed that Buchanan suffered a "paralytic stroke" during the ten miserable days he spent at Moyamensing. This assertion seems more hyperbole than fact. No one on the *Philadelphia* that night commented on anything unusual in Buchanan's gait, speech, or appearance supporting the claim of a stroke. Still, Buchanan had apparently felt so unwell that the day before boarding the ferry, August 16, he had been unable to join his attorney, a former Philadelphia judge named William Mann, before the district court for delivery of the indictment. The judge had expressed extreme displeasure at Buchanan's absence, but Mann had placated him with the promise that his client would appear in court before noon the next day, August 17.[5]

The federal mail fraud charges against Buchanan were the culmination of a long spring and summer of exposé reporting and heightened scrutiny that drew even the attention of federal officials. During this period, John Norris and the *Philadelphia Record* had worked tirelessly to secure key evidence leading to Buchanan's arrest and indictment; Norris had even used the U.S. Postal Service to purchase several bogus diplomas from Buchanan. That same spring, various journals and newspapers throughout the country had published a letter from Andrew White, the American ambassador to Germany, drawing more attention to Buchanan and his school. White was a reform-minded educator and the driving force behind the establishment of Cornell University, and his experiences in European institutions in the 1850s had made him a staunch advocate for modern, "scientific" educational methods.[6] White had written to the U.S. secretary of state detailing German authorities' mounting frustration with the number of dubious diplomas originating from America and presented as *bona fide* credentials in their country. Prominent among these were many diplomas signed by "John Buchanan, M.D." White's letter also related his own experiences in Berlin, where he personally examined these "sham" diplomas. He claimed they were so common that they had entered German popular culture as a feature for comic and melodramatic effect in contemporary plays and novels. The American ambassador failed to share the amusement of German audiences at this new literary conceit featuring America as the refuge of pompous frauds and unscrupulous scoundrels.[7]

John Buchanan viewed matters differently, asserting that local authorities had long been engaged in a campaign intended to harass, intimidate, and persecute him. One sign of Buchanan's increasing desperation occurred on August 9, just days before he boarded the *Philadelphia*. On that day, his brother-in-law, Martin V. Chapman, met with the *Record's* John Norris. Acting as Buchanan's intermediary, Chapman made Norris an offer: if Norris would drop the matter and refuse to testify as a state witness, Buchanan would transfer the deed for the EMC's building at 514 Pine Street, valued at $20,000, to Norris and surrender the school charter to state authorities. Norris refused the offer. This overture not only had been futile but also signaled Buchanan's desperation and the weakness of his position. If John Buchanan regretted anything at that time, it was probably extending the offer to Norris.

According to Vanduser, John Buchanan boarded the ferry that night headed to his daughter's home in Magnolia, situated a few miles below Camden. Now he stood at the rail, silent and seemingly contemplative as the boat crossed the Delaware River. Ahead, the dim outlines of Ridgway Park on Smith Island appeared. The popular site boasted a fine new hotel, public baths, and a dancing pavilion. The island was quiet, with only the park watchman, Davis Edwards, awake at that hour. As the ferry neared the canal between Smith and Windmill Islands, Edwards heard a commotion on the water. Grabbing his lantern, he raced toward the canal, where the ferry had stopped its engine. Passengers and crew aboard the ship hollered that someone had gone overboard. Edwards later testified he had a "clear view," but saw nothing in the water.

Facing arraignment later that day and, according to friends, now dangerously despondent, John Buchanan had apparently clambered over the boat railing, uttered an audible "Good-bye," and dropped overboard. His companion, Vanduser, raised the alarm among startled passengers and crew. "My God, Dr. Buchanan has jumped overboard!" Reporter W. R. Hamilton had been standing nearby and just happened to look over in time to see a man going over the railing. Unaware at the time of the identity of the jumper, newspapers later quoted Hamilton as saying he believed the man had drowned. Like several others scrambling to the railing, he felt certain that the river had taken Buchanan under, as he saw nothing on the water's surface. Holton, the boat engineer, heard the commotion on deck and stepped toward the stern to ascertain what had happened. He claimed that he saw someone struggling in the water and then ran back to stop the ferry. The boat fireman, Middleton, said that he saw Buchanan shed his coat and jump overboard. He next spied the man struggling in the water and asserted that he kept a "constant" eye on him as he thrashed about. He then heard several cries of "Oh!" before the drowning man went under for good. One of the deckhands, William Wood, also saw Buchanan go overboard and later said he was certain that the man had drowned. According to Middleton, the river ran to a depth of more than forty feet in that area and the spot where Buchanan leaped into the water was roughly sixty to seventy feet from Smith Island and had a strong, swift current. Middleton stated that while he considered himself a strong swimmer, he "wouldn't have dared to jump" in at that point in the river.

Despite the quick alarm from passengers and the crew's speedy response in backing the ferry to keep the man in sight, rescue efforts proved futile. Multiple eyewitnesses—Vanduser, Hamilton, Middleton, and Wood—reported not only seeing Buchanan leap into the river but also watching him struggle in the water. Despite variances in the details, their accounts agreed in the main: the tide-driven waters had done their work, drawing John Buchanan to his death. One passenger picked up the coat shed by Buchanan as he clambered overboard. Inside a pocket he discovered a crumpled newspaper with "disjointed sentences" written in the margins. The jottings revealed nothing except perhaps the doctor's troubled state of mind. Newspapers outside Philadelphia quickly picked up the story of the suicide, deeming it a fitting end to a sad and sordid tale.

As it turned out, the events of that night were far from the end of the story. Within twenty-four hours, Philadelphians opened the *Record* and the *Inquirer* to read another twist in the saga of John Buchanan and the EMC.

The story would feature an imposter, a faked suicide, and, soon enough, a manhunt across international borders and the demise of the EMC. For a brief period, it seemed that John Buchanan, dean of the Eclectic Medical College of Pennsylvania and the driving force behind America's largest medical diploma mill, had once again eluded authorities—this time in a spectacular fashion.

Part One

Rise

One

The Rise of Eclectic Medicine

The Eclectic Medical College of Pennsylvania presents the researcher with numerous contradictions and false leads in attempting to recreate its story. The school's prospectus materials routinely blended fact and fantasy in a self-portrait providing all the retrospective clarity and precision of an Impressionist painting. Just when the school appeared to be dead and buried, with its charter annulled in 1872, it rose like Lazarus by courtesy of the Pennsylvania Supreme Court. For nearly another decade, under John Buchanan's leadership, the school carried on its questionable practices unimpeded by official efforts from either state or local authorities to close it permanently.

In exploring the EMC's path from its modest founding in 1850 to its spectacular demise thirty years later, such inexplicable events complicate efforts to answer fundamental questions about the school. Did the EMC originate as a legitimate institution? If so, when did it adopt its dubious practice of selling diplomas? Did this practice originate as a deliberate attempt to monetize the school's legal right to issue diplomas? Or did the school drift into the diploma trade, bastardizing otherwise commonly accepted practices such as issuing honorary and *ad eundem* diplomas? What was John Buchanan's part in all this? Was he, as the newspapers characterized him, the mastermind of the diploma trade? Or did he simply have the bad luck to be the school's primary leader when a new era inaugurated previously unseen levels of scrutiny in the form of medical regulation and licensing laws?

The answers to these questions are nuanced and, at this late date, somewhat speculative; since the college's official records have long since been lost, scholars seeking such answers must draw heavily on information in contemporary journals and newspapers. While these sources certainly suffice for drawing the main contours of the story, many of them were partisan and must be sifted accordingly. Those writing such accounts often represented distinct perspectives, such as those of medical educator, medical regulator, or medical professional; moreover, many were competitors or critics of Buchanan and the EMC. This chapter and those following in Part 1 attempt to trace the EMC's origins within the context of reformed or eclectic medicine, its devolution into a medical diploma mill, and John Buchanan's role in this process.

THE REFORM MOVEMENT IN AMERICAN MEDICINE

A reasonable argument can be made that during the first decades of the nineteenth century, the understanding of disease and its causes held by most American physicians had evolved relatively little beyond the conjectures of the ancient world. Many, if not most, physicians still held by Galen's humoral theory, itself based on Aristotelian doctrine. This theory maintained that the human body was composed of four cardinal elements (water, fire, air, and earth), that in turn produced four principal humors (phlegm, blood, bile, and black bile). Galenic theory had been taught for centuries throughout Europe and beyond. Avicenna's celebrated eleventh-century *Canon of Medicine*—one of the Western world's premier medical texts for fully six centuries—further popularized Galen's system. Galenic theory held that all disease arose from excessive quantities or improper temperatures of these humors; physicians therefore routinely sought to treat illness by balancing the humors through dietary measures, herbal remedies, and phlebotomy.[1] The long persistence of this theory is staggering. As one medical historian put it, "The Roman Empire would fall . . . the Middle Ages would pass . . . the Renaissance would come and go, before humanity conceived of better explanations."[2]

By the early nineteenth century, the restrictive intellectual confines of Galenic theory were under attack in both Europe and America. The writings of influential French physicians such as Pierre Charles Alexandre Louis and Philippe Pinel represented an emerging Parisian school of medicine, one that rejected rationalist, speculative systems that placed greater primacy on textual authority than on the realities presented by the human body. Adherents of the Parisian school of thought asserted that the key position for all physicians was at the bedside, usually in a hospital, directly observing the patient and the symptoms accompanying his or her illness. This physical and intellectual repositioning grounded physicians in a perceptual and sensory encounter with their patients. It also reoriented medical discourse away from the "language of fantasy" (e.g., humoral theory) and toward more precise, qualitative, and descriptive terminology. The ideas emerging from the Parisian school reached America through the writings of Elisha Bartlett (*An Essay on the Philosophy of Medical Science*, 1844), John Godman (editor of the *Journal of Foreign Medical Science*), Samuel Jackson (*Principles of Medicine*, 1832), and Jacob Bigelow (*Discourse on Self-Limited Disease*, 1835), as well as through the experiences of the estimated six hundred Americans studying in Paris before 1860.[3]

This is not to imply that dissent from medical orthodoxy in the United States stemmed wholly or even primarily from the French experience. Many contemporary references within the country likewise expressed dissatisfaction with medicine's status quo. In 1807, for example, the secretary of New York's Medical Society, David Arnell, lamented the deadening effect of "absurd systems of ancient physicians" and the equally "preposterous" theories of some of his own contemporaries, who dismissed the need for "experimentation . . . to precede conjecture." Arnell questioned his colleagues' blind adherence to any overarching philosophy of medicine when our "knowledge of Nature is too limited and our collections of materials too scanty to enable even the most diligent and ingenious to form a correct theory."[4] Arnell's assessment of and doubts concerning the state of medicine exemplified a growing realization among American physicians that standard or orthodox medicine, as commonly understood and practiced, no longer provided a satisfactory account or therapeutic regimen for treating disease.

Not surprisingly, those questioning the status quo faced considerable opposition. This was true whether they were inspired by the writings of French clinicians or by their American colleagues responding to direct experiences in treating patients. Challenges to medical orthodoxy were often barely palatable even when coming from within the community of established physicians and were fraught with risk to one's reputation and standing among contemporaries. Challengers from outside this community fared even less well, drawing the most contemptuous responses and harshest criticism. The first major challenger to America's medical orthodoxy, Samuel Thomson, was just such an outsider, and his teachings forged a trail leading to John Buchanan and the Eclectic Medical College of Pennsylvania.

Historians of nineteenth-century American medicine have consistently pointed to Samuel Thomson as mounting the first significant challenge to America's medical orthodoxy. Thomson, a self-taught healer from New Hampshire, was deeply suspicious of "orthodox" physicians and their mineral-based treatments (e.g., mercury and arsenic). Working from the theory that all disease stemmed from cold, Thomson developed a botanically based theory of medicine, proposing heat as the key therapeutic treatment and offering it often in the form of steam baths and "hot" botanicals like cayenne pepper—though he also favored purgatives, such as lobelia powder and bayberry root bark. In 1822, Thomson published his *New Guide to Health; or Botanic Family Physician*; this not only sold well, it created a mass following for Thomson in rural America where adherents embraced his call to reclaim medicine from the privileged and place it in the hands of the people. Thomson's theories spawned a range of intellectual "descendants," including eclectic physicians such as John Buchanan, who identified themselves as inheritors of Thomson's botanical system.[5]

While Samuel Thomson did much to popularize botanically based medicine in the first quarter of the nineteenth century, his efforts succeeded in large part because of Americans' familiarity with the commonsense herbal medicine and folk remedies many had brought with them from England or learned or adopted from Native Americans. Figures as diverse as Methodist founder John Wesley (1703–1791) and English botanist Nicholas Culpeper (1616–1654) contributed to native and adapted medico-cultural approaches in America by touting the virtues of single plants that ordinary men and women could administer themselves and promoting indigenous flora as those most likely to support health.[6]

Despite this robust botanic tradition, however, Thomson's efforts also drew tremendous criticism. There were several reasons for the intensity of this reaction. His rejection of mineral-based treatments alone roused the ire of most physicians comfortable with the era's typical therapeutic arsenal; that the messenger (Thomson) was a self-taught healer rather than a man of formal education further undercut his message. Jealousy over Thomson's thriving practice most likely aggravated such criticism and may have contributed to murder charges brought against Thomson by a local physician for the death of a patient in 1808. Another complicating factor was Thomson's decision to patent his system of botanicals for direct sale to the public through a network of agents. In setting up this system, Thomson was mixing New England pragmatism and business acumen with the zeal of a true believer determined to harness and promote the power of botanicals. Given that more than 160 authorized agents were selling his botanicals in 1833 alone, garnering tremendous success in areas such as Ohio and Indiana, physicians' harsh reactions to Thomson were hardly surprising. Some physicians were willing to acknowledge Thomson for his recognition of the medicinal properties of *lobelia inflata* ("pukeweed") and to ask that he be given a fair hearing, regarding him not as a quack but as an "Experimenter, who accumulates knowledge by his own experience." Most condemned him, however, for his lack of learning, characterizing him in derisive terms as a "steam and puke" doctor.[7]

In some ways, the success enjoyed by Thomsonism in the 1820s and 1830s was not surprising. American medicine in the early nineteenth century remained largely a domestic affair, administered by family, friends, and neighbors. Physicians were seldom at the center of this experience for most Americans, who relied instead on informally trained healers who used their senses to diagnose the "imbalance" affecting the patient.[8]

Historians have long been drawn to this era as the start of a period of experimentation and rupture characterizing much of American life. From the religious experiments of Joseph Smith and William Miller and the broadening of the political electorate during the presidency of Andrew Jackson (1829–37), to the rise of abolitionist and other social reform movements and the beginnings of a market economy, American society seemed not only in flux but immensely receptive to new ideas coming from all quarters of society. In the field of medicine, such currents of change not only resulted in Thomson's great popular success but produced other quasi-medical ideas and movements that captured the interest and imagination of Americans. During the 1830s, Johan Spurzheim popularized phrenology in America, asserting that the shape of the skull mirrored the brain itself, the organ of human consciousness and emotion. Only a few years later, Charles Poyen de Saint Sauveur toured America, enthralling audiences with his demonstrations of "mesmerism" (hypnosis), a technique that some physicians were exploring as the basis for alleviating pain through somnambulistic surgery. In similar fashion, Joel Shaw, Russell Thatcher Trall, and later Mary Gove popularized hydropathy (i.e., the water cure) as the key to health. Sylvester Graham introduced ideas for diet and hygiene mixed with his notions of social and moral development, a combination that fostered a massive following of advocates identifying themselves as Grahamites.[9]

Within this receptive environment, a second major challenge to the American medical orthodoxy—homeopathy—arose contemporaneously with, but wholly unrelated to, Thomson's botanical philosophy. The principles of homeopathic medicine were established by Samuel Hahnemann, a highly educated German physician, and reached the United States through the agency of the Dutch-born doctor Hans Burch Gram in the 1820s and were spread more broadly a decade later by Constantine Hering, a German doctor who relocated to the United States in 1833.[10] Gram's labors in translating key Hahnemann works and Hering's teaching at the Homeopathic Medical College of Pennsylvania proved critical to homeopathy's popular acceptance in New York and Philadelphia. Hahnemann's homeopathic philosophy built on two concepts: the idea that "like cures like" and a so-called law of infinitesimals in the administration of drugs—the belief that only the minimum dose of a medicine should be given a patient to stimulate healing from within. The drug therapies stemming from these principles involved administering drugs in such small doses as to have minimal effect—in essence, leaving nature to do the work of healing.[11] As the historian William Rothstein observed, Hahnemann's great insight (whether he recognized it as such or not) was that in the first decades of the nineteenth century, no therapy at all was far better than heroic therapy in medicine.[12] One might argue that the botanic and homeopathic approaches to medicine were more closely aligned than either would have been willing to admit at the time. However, homeopaths' insistence on the efficacy of extremely diluted doses of drugs provoked vociferous criticism. Their opponents asserted that the theory and practice behind such dilutions stretched beyond "human credulity" to border on the fantastical.[13]

In one regard, homeopathy diverged significantly from the botanical movement. Where Thomson's followers and his intellectual heirs found fertile ground in the countryside and among less affluent Americans, homeopathy took a pronounced hold in larger cities among regular physicians disaffected by conventional therapeutics and eager to attract a middle- and upper-class clientele. New York and Philadelphia, for example, became strongholds of homeopathic medicine. That this sociofinancial success came without resort to purgatives and bloodletting further intrigued some medical regulars. This is not say that medical biases and sectarian loyalties disappeared with the growing popularity of homeopathy. The Philadelphia Medical Society offered a cautionary example when it ousted homeopathic members in 1843. Several years later, in reaction to such slights and to increased measures by medical regulars to eliminate the role of homeopathic physicians in medical education, proponents of homeopathy established the Homeopathic College of Pennsylvania. Homeopathic physicians later became uneasy allies of eclectic physicians like John Buchanan in attempts to forestall a campaign by allopathic physicians to establish medical licensing laws that would marginalize both groups as irregular practitioners.[14]

While both homeopathy and the botanical movement presented distinct challenges to the medical orthodoxy of the day, they differed in one important aspect. Unlike homeopathy, which consciously tried to formulate a coherent, well-defined system for educated practitioners of medicine, the botanical movement, reflecting the values of its popularizer, Samuel Thomson, advocated a more populist approach. Its members were wary of higher education, instead championing the practical good sense of the common man; eschewed the rigid, formal system of orthodox medicine in favor of straightforward instructional manuals showing every family how to harness nature's *materia medica;* and espoused botanical over mineral treatments. This approach initially proved advantageous to the botanical movement, since the "democratic appeal" at its core proved highly popular with Americans in the 1820s and 1830s.[15]

Over time, however, this same populism undermined the botanical movement's unity of purpose. Many physicians who embraced botanicals as a viable treatment alternative to allopathic practice balked at Thomson's rigidly anti-intellectual pronouncements and his insistence upon adherence to his patented system for administering prescribed medicines. The result was an inevitable splintering. One group, remaining closest to the spirit of Thomson, aligned with leaders like Alva Curtis under the umbrella of what came to be known as the Physio-Medicals. Another branch, drawing on the work of Wooster Beach, Thomas Cooke, and others, evolved into a loose association that initially identified itself as the American reformed system of medicine, later adopting the name eclectic.[16] While the two names were used synonymously for a period, ultimately the latter prevailed. The term *eclectic* derived from the Greek (*eklego*), meaning "to choose from." Eclectic physicians saw virtue in the perceived freedom to select from multiple sources implied in the name.[17] It was this group, basing their approach on the work of Beach and Cooke, that led directly to John Buchanan and the EMC.

THE RISE OF ECLECTIC MEDICINE

While John Buchanan and other physicians donning the mantle of medical eclecticism acknowledged their Thomsonian roots, their deference to his views had limits. Thomson's commitment to providing all Americans with the unfettered ability to practice medicine for themselves and their families carried a corollary less palatable to many otherwise sympathetic physicians—staunch opposition to formalized medical schools as the sole legitimate sources of medical education for physicians. Thomson's rigid stance on this point underscored inherent strains of self-sufficiency and anti-intellectualism in his theories that most eclectics were unwilling to accept, since such attitudes undermined their own professional aspirations. Eclectic writers labored to draw the appropriate distinction without entirely refuting their intellectual debt. As one writer aptly described the relationship, eclecticism was not so much "an offshoot" of Thomsonism as it was a "fellow laborer . . . in dissent."[18]

Most eclectics drew instead on the teachings of a contemporary of Thomson's in the 1820s, Wooster Beach, as the immediate inspiration for American reformed or eclectic medicine. Labeled by some as a "medical agitator," Beach first learned medicine from a German herbalist and physician before entering the New York College of Physicians and Surgeons. Fiercely critical of bloodletting and mercurials, Beach became a staunch advocate of botanic medicine, establishing in the 1820s the first sectarian medical school in the United States, one that after a name change became known as the Reformed Medical College of New York.

The founding of this school came in the midst of a boom period in the creation of U.S. medical schools. While only a handful of medical schools existed in 1800, twenty-six new schools were established between 1810 and 1840, and a second boom more than doubled that number between 1840 and 1876. Despite (or perhaps because of) his ostensible success in treating patients at New York City's Tenth Ward hospital in 1832 and the early popularity of his school, Beach failed to obtain the charter for his school necessary to secure its legal standing. In the face of staunch opposition from orthodox practitioners, Beach closed his New York school and then reorganized it in Ohio as Worthington College. There the school flourished for a decade before the political aftermath of an antidissection riot in 1839 resulted in the state legislature's repeal of the school charter.[19] Through the efforts of a Beach disciple, Thomas Vaughn Morrow, the eclectic movement in Ohio gained its greatest strength in 1845, with the legally chartered establishment of the Eclectic Medical Institute (EMI) of Cincinnati. Almost immediately, "Old EMI" became the fountainhead of eclectic medicine, as symbolized by its selection of Beach as chair of internal medicine and surgery.[20]

In considering the American reformed or eclectic movement in medicine, one quickly realizes that its greatest strength and greatest weakness sprang from the same source. As a group, physicians like Beach, Vaughn, and Cooke rejected the confining strictures of any rigid system for the practice of medicine. Instead, they championed the idea that scientific truth was to be found beyond the confines of any one system. They felt morally and professionally bound to follow scientific truth wherever it might take them. Critics like Alva Curtis derided this hedging philosophy as "non-commitalism."[21] Eclectics, on the other hand, saw their approach as praiseworthy, reflecting intellectual openness and a receptivity to new

Table 1: Select List of Eclectic Medical Schools Established Prior to 1880

School	Year Established	Year Closed	Notes
New York Reformed Medical College	1826	1840	Established by Wooster Beach.
Botanic College of Medicine in New York City	1836	1846	
Georgia Eclectic Medical College	1839	1919	Originated as Southern Botanico-Medical College; renamed Reformed Medical College of Georgia, 1845; inactive during Civil War; renewed as American College of Medicine & Surgery, 1874; merged to become Georgia Eclectic Medical College, 1881.
Eclectic Medical Institute (Cincinnati)	1845	1939	Originated as Worthington Medical College, 1833; inactive 1839-43; relocated with new name to Cincinnati, 1845; absorbed American Medical College of Ohio (1857) and Eclectic College of Medicine and Surgery (1859).
Eclectic Medical Institution of New York (Rochester)	1847	1852	Organized as Medical School of Fredonia; took EMI title in 1848; merged with Randolph EMI (1849) to become Central Medical College of New York.
Memphis Institute (Tennessee)	1847	1851	Faculty included R. S. Newton.
Eclectic Medical College of Kentucky	1848		Based in Louisville.
Boston Female Medical College (Massachusetts)	1848	1874	Chartered in 1850 as New England Female Medical College. Original faculty eclectic. Later absorbed into Medical Dept., Boston University.
Worcester Eclectic Medical College (Massachusetts)	1848	1859	Organized as New England Botanic Medical College; reorganized as Worcester, 1852.
American Reform Medical Institute (Louisville)	1849	1850	Faculty included eclectic and botanic physicians.

Eclectic Medical College of Pennsylvania	1850	1880	Charter revoked.
Female Medical College of Pennsylvania	1850	1852	Eclectics among the original faculty.
Metropolitan Medical College (New York)	1852	1862	Operated in New York City.
Philadelphia University of Medicine and Surgery	1853	1880	Chartered as the American College of Medicine in Penn.; renamed Eclectic Medical College of Philadelphia, 1860; renamed Philadelphia University, 1865.
Eclectic Medical Institute of Tennessee (Memphis)	1857	1861	Organized as Botanic Medical College; renamed in 1859.
Brooklyn Academy of Medicine	1861	1888	Charter revoked.
Bennett College of Eclectic Medicine and Surgery	1868	1908	Located in Chicago; "eclectic" dropped from title after 1908.
Eclectic Medical College of New York City	1866	1913	Incorporated by act of New York legislature.
Eclectic Medical College of New Jersey	1871	1888	Never fully operational before charter repealed.
American Medical College (St. Louis)	1873	1918	Dropped eclectic affiliation in 1910.
American Medical University (St. Louis)	1874	1883	Split from American Medical College; name change 1875 to St. Louis Eclectic Medical College.
American Eclectic Medical College (Cincinnati)	1876	1896	Successor to Physio-Eclectic Medical College.
Georgia Eclectic Medical College	1877	1886	Later operated as Georgia Eclectic College of Medicine & Surgery until 1916.
United States Medical College	1878	1882	Operated in New York City; faculty included Alexander Wilder.
California Eclectic Medical College	1879	1915	Organized in Oakland; relocations to San Francisco (1887) and Los Angeles (1907).

Sources: AMA Council on Medical Education and Hospitals, *Medical Colleges of the United States and Foreign Countries* (Chicago: American Medical Association, 1918), 6–9, 11, 13–15; John S. Haller Jr., *Medical Protestants* (Carbondale: Southern Illinois University Press, 1994), 75, 82, 145–46, 150–51, 239; John S. Haller Jr., *A Profile in Alternative Medicine* (Kent: Kent State Univ. Press, 1999), 19, 21; Lloyd Library and Museum, Cincinnati, Ohio. Database of Reform Medical Colleges http://www.lloydlibrary.org/reformmedicine.html.

ideas whatever their origin. A resolution adopted at the May 1849 meeting of the National Eclectic Medical Convention captured this view: "We regard it as one of the most important duties of the medical profession to investigate truth from whatever source it may come, and . . . to encourage the fullest and freest investigation by all."[22]

The challenge for eclectics was often one of differentiation. They embraced the notion of a botanically based *materia medica* but felt no restrictive allegiance to it or its intellectual heirs as an exclusive pathway to treatment. They disavowed bleeding, blistering, and heroic mineral treatments but they also rejected the extreme sweating and vomiting regimens of some early botanics. They might ridicule homeopathic notions of the infinitesimal, yet eclectic stalwarts like John King and later John Scudder championed such related concepts as "concentrated medicines" and "specific medication"—a development that left some critics labeling them as "pseudo-homeopaths."[23]

The fundamental tenets of eclecticism were laid out in an "eclectic platform" written years later by eclectic physician Alexander Wilder, who was a prolific historian of the group. According to Wilder, eclectics embraced a handful of key principles:

- Eclectic medicine represented "reform" and "protest" against dangerous medical practices, such as the use of mercurials and bloodletting;
- The physician's role was that of "minister and auxiliary," assisting nature and the body's natural functions to return a patient to health;
- The botanical focus of the founders of eclecticism was sound, and the intellectual origins of the movement should not be "eradicate[d]";
- The "interest of science and humanity" should be placed above that of sectarian exclusivity.[24]

Wilder wrote also of the libels and "persecution" allopathic practitioners imposed on eclectics directly and through their journals. The Physio-Medical physicians who most closely adhered to Thomson's legacy delivered equally harsh criticisms of the eclectics. Their leader, Alva Curtis, could be withering in his portrayal of the eclectics. In an 1856 article, for example, he proclaimed them hypocrites, claiming that they played on public fears of allopathic treatments while secretly resorting to the same remedies at the bedside. He also mocked eclecticism's vaunted liberality of thought, observing derisively that freethinking ragpickers must be ideal candidates for eclectic schools. Asserting that eclectics were little better than "literary leeches" and "scientific pilferers," he argued that the movement arose from "willful dishonesty" and claimed that Drs. Beach and Morrow had stolen the Thomsonian birthright. The animus displayed in Curtis's attacks is all the more surprising given his apparently friendly relations with the National Eclectic Medical Association only two years earlier, when he had expressed his "regret" at being unable to attend their annual meeting.[25]

Criticism of this nature, coming from an intellectual cousin of eclectic medicine, brings to mind the adage that a subject's importance stands in inverse proportion to the ferocity surrounding its debate. This adage—widely applied to academia in the twentieth century, as in the statement "Academic politics are vicious precisely because the stakes are so small"—proved particularly apt for American medicine throughout most of the nineteenth century, especially given the prevelance of competing theories of medicine during that period. The best evidence of this contested ground was the splintering of the medical profession into various camps (regulars and irregulars) and sects (e.g., allopathic, homeopathic, eclectic, botanical).

While the human physical form had been fully described and depicted for centuries, the functions and operations of its parts had barely been explored by the first half of the nineteenth century. The underlying interaction between an organ's form and function—the liver and its roles in filtering blood and secreting bile, for example—remained obscure until better tools allowed a clearer understanding. Only with improvements in the microscope did it become clear that cells formed the basic chemical and biological building blocks for life—an appreciation ultimately leading to the revolutionary notion of germ theory and its later study, bacteriology.[26] In the mid-nineteenth century, when John Buchanan took up medicine, most American physicians still lacked the critical tools needed for a truly scientific understanding of disease and its pathways into or within the human body. Consequently, their therapeutic arsenal remained limited at best.

Lacking such critical information, as well as viable options for treatment even after such information was gained, American physicians remained locked in the rational, but ultimately wholly speculative, philosophical systems they had embraced while studying to become doctors.

Here the "vicious debate because the stakes are small" adage springs to life: lacking any solid, scientifically based common ground beneath them and with little basis for proving the merits of their respective approaches to medicine, American physicians engaged in bitter debates about the virtues and efficacy of the particular system they espoused (e.g., allopathy, homeopathy, eclecticism) and the deficiencies of all the other systems.

Moreover, as we look back at that period from a vantage point of greater knowledge, it is clear that the specific therapeutic approach a physician applied (provided it did not involve excessive bleeding or the administration of poisons such as mercury or arsenic) made little difference, since few of the treatments applied at the time were effective. Consequently, those physicians who most faithfully applied the maxim "First, do no harm" offered patients the best care. In an era when the operations of the body were so little understood, the less invasive and dangerous treatments of alternative practitioners—the milder botanical treatments of eclectics or the infinitesimal dosages offered by homeopaths—were generally safer and more palatable for patients than the treatment options prescribed by many of their allopathic colleagues.

With a staunch belief in their approach to medicine and the mindset of an embattled minority arising from their relatively small numbers, eclectic physicians were not shy about defending their faith in a reformed system of medicine. They were often combative, willing to trade verbal blows with their allopathic contemporaries. EMC faculty member William Paine presents a good example. Shortly before John Buchanan's arrival at the college, Paine delivered a formal address to the school's 1859 graduating class. His speech included a poem describing his personal evolution from idealistic youth to a hardened practitioner, coarsened by allopathic criticisms.

> "But now so callous grown—so changed from youth,
> I've learned to think and plainly speak the truth.
> Learned to deride the critic's stricted ire,
> And break him on the wheel he meant for me.
> I spurn the rod the scribbler bade me kiss:
> Nor care if allopathic doctors applaud or hiss."[27]

FAILURES AND SCANDALS OF ORTHODOX MEDICINE

Many eclectics were not content with merely defending their faith in eclecticism. They relished opportunities to attack the methods of allopathic practitioners, and therefore welcomed publicized treatment failures by practitioners of orthodox medicine. The final illness of President William Henry Harrison in 1841 provided a golden opportunity of this type. Eclectics leapt at the opportunity to critique the orthodox medical treatment he received, especially in light of his death only one month after his inauguration. The president's attending physicians attributed his death to complications from pneumonia, and published a description of his illness and their treatment regimen, which included bloodletting (through cupping, not the lancet), the administration of several mercury-based medicines (Calomel and Blue Mass), the use of Tartar Emetic to induce vomiting, and the application of a series of mustard poultices to induce blistering.[28]

This regimen was relatively conventional by the standards of the day, but eclectic physicians pounced on the details as evidence of misguided therapeutics. Thomas Cooke, editor of the *Botanic Medical Reformer* and later a founding faculty member at the EMC, characterized the entire approach to treatment as "wrong," claiming that Harrison's doctors had "bled, blistered and cupped, thereby reducing . . . his strength." Cooke asserted that the treatment regimen clearly demonstrated the "fallacy of the old mineral and bleeding system." Lest anyone miss the magnitude of what had transpired, he blasted the president's doctors for their blind adherence to conventional but dangerous treatments, concluding: "They know not what they have done—BUT THEY HAVE KILLED HIM."[29]

Eclectics were hardly alone in questioning the attending physicians for the first death in office of a sitting American president. An allopathic contemporary leveled his own criticism—but on a very different basis. He claimed that Harrison's doctors had showed insufficient commitment to mercury-based treatment and bloodletting, insisting that " . . . more mischief is done by bleeding too little, than by bleeding too much."[30] In hindsight, according to several doctors looking at Harrison's case in 2014, it is unlikely that any treatment could have saved the life of the sixty-eight-year-old president. In their retrospective diagnosis, the doctors in 2014 concluded that Harrison was suffering from enteric fever—a disease wholly consistent with the unsanitary, typhoid-producing conditions in the "fetid marshes" near the White House, where drinking water and human waste pooled in close proximity. Not surprisingly, at least two later presidents (James Polk and Zachary Taylor) also suffered from gastrointestinal ailments during their terms of office, while Abraham Lincoln's son Willie succumbed to typhoid fever in 1862.[31]

The vehemence of Cooke's reaction to Harrison's medical treatment stemmed primarily from the fact that only four months earlier, he had written on the medical treatment George Washington received during his final illness in 1799. Washington had apparently suffered from an acute case of bacterial epiglottitis, a condition causing swelling and obstruction of the airway that, in essence, suffocates the patient.[32] Washington's physicians (James Craik, Gustavus Brown, and Elisha Dick) treated him with established allopathic protocols: calomel, blistering poultices, and "copious" bloodletting. In fact, they bled him four times in less than ten hours, removing approximately eighty ounces of blood, a staggering amount even for a tall and physically strong man (Washington was 6'3" and weighed 230 pounds).[33] Cooke argued that a syrup of *lobelia inflata* under a "milder" botanic treatment would have spared the patient. From a modern perspective, it is clear that this would have done nothing: the only measure that *might* have saved Washington was a tracheotomy. Elisha Dick did suggest this procedure, but one can hardly fault Drs. Craik and Brown for refusing to perform such a drastic, largely unknown procedure on the most prominent living American of the day. Cooke lamented Washington's medical treatment as "barbarous" and held up his case as a "warning" to both physicians and patients on the perils of the bloodletting regimen favored by allopathic physicians. "Let them shun those deadly instruments, the Lancet, Calomel, and all similar poisons," he demanded, "as they would the fatal sting of that reptile which has been chosen as the emblem of the Mineral School of Medicine."[34] Cooke must have especially relished this last dig: the chance to turn the era's commonly accepted emblem of regular medicine—the Rod of Asclepius—into a serpentine symbol of death.

In critiquing the medical treatment received by these two presidents, Cooke and his fellow eclectics hoped to show the public the virtues of their approach to medicine by exposing what they saw as the dangers inherent in allopathic regimens. However, since so little in medicine could be conclusively proven, attacks and rejoinders by the various schools of thought drifted invariably into hyperbole, once again producing vicious debate for small stakes. It should be made clear, however, that the stakes were small only in the sense that physicians were choosing from a limited array of suboptimal therapeutic options. In terms of patient health and wellness, the stakes were enormous.

Unfortunately, physicians of the day remained captive to a limited scientific framework for adjudicating the best methods of diagnosis and treatment. Eclectic leaders like Thomas Vaughn Morrow and Joseph R. Buchanan explicitly acknowledged the "limited" and "imperfect" resources available to contemporary physicians, lamenting the absence of an "infallible standard" for settling contentious questions.[35] Lacking this, medical disagreements often degenerated into passionate, rancorous arguments that were largely speculative and unprovable—the nineteenth-century equivalent of medieval theologians arguing over the nature of angels. During the debate over Harrison's medical treatment, one anonymous writer for the *Boston Medical and Surgical Journal* acknowledged the speculative terrain in which all physicians practiced and the lack of any definitive arbiter: "The profession of medicine is singularly situated. When differences occur among its members, there is no power to settle and adjudicate them . . . in medicine caviling is endless." The same writer further portrayed medicine as "a true democracy," in which all physicians stood upon "equal ground" in receiving the praise or condemnation of their peers. Even so, he acknowledged that the profession acted in the manner of a "tribunal" while ultimate authority rested with the "controlling power [of] the public."[36] Sociologist Owen Whooley would concur. In his study of cholera's impact on nineteenth-century medical practices and medical regulation, Whooley characterized medicine during this period as an "exercise in philosophizing rather than scientific researching."[37]

Though physicians across all the major schools of medicine willingly engaged in speculative debate, there was no escaping what one historian characterized as the new "reality of science"—that is, statistical data as the underlying foundation for a new empiricism.[38] Once again, the work of the Parisian school of medicine helped bring about this change. French physicians like Pierre Charles Alexandre Louis promoted the "numerical" or statistical method. Louis's 1835 work *Recherches sur les Effets de la Saignee* (republished in Boston the following year) showcased his statistical findings on bloodletting and tartar emetic, which demonstrated the former's irrelevance to outcomes in treating pneumonia and the latter's lack of value in treating pneumonitis.[39] Eclectic and homeopathic physicians seemed to welcome opportunities to present statistical data, not simply to demonstrate their commitment to science but as a means of defending their approach to medicine. A major opportunity to display the usefulness of compiling and analyzing statistical data arose in the wake of a major cholera outbreak in 1848–49, the second major cholera epidemic to strike America in the nineteenth century. Just as it had in 1832, cholera swept across the country, starting from port cities like New York and Philadelphia and following river and transportation routes further inland. Treatment options in 1848–49 were little better than they had been seventeen years earlier, generating considerable fear among Americans old enough to remember the devastating impact of the earlier outbreak and the futility of medical treatments then, particularly those of allopathic practitioners.

Eclectics understood that the new outbreak posed a potentially devastating health threat, yet some also sensed an opportunity within the threat to boost their status relative to that of conventional doctors, given the heated criticism orthodox medical treatments had garnered in 1832.[40] In consequence, eclectics consistently attacked the use of calomel and bloodletting by their allopathic colleagues. While eclectics' treatments may have been little better (Morrow proposed a "tincture of Lobelia and Sanguinaria"), they certainly did none of the harm perpetrated by doctors relying on mercury-based products or the lancet.[41] The minimalist, herbal approach employed by eclectic physicians, while largely ineffective *per se*, still provided a safer approach to treating cholera patients than conventional regimens—even if only by not further weakening patients already dangerously debilitated by cholera.

Eclectic physicians vociferously proclaimed their successes in treating cholera victims in their journals, specifically claiming much lower mortality rates than among patients treated by conventional means. Eclectics seem to have found a new confidence in their experiences with cholera, resulting in strong assertions of their success. One eclectic writer, L. C. Dolley, claimed that they had "disarmed [cholera] of its terrors," making the "dreaded disease" more "manageable." Their journals offered statistics from individual eclectic physicians in Ohio and New York, as well as statistics from hospitals supervised by eclectics proclaiming their success in reducing morbidity. They trumpeted mortality rates of less than 10 percent (and sometimes as low as 3 percent), and contrasted them with mortality rates they claimed were close to 50 percent among patients treated by allopathic colleagues. In an 1849 editorial at the height of the cholera epidemic in Cincinnati, Joseph Buchanan and Thomas Morrow lamented that more comparative data were not available, hinting that allopaths feared supplying data that would document their "awful catalogue of death" relative to the much better rates achieved among patients of eclectic physicians.[42]

More than a decade later, eclectic physicians like William Paine continued to reproduce the data supplied by J. H. Jordan, Thomas Morrow, and other eclectics during this period as part of an ongoing effort to bolster the appeal of eclectic medicine to prospective students and to the public. Such data resonated especially with Paine, who began his medical practice in Ohio as a practitioner working in "exact accordance with . . . Old School" therapeutics for three years before taking up the eclectic regimen. As early as the 1851 meeting of the National Eclectic Medical Association (NEMA), Paine shared statistical evidence of his improved patient outcomes once he abandoned bloodletting and mercurials.[43] Although eclectics did not fully sustain this emphasis on statistical data, they clearly understood the potential this more scientific approach provided to bolster their cause. As a result, at its second annual National Eclectic Medical Convention, held in May 1949, NEMA adopted a constitution that, among other provisions, established in Article 4 a standing committee on medical statistics, and passed a resolution asking "all eclectic physicians" to forward their statistics for the year to that committee.[44]

Given that eclectics remained a relatively small minority of physicians in mid-nineteenth-century America, leading members of the movement like John Buchanan and William Paine often felt themselves on the defensive. It is not surprising that the analogies eclectics commonly drew upon were those of religious and political dissent. They saw themselves as "free and fearless inquirers" facing opposition from "medical bigots" determined to enforce a medical orthodoxy that labeled all who failed to conform as quacks and charlatans. When circumstances arose that gave eclectics an opportunity to strike back at the medical orthodoxy for its deficiencies, both real and perceived, they were eager to take the offensive.[45] Evidence from President Harrison's conventional treatment in his final illness and statistical data from the 1848–49 cholera epidemic provided two valuable, high-profile opportunities for eclectics to put their case to the profession and the public. Eclectics were not loath to pick up these weapons, as they believed themselves engaged in a "great struggle" between "the spirit of freedom" and that of "conservative despotism."[46]

Eclectics and Antebellum-Era Medical Regulation

Eclectics' self-professed struggle in support of scientific and medical freedom was being waged on another front as well—medical regulation through licensing laws. By the 1830s, when the Thomsonians were at their peak of popularity and medical eclectics were slowly coalescing into a reform movement of their own, states had haphazardly adopted the practice of licensing physicians, although in many states such laws were seldom enforced.[47] In the postrevolutionary era, state legislatures often vested *de facto* licensing authority in state and local medical societies, most of which reflected the interests and ambitions of the small minority of physicians who joined these groups. The powers granted these societies varied, but generally they were empowered to control their own membership, giving them legal control over individuals' entry into the lawful practice of medicine. In several states (Connecticut, Maryland, Massachusetts, New Hampshire, and Rhode Island), medical societies did in fact maintain control of medicine by virtue of this *de facto* licensing, represented by society membership. In others, however, the ostensible control and oversight formally granted these societies by the language of the law was undermined by the reluctance of state legislatures to curb unlicensed practice.[48]

The first challenge to medical societies' control of licensure came in Massachusetts, when Harvard asserted the right of its medical school graduates to practice without the subsequent imprimatur of the state's medical society. The legislature resolved the issue by adopting what amounted to a "dual" system, in which either a medical degree or membership in the state medical society sufficed to meet the legal requirements for practice. Whether appropriate or not, state legislatures seemed more "impressed" by a medical degree than by the collective judgment of a medical society on an individual physician's fitness to practice. A medical degree conferred a perceived "prestige," perhaps harking back to European scholarship.[49]

Over time, several other states developed similar dual systems of licensure, but the small number of medical schools meant that medical societies remained the primary licensing entities on behalf of the state.

This state of affairs changed rather quickly in the second decade of the nineteenth century, when the first wave of new medical schools "unbalanced" the system by presenting medical societies with a wave of challengers to their traditional authority. A few numbers from the state of New York illustrate this change. In 1820, only 38 physicians were licensed in that state by virtue of a medical degree, compared with more than 100 licensed through admission to the state medical society. By 1846, this dynamic had reversed completely: in that year, more than 250 individuals were granted licenses based on a medical degree, while fewer than 10 physicians were licensed through the state medical society.[50]

At much the same time that the medical degree became the key credential in licensing a physician, the public became increasingly skeptical of, and in some cases openly hostile to, the general concept of licensing and regulation. During the Jacksonian era, the notion of licensing came under critical scrutiny as a monopolist practice, antithetical to democracy. Individual physicians and medical societies began to question the system as well. They recognized the limitations of state licensing laws, which were generally ineffective in curbing unlicensed practice and often went unenforced. Just as important, with the rise of irregular practitioners, these laws presented a "no win" scenario for medical regulars. The mere existence of these laws invariably drew cries of persecution from irregulars, who could deftly play the sympathetic role of an oppressed minority, a posture easy to adopt and maintain as public interest grew in such alternative medical theories as Thomsonianism. By 1845, a coalescence of factors prompted eighteen states to either repeal their medical licensing laws entirely or, in the case of newly established states, opt not to enact any regulating legislation at all.[51]

The licensing laws put in place in the early years of the republic were slowly being dismantled in the 1830s and 1840s, as state legislators grew exasperated with the wrangling among physicians. New York was the epicenter for much of this prolonged legislative battle. "Men cannot be legislated out of one religion and into another," one legislator remarked, expressing a growing sentiment among his colleagues, "nor can the Legislature thrust calomel and mercury down a man's throat while he wills to take only cayenne or lobelia."[52] However, legislative fatigue and the retreat of licensing laws provided little solace to eclectic physicians facing challenges from medical regulars on multiple fronts. Eclectics remembered the legal challenges thrown earlier at Samuel Thomson and his followers in New York and elsewhere, and they were not as sanguine as Thomson in dismissing such legal barriers. They prepared to defend their right to practice by challenging discriminatory legislation. At the eclectics' 1848 national convention, attendees established a committee on the "legal rights of reformed physicians." Two years later, they adopted a resolution protesting "unequal and oppressive laws" that hampered their ability to practice and to gain faculty and hospital positions.[53]

The resolve of eclectics to fight for their legal rights was in part a reaction to the experience of Ohio eclectics facing stiff opposition from that state's medical regulars. Ohio's eclectics waged a fierce legal battle to "open" the Cincinnati hospital to "all students upon equal terms to the medical lectures," including students at the EMI. Cincinnati's efforts to establish and run a board of health during and after the 1848 cholera outbreak provoked similar confrontations. Pointing out that Old School physicians controlled the Health Board, eclectics condemned as unethical the precedent these medical regulars had set in turning away a patient from the city's cholera hospital who insisted upon treatment by his homeopathic physician. Equally galling was a selective recognition tactic used by Old School practitioners during the cholera outbreak. Regulars harped on the failure of any eclectic to report cholera cases during the outbreak as a breach of the city's protocols for physicians, despite the fact that in all other circumstances, the regulars had steadfastly refused to recognize the eclectics as physicians at all.[54]

Even though the collective demise of state medical licensing laws left eclectics in Ohio and elsewhere in a stronger position than ever, they remained mindful of the ongoing animus and disdain of the orthodox medical establishment. Although the small membership of the American Medical Association (AMA) in its first decade (1847–57) mitigated its ability to impact legislative issues, the association's organizational reports and the sentiments expressed by its leaders kept irregular practitioners on the alert for new attacks. The AMA's early focus on raising standards of medical education as a way to limit the number of physicians and control the market ensured its disdain for homeopathic and eclectic schools like the EMI in Cincinnati and the EMC in Philadelphia. One report by an AMA Committee on Educational Standards lamented that irregular schools' graduates contributed to an "army of Doctors" whose flooding of the marketplace undermined fees to the "merest pittance in the way of remuneration." The AMA derided these schools' graduates as a "swarm of locusts" that, if they could not be eradicated, must be kept at arms' length through a rigid application of the association's controversial consultation clause, which prohibited regular physicians' interactions with them.[55]

The efficacy of this prohibition remains debatable. Medical regulars hoped the prohibition would marginalize and contain irregular practitioners, but any success in this regard was balanced by a clear trade-off that made the tactic of questionable value. This policy and other efforts of containment by the medical regulars allowed eclectic and other irregular practitioners to argue that they were victims of medico-legal oppression and to don the role of the persecuted minority seeking only an equitable playing field. More importantly, it placed eclectic practitioners in the enviable position of swimming with the historical and popular tide as licensing laws collapsed prior to the Civil War. Unfortunately, the rising tide eventually gives way to an ebb tide. As will become evident, the fashion of one generation gives way to others as inherited notions, including perceptions of the proper role of government and of licensing laws, give way to the next generation's fears and priorities.

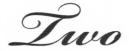

The Rise of the Eclectic Medical College of Pennsylvania

The roots of the Eclectic Medical College of Pennsylvania emerged from deep in the soil of mid-nineteenth-century American medicine and grew into several contributory branches. One main branch is rooted in the history of medical education in Philadelphia; another arose farther west in Ohio, where the first chartered eclectic medical school, Worthington College, was founded only a few years earlier. Yet another branch can be traced back to growing popular dissatisfaction with orthodox medicine and the consequent rise of alternative approaches. All of these factors contributed to the creation of the EMC, but the best explanation is the simplest: like many institutions, the EMC began with an idea.

In the mid-1840s, Thomas Vaughn Morrow, the driving force behind Cincinnati's Eclectic Medical Institute, took note of the efforts of Philadelphia physician Thomas Cooke to organize reformed medicine. Cooke had successfully established and sustained a relationship with the

Pennsylvania Medical Society of Botanic Physicians, an assortment of Thomsonian and herbalist practitioners dedicated to "uniting" all botanic physicians, and in 1840 Cooke persuaded the group to change its name to the Eclectic Botanic Association of Pennsylvania.[1]

Intrigued and inspired by Cooke's efforts, Morrow sought to mirror and expand on them by organizing a national meeting of eclectic physicians as the springboard for what he envisioned as a national medical university. Morrow contacted Cooke and shared his vision of creating a centrally located eclectic medical school capable of handling more than five hundred students annually. Morrow's ambitious efforts never came to fruition, but Cooke never forgot the idea of an eclectic medical college and, inspired by the success of the EMI in Cincinnati, began imagining what might be possible in Philadelphia. Supported by others in Philadelphia seeking to advance the cause of reformed medicine, Cooke and several colleagues soon became active in a group called the Middle States Reformed Medical Society, which routinely met in Philadelphia. Here he came into contact with Drs. Perkins Sweet and Joseph Sites, who shared his aspirations for a reformed medical school there.[2]

By 1850, these three men had become the primary agents in establishing an eclectic medical college in Philadelphia. Their timing proved fortuitous. For many years, the University of Pennsylvania had held the field as the sole medical school in the region. In 1826, Jefferson Medical College broke this hegemony when it gained legal standing from the state legislature, although it did so only after a protracted battle with both unsympathetic legislators and officials of the University of Pennsylvania. Once breached, Philadelphia's bastions of medical orthodoxy steadily crumbled. In 1839, the state legislature chartered the Medical Department of Pennsylvania College. Additional players arrived in the late 1840s—Franklin Medical College in 1846, the Philadelphia College of Medicine in 1847, and the Homeopathic Medical College of Pennsylvania in 1848.[3] Then 1850 saw the founding of the Woman's Medical College in Philadelphia.[4] These developments meant that, at the time Cooke and Morrow were corresponding about the prospects for a national eclectic university in Philadelphia, the politico-legal environment in Pennsylvania seemed amenable to the founding of another medical school. When Morrow's hopes for a national school proved too ambitious to garner serious support, Cooke looked closer to home for collaborators.

At some point in 1849, Cooke, Sweet, and Sites commenced negotiations to secure the necessary support of a state legislator to sponsor a bill. On February 25, 1850, their efforts resulted in success: the Commonwealth of Pennsylvania issued a charter establishing the "Eclectic Medical College of Pennsylvania." Under section three of the enabling legislation, the EMC was given the "power to grant the degree of Doctor of Medicine to any such persons as shall have attended two courses of medical lectures, and completed a course of study, and possess the qualifications necessary for the same."[5] The EMC joined the ranks of several other eclectic schools operating at that time: the Reformed Medical College of Georgia (1845–61), the Eclectic Medical Institute in Cincinnati (1845–1939), and the Central Medical College of New York (1849–52), as well as a half dozen more that appeared briefly before and after the launch of the EMC.[6]

Twenty years later, the report of a Pennsylvania state senate committee cast aspersions on the school's origins by characterizing the enabling legislation as "complicated and mysterious."[7] That characterization seems more a retrospective application of questionable motive to the school's founders than the evidence then or now would seem to suggest. Despite this insinuation, the impetus for founding the EMC stemmed from the genuine desire of eclectic physicians to establish a school along reformed medical principles as part of a larger collective effort to organize at the state, and later national, levels. The success of Cooke, Sites, and Sweet in gaining the support of a state legislator to introduce and shepherd a bill through the legislature in 1850 was neither mysterious or unique. It followed similar successful applications for charters to found several other Philadelphia schools, each representing a legitimate effort in medical education. Hence it seems reasonable to conclude that there was nothing duplicitous about the school's founding. The best evidence indicates that the Eclectic Medical College of Pennsylvania began as a legitimate institution seeking to educate prospective physicians.

Contemporary nineteenth-century writers like Alexander Wilder noted the EMC's reputable beginning as part of their accounts of how far the school had fallen from its original inspiration. Even harsh critics of the EMC, such as the prominent Philadelphia physician Daniel Garrison Brinton, implied such a fall from legitimate origins in their portrayals of Buchanan and the school.[8] While some critics may have doubted the school's legitimate origins, assuming its respectable origins lent even greater force to their narrative by casting John Buchanan as the villain behind its subsequent downfall.

EARLY OPERATIONS AT THE EMC

Once they had secured the necessary charter, Cooke and his colleagues moved quickly to begin operations. A September 1851 advertisement in the *Philadelphia Inquirer* announced the opening of a four-month session of the EMC beginning in October. The school's five original faculty members were Drs. Thomas Cooke (serving as dean), Stephen H. Potter, Henry Hollembaek,[9] Joseph Sites, and St. John Watkins Mintzer. (In his 1901 work covering the rise of eclecticism, *The History of Medicine*, Alexander Wilder identified these same individuals, along with Thomas G. Chase, as the original faculty.) In general, these physicians all possessed solid, respectable reputations within the medical reform movement. Four of these men—Cooke, Potter, Sites, and Hollembaek—appear in the records of the National Eclectic Medical Association (NEMA) during the organization's earliest annual meetings from 1850 through 1853. In fact, this cohort of EMC faculty served on multiple committees for the national association.[10]

While we have relatively limited information about these men, what we know does not point toward dubious motives or suspect practices in the school's first decade. Cooke's pedigree in the reform movement was impeccable. He trained in Philadelphia under an English botanic physician, John Howell, and later founded the *Botanic Medical Reformer and Home Physician*. He was an original member of the NEMA and one of the signatories of an 1848 resolution calling for a national convention of eclectic physicians. Cooke may have been the originator of the term *eclectic* as it applied to the reform movement in medicine, a distinction supported by his renaming of Pennsylvania's botanic society.[11]

Stephen Potter had similarly deep roots in the medical reform movement. He graduated from Worthington College, the predecessor school of the EMI in Cincinnati, the flagship of eclectic medical schools. Potter also played a role in establishing several short-lived eclectic schools during the mid-nineteenth century, including the Central Medical College of New York (Randolph), the Syracuse Medical College, and the

American Medical College (Cincinnati). Potter's tenure at the EMC appears to have been fairly brief. Perhaps this reflected the inevitable tensions with colleagues arising from Potter's temperament, which even a sympathetic fellow eclectic described as "ambitious of superiority and fond of notoriety."[12]

Henry Hollembaek was a graduate of Jefferson Medical College and a collaborator with Cooke in publishing the *Botanic Medical Reformer.* He spent most of his adult life in nearby Burlington, New Jersey, where he earned sufficient respect from his community to serve on the town's Common Council and as city mayor in the 1850s and 1860s.[13] Further evidence of Hollembaek's political connections can be deduced from his appointment for many years as postmaster for that city.[14]

Joseph Sites maintained a successful obstetrical practice in Philadelphia beginning in the early 1840s. He, too, carried some local influence as evidenced by his years as a trustee for Girard College and his multiple terms serving on the Philadelphia Common Council. Like their colleagues among the original faculty, Sites and Hollembaek were active participants in the NEMA, serving on committees, delivering reports, and sometimes offering dissenting opinions.[15] The other members of the early faculty, Thomas Chase and St. John Mintzer, did not appear to have engaged directly with the NEMA or otherwise participate in organized efforts to foster eclectic medicine.

The EMC held classes at a building on Haines Street, just west of Sixth at the time of its opening in October 1851. The facilities of the three-story structure were probably modest, but adequate by the standards of the day. The first floor held lecture rooms and a chemistry lab, the second floor housed a medical museum, and the third floor offered an amphitheater for surgery and dissection. Remodeling in 1855 gave much of the building fresh paint and wallpaper, along with the installation of water and gas.[16] This upgrade was not merely aesthetic. One faculty member stressed that securing a stronger foothold for eclectic medicine meant that schools like the EMC must be as "desirable in appearance" as in the "science" they were teaching. In his assessment, many students flocked to allopathic schools simply because of their familiarity with the institution and not their "belie[f] in its teachings."[17] This contemporary assessment highlights the strong competition for students among medical schools of the era. One historian characterized the environment as one of "contentious rivalry, deep-seated jealousy, . . . and uncontrolled competition."[18]

The ambitions of some EMC faculty extended beyond the school. Two faculty members, Chase and Mintzer, established the American Medical Museum in Philadelphia. From the evidence in his surviving correspondence to a state senator, the museum appears to have been largely Mintzer's idea. This initiative offers another example of how a "private" bill was navigated through the state legislature and demonstrates the political acumen and legislative connections of the EMC leadership during its first decade. In only thirty days and for what Mintzer characterized as a reasonable sum ($485), the bill passed the legislature as an amendment to another bill. In its final form, the legislation incorporating the museum listed its purpose as the "encouragement of medical science in the profession and the dissemination of physiological and hygienic laws . . . to the public." Mintzer apparently felt strongly on the latter point. He hoped the museum's educational focus would "disarm Mystery and Quackery of its power" and help the public avoid being "duped."[19] Though the museum never operated as a separate, stand-alone entity, any acquired holdings probably bolstered those of the EMC's medical museum, if nothing else.

From the very beginning, the EMC's printed materials made clear its philosophical orientation within the medical reform movement. A school circular published just before the first term struck the main chords associated with eclectic medicine: The EMC would avoid the rigid, dogmatic adherence to "pathy" and "ism" that characterized the extremists within allopathy and homeopathy; the school would "select from all other systems that which we deem good and useful, and discard that which is deleterious"; it disavowed the harsh treatments favored by allopathic practitioners, notably bloodletting, blistering, and the use of toxic minerals; and it would instead promote "innocent agents" (i.e., botanicals) for their less traumatic impact on patients.[20]

Valedictory addresses made in 1854 and 1855 by faculty members Henry Hollembaek and Marshall Calkins give further insights into the EMC's philosophy, describing the school's intent to teach a therapeutic regimen dominated by indigenous, natural remedies. Noting the Thomsonian success in promoting and popularizing botanic therapies, Hollembaek interpreted this as a sign of Americans' growing rejection of allopathic treatment, observing that they were beginning to "question the propriety of dying . . . in a scientific mode."[21] Calkins developed this same theme by making the case for replacing dangerous minerals with "indigenous" botanic remedies, and promising that the school would teach its students to "expel disease through . . . *natural* avenues."[22] Fellow faculty member John Fondey echoed these ideas, asserting that they formed the bases for eclectics' success because they "appeal[ed] to the common sense and reason" of not only the public but a growing number of American physicians.[23]

Cooke and his fellow faculty members created a school calendar and curriculum mirroring conventional approaches. The EMC commenced instruction with a fall session running approximately four months, from mid-October to March 1. This academic calendar remained in place until 1857, when the school shortened the fall session to end in January, with a spring session immediately following. In 1868, the EMC again revised its academic calendar to include a summer session, running from May through July, ostensibly to offer a truncated set of lectures designed to prepare students for the fall session. Financial considerations probably weighed equally in the decision.[24]

Didactic instruction remained the norm in all American medical schools of the day. Regarding their primary job as helping students acquire, retain, and apply medical knowledge, faculty members generally demanded a foundation of rote memorization from students, while presenting them with a series of lectures in the fall and repeating the lectures in the spring. Pedagogical innovations, such as a sequential introduction of content with scored examinations over a three-year curriculum, did not arise until the 1870s, and even then only a few schools—e.g., Harvard, Penn, Syracuse, and Michigan—employed them.[25]

By the mid-1850s, the list of subjects covered in the EMC curriculum expanded to cover an impressive array of medical content: anatomy (descriptive, surgical, comparative, and microscopic), physiology, pathology, histology, embryology, botany, *materia medica*, therapeutics, organic chemistry, toxicology, surgery, hygiene, obstetrics, diseases of women and children, and the theory and practice of medicine. Beginning in 1864, the EMC began offering lectures in military and dental surgery. The EMC's announcement for the 1863–64 academic year set forth an ambitious schedule for students, claiming to offer six lectures daily. These included clinical lectures on Wednesdays and Saturdays, augmented by extensive

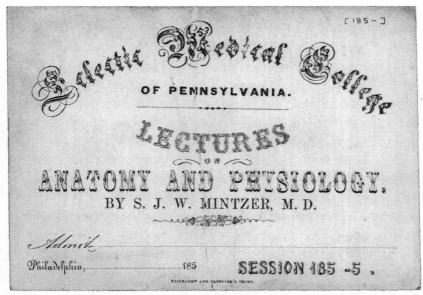

Fig. 1. Lecture card from the Eclectic Medical College of Pennsylvania. Lecture cards served both as an entry ticket and as documentation of a student's progression through medical education. This card for Dr. St. John Watkins Mintzer dates to the 1850s, when the EMC operated as a legitimate educational institution. Image MSS2_0019_01, lecture card, courtesy of the College of Physicians of Philadelphia.

clinical instruction through accompanying faculty on their "daily rounds" and dissection.[26] Although this was unstated, the "rounds" must have involved seeing patients at faculty members' personal offices or at smaller neighborhood hospitals, since the EMC undoubtedly would have heavily promoted any relationship with one of Philadelphia's major hospitals.

Despite the conventional course offerings and the semblance of a shared vision among the faculty in the EMC's early days, tensions lurked beneath the surface. According to Alexander Wilder, a contemporary with knowledge and familiarity of many of the players in eclectic medicine, the Middle States Reformed Medical Society (and especially one of its members, Dr. William F. Smith), which had been an early supporter of the EMC, soon became dissatisfied with the "management" of the school and the "controversy" refused to die. The issue was brought before the NEMA without success in 1851, only to be resurrected the following year. The national association decided the matter in favor of the EMC. Rather than settling the dispute, however, the decision left the society so indignant over the perceived injustice that it approached the Pennsylvania legislature to seek a charter for another medical school. This effort succeeded in 1853, when the society secured a charter for the American College of Medicine. One source claims that the new college secured a building and faculty and attracted more than two dozen students, who attended the fall 1853–54 session of the school. However, most of the evidence suggests that the school never became operational; perhaps cooler heads prevailed or concessions were offered. Regardless, Wilder reported, the "difficulties were adjusted."[27] This minor squabble would not ordinarily merit discussion except that the 1853 charter for the American College of Medicine provided the legal basis for a later, more consequential split among the EMC's faculty.

During its first decade, significant changes occurred at the EMC. In the mid-1850s, Drs. James M. Buzzell, Marshall Calkins, John Fondey, Joseph B. Holland, and William Paine were added to the faculty to replace Cooke, Potter, and Mintzer. Cooke died in 1855, while Potter and Mintzer moved on to other ventures.[28] Like the original faculty, the new faculty members possessed strong credentials in eclectic circles. Buzzell had acquired his medical education at Dartmouth and apparently had dabbled in homeopathic medicine for a time, publishing several issues of *The Homeopathist* before embracing the eclectic philosophy at another early eclectic school, Worcester Medical College in Massachusetts. Buzzell later helped to establish the short-lived Eclectic Medical College of Maine.[29]

Calkins's bona fides in reformed medicine included a period of study with Calvin Newton at the Worcester Medical Institution, from which he graduated in 1848. If his published addresses to EMC students are indicative, Calkins possessed a shrewd sense of the opportunities open to eclectic physicians willing to commit themselves unreservedly to evidence-based science as the basis for their practice. Calkins's shrewdness in measuring the historical tide can also be seen in his post-EMC career. He later took a second medical degree from Dartmouth (1868) and made a conscious decision to move away from eclecticism back into orthodox medicine. It was probably no accident that his 1922 obituary in the *Boston Medical and Surgical Journal* omitted all reference to his time at the EMC.[30] Whether this embarrassed silence stemmed from his association with the by-then long discredited school or from his early role in eclectic medicine in general is hard to say. The third new addition to the faculty, John Fondey, was a native Philadelphian and a graduate of Penn. Like Cooke, he proclaimed himself an eclectic physician by choice and professional "conviction" on the merits of reformed medicine.[31]

The most significant addition to the faculty in shaping the history of the EMC was William Paine, a former graduate of the Berkshire Medical College. Like many of the EMC faculty preceding him, Paine held impeccable credentials in the reformed movement. He had practiced for many years in Warren, Ohio, where he had helped "organize" the eclectic medical college in Cincinnati.[32] He knew many of Philadelphia's eclectics through his participation with the Middle States Reformed Medical Society, and had become particularly well-acquainted with Stephen Potter while the two had served on the faculty of Syracuse Medical College. Paine appears to have had an intense personality, holding equally strong opinions of his own abilities and those of his colleagues. An unspoken ambivalence about Paine is noticeable in even the accolades given him by his supporters. One commented favorably on his leadership skills, describing him as liberally endowed with those "qualities that persuade and *control*" (italics added).[33] Friends and critics alike acknowledged him as keenly "ambitious." As one contemporary put it, Paine wanted always to be in charge of affairs, whether circumstances warranted it or not.[34] Writing later in his *History of the American Eclectic Practice of Medicine*, Paine boastfully listed his contributions to the EMC. These included inaugurating the school's *Eclectic Medical Journal*, and securing the site for the college's move to a new, more spacious location at Sixth and Callowhill. He also wrote his own tome on eclectic medicine in 1857, *The Epitome of the Eclectic Practice of Medicine*, and summarized his labors in Philadelphia as nothing less than "assum[ing] the arduous task of re-organizing the Eclectic College and engaging competent teachers."[35]

MOUNTING TENSIONS AND A FACULTY SPLIT

In addition to faculty tensions, monetary woes exacerbated conditions at the EMC. In 1857, the school discounted the price of "professors' tickets" and signaled a strong interest in attracting students of modest income as a means of expanding enrollment. The following year, the school offered only a fall-winter session, foregoing a spring session in 1858.[36] This mix of ongoing financial pressures and strong personalities proved too combustible to remain stable for long.

Evidence of these pressures can be found in the school fees published regularly in the EMC's *Eclectic Medical Journal of Pennsylvania*. In reviewing the published fees for each session over more than a decade, two points emerge. First, the EMC's fees appear to have been comparable to those of other Philadelphia medical schools.[37] Competition for students limited the potential ceiling for student fees in Philadelphia's medical schools. However, the actual number of attending students at the EMC was probably lower than the published figures; certainly this was the case by the 1870s, when the school's prospectus materials had become far less reliable. Thus, simply offering competitive fees could not by itself make the school financially competitive with larger, better-known institutions like Penn and Jefferson. Second, new practices introduced after the Civil War indicate a growing scramble for revenues in the short term. The first of these was the EMC's introduction of a flat "scholarship" fee (discussed in chapter 3), which not only signaled mounting financial pressures but also a shift toward the questionable diploma practices that would later make the school infamous. The second practice introduced by the mid-1860s was the sale of textbooks. While assigned medical texts still included such standard fare such as Gray's *Anatomy*, Dalton's *Physiology*, and Brandt

Table 2: Published Fees Charged by the EMC, 1863–1877

	1863–64	1866–67	1869–70	1870–71	1877–78
Matriculation fee	$5	$5	$5	$5	-
Lecture fee	$60	$60	$60	$40	-
Demonstration fee	$5	$5	$5	$10	-
Fee for graduation or Diploma	$25	-	$30	-	$30
Dissection fee	-	-	-	-	$10
Scholarship	-	$100	-	$60	$100

Sources: "Thirteenth Annual Session, 1863–64," *Eclectic Medical Journal of Pennsylvania* (March–April 1863), 64ff.; "Sixteenth Annual Session, 1866–67," *Eclectic Medical Journal of Pennsylvania* (March–April 1866), 104ff.; "Sessions 1869–70," *Eclectic Medical Journal of Pennsylvania* (July 1869), 336ff.; "Sessions of 1877–78," *Eclectic Medical Journal of Pennsylvania* (July 1877), 173ff.

and Taylor's *Chemistry*, additional texts written by EMC faculty members (Buchanan, Sites, Hollembaek, and Cochran) featured heavily in the curriculum, with each volume selling for three to five dollars.[38]

John Buchanan arrived at the EMC in 1860, around the time of a major fracture among the faculty. The reasons for the rift are no longer entirely clear, although one author, writing many years later, claimed William Paine's insistence on giving "public lectures on sexual diseases" prompted the final disagreement leading to an irrevocable breach among the faculty.[39] This explanation is plausible, but it rather conveniently placed the blame on Paine, a figure by then long discredited for his role in the diploma scam. Since the practice of public lectures had become common, the controversy over Paine's lectures, if true, concerned their content rather than their method of delivery.[40] Paine had become dean of the school in 1859 and had proved to be a powerful force within it after the departure of Marshall Calkins. Paine brought with him to the faculty James McClintock, a Jefferson graduate and former student of that school's founder, George McClellan, whose son later commanded the Army of the Potomac during the Civil War. McClintock and Paine first crossed paths as instructor and student at the Berkshire Medical College in the early 1840s. McClintock was well known in Philadelphia's medical circles as the founder of the highly successful Philadelphia School of Anatomy and later of the Philadelphia College of Medicine. The closure of the latter in 1859 probably prompted McClintock's move to the EMC with Paine.[41]

McClintock's addition to the EMC faculty represented a minor coup for the school. McClintock enjoyed a solid though somewhat controversial reputation in medical circles. He and the Philadelphia College of Medicine had raised eyebrows by instituting a two-term curriculum: a four-month session beginning in October and a second nonrepeating four-month term commencing in March. This format, discontinued in 1854, allowed students to graduate in one year rather than two.[42] He felt a kinship with medical "irregulars" and told his students numerous anecdotes of the many slights and slanders he had endured for his independent approach, such as the destruction of cards announcing his lectures and the spread of rumors that cadavers he used for dissection had died of smallpox. He dismissed such harassment as a minor nuisance and evidence of Philadelphia's "medical fogyism." Given his past associations with Paine, it was not surprising that McClintock quickly aligned himself with his former student in the burgeoning disagreement among faculty at the EMC.

Paine's and McClintock's dissatisfaction with the state of affairs at the EMC led them to begin a behind-the-scenes movement that culminated

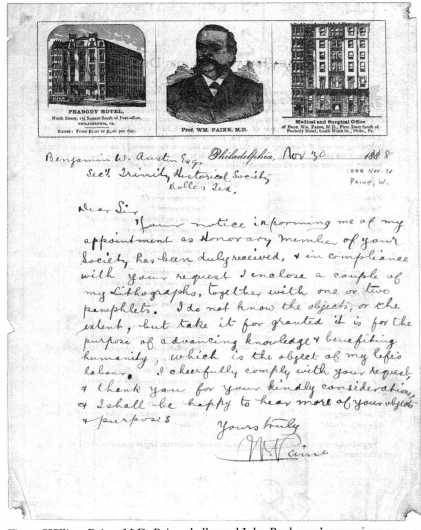

Fig. 2. William Paine, M.D. Paine challenged John Buchanan's preeminence on two fronts: leadership in the Philadelphia eclectic community and the sale of medical diplomas. Image MSS2_0268_01, William Paine letter, courtesy of the College of Physicians of Philadelphia.

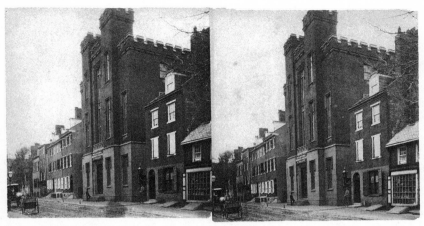

Fig. 3. Philadelphia University, located at Ninth Street south of Walnut. In 1865, William Paine dropped the label eclectic from his school, renaming it Philadelphia University of Medicine and Surgery. Image courtesy of the Library Company of Philadelphia.

in the establishment of a rival eclectic school in Philadelphia. They did so by acquiring the charter for the American College of Medicine. This charter had originally been secured in 1853 by members of the Middle States Reformed Medical Society, but the school had never gone into operation. Now Paine and McClintock arranged for Pennsylvania's legislature to pass a bill on February 15, 1860, amending the name of the school allowed by the charter to an ungainly new form: the American College of Medicine in Pennsylvania *and Eclectic Medical College of Philadelphia* (italics added). Paine moved rapidly to secure a building for the new school, finding a location near Race Street between Fourth and Fifth Streets. Several years later, the school relocated to Ninth and Locust, where it remained until its closure in 1880. In modifying the school's name to mirror so closely that of the EMC, Paine signaled his intention to establish a school that would compete with the EMC for pride of place and even survival in Philadelphia. By 1865, however, Paine relinquished the fight, eliminating *eclectic* from the name entirely in favor of a new title, Philadelphia University of Medicine and Surgery.[43]

Given these events, John Buchanan's arrival at the EMC in 1860 came at an inauspicious juncture in the school's history. The city now had two competing eclectic medical schools with nearly identical names: the

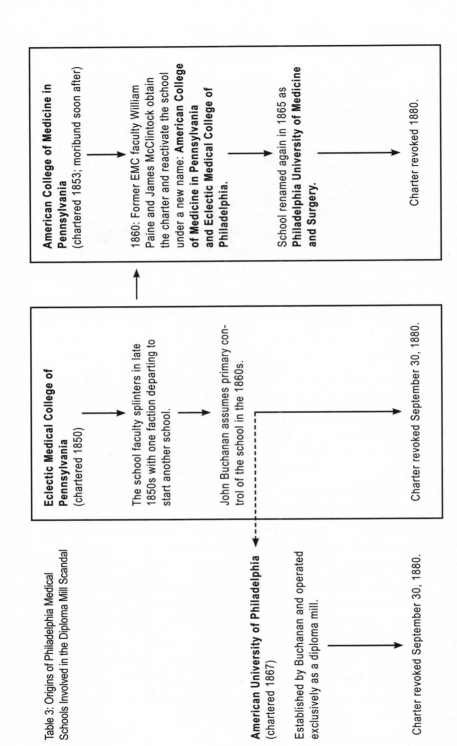

Table 3: Origins of Philadelphia Medical
Schools Involved in the Diploma Mill Scandal

Eclectic Medical College of Pennsylvania
(chartered 1850)

The school faculty splinters in late 1850s with one faction departing to start another school.

John Buchanan assumes primary control of the school in the 1860s.

Charter revoked September 30, 1880.

American University of Philadelphia
(chartered 1867)

Established by Buchanan and operated exclusively as a diploma mill.

Charter revoked September 30, 1880.

American College of Medicine in Pennsylvania
(chartered 1853; moribund soon after)

1860: Former EMC faculty William Paine and James McClintock obtain the charter and reactivate the school under a new name: **American College of Medicine in Pennsylvania and Eclectic Medical College of Philadelphia.**

School renamed again in 1865 as **Philadelphia University of Medicine and Surgery.**

Charter revoked 1880.

Source: Adapted from Harold J. Abrahams, *Extinct Medical Schools of Nineteenth Century Philadelphia* (Philadelphia: University of Pennsylvania Press, 1966), 245.

Eclectic Medical College of Pennsylvania (Buchanan) and the Eclectic Medical College of Philadelphia (Paine). However it transpired, the disruption among EMC faculty created an opportunity for John Buchanan. He moved quickly into a leadership role at the school, including serving as editor for the EMC's journal. Buchanan and Paine took turns lobbing verbal assaults against each other and their respective schools. Paine labeled the EMC faculty an "embarrassment" to the profession, calling them "ignorant pretenders" practicing a "steam and pepper system of Thomson[ian]" medicine. Buchanan responded in kind, characterizing Paine's school a "one-horse, unchartered humbug" and, in more crass language, as the delivery of a "great abortion" into medical education. From there, Buchanan launched into a point-by-point recitation of Paine's alleged transgressions—from operating under an invalid charter to poaching students and absconding with EMC funds.[44]

Unfortunately, conflicts of this nature seemed endemic to much of nineteenth-century American medicine, whether they were waged along the more common sectarian lines of allopath versus homeopath and eclectic or within the ranks of irregular practitioners. The EMC was hardly alone in experiencing a significant episode of faculty infighting. Philadelphia's Homeopathic Medical College split as a result of faculty dissension in 1867, resulting in a two-year period in which two homeopathic schools competed for students.[45] At the EMC, the faculty infighting contributed to a dysfunctional environment that destabilized the school, leaving it vulnerable to ethical lapses and a drift toward unsavory practices around the issuance of diplomas. On a purely practical level, the formation of Paine's eclectic school only blocks away put the two schools into direct competition for students at a time when enrollment numbers were beginning to plummet, threatening financial ruin. Only one year later, this strain was compounded by the outbreak of the Civil War. A significant number of medical students in Philadelphia came from Southern states, Virginia in particular, and many of them dropped their studies and rushed home in the spring of 1861.[46] It was at this point that John Buchanan became immediately integral to the EMC story. Buchanan's personal and professional background, as well as his activities at the EMC, directly influenced the school's descent into the medical diploma trade.

" . . . no waste is so extravagant as
the waste of human life."

—John Buchanan, *Family Physician and
Domestic Practice of Medicine*, 1884

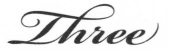

The Rise of Dr. John Buchanan

Little can be stated definitively about John Buchanan's early years or even about his adult life before he joined the EMC faculty in 1860. Multiple records from the U.S. federal census indicate that John Buchanan was born in Scotland. However, these same records are contradictory on several other fundamental facts. For example, these records variously list Buchanan's date of birth as 1826 (1860 census), 1827 (1900 census), and 1829 (1880 census).[1] Little is known about Buchanan's family or the circumstances of his life in Scotland. From references later appearing in journal articles and newspapers, Buchanan had at least two brothers (James and Peter), who immigrated to America and may have had some minor involvement with him at the EMC. His parents apparently joined him as well. In a confession reported in the Philadelphia newspapers in spring 1881, John Buchanan alluded to the financial pressures laid on him by his efforts to support multiple households in the United States: two of his own (in Philadelphia and New Jersey) and one for his aged parents.[2]

A similar confusion exists regarding Buchanan's immigration to the United States. The 1900 census lists the year of his arrival as 1850, but

Fig. 4. Portrait of John Buchanan, M.D. This likeness appeared in Buchanan's *Practical Treatise on the Diseases of Children* (1866). Image reprinted with the permission of the Library Company of Philadelphia.

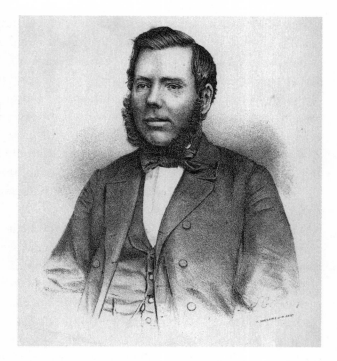

this date seems likely to have been an approximation provided to the census taker by a then-elderly Buchanan. Information from the 1860 federal census, a source more contemporaneous to his arrival, lists the ages and birthplaces of his children, which help to narrow the date of Buchanan's arrival in America. Buchanan fathered four children with his first wife, Isabella—James, born in 1852; John, born in 1855; Isabell, born in 1857; and George, born in 1859—all of whom, except for the eldest, were born in Pennsylvania.[3] This makes it likely that Buchanan arrived in the United States between 1852 and 1855.

The date of Buchanan's arrival is significant in that it would provide some insight into how quickly he made the transition to practicing physician in the United States. Soon after arriving from Scotland, Buchanan worked for a time as a porter in the Philadelphia oilcloth factory of Thomas Potter on Arch Street.[4] Journals and newspapers later harped repeatedly on this snippet from his life story. Their intent was clear: to discredit Buchanan by insinuating a suspiciously rapid rise from porter to physician. That critics latched onto this piece of Buchanan's personal history is not surprising, as this biographical fact perfectly fit their narrative needs by portraying him as an illegitimate member of the medical profession and a scoundrel from his earliest years. A less partisan—and perhaps more realistic—interpretation of his life history might hold that Buchanan's time as a porter reflected nothing more than the economic need of a recent arrival to provide for himself and his family. A physician newly arrived in America might well find it difficult to immediately set up a financially viable medical practice, and thus would accept whatever employment was available until he could establish himself professionally. Such a course of action in Buchanan's early career seems entirely understandable rather than suspicious.

This leads next to the question of Buchanan's medical education and training. Philadelphia newspapers and journals provided considerable contemporary coverage of Buchanan beginning around 1872. The events of 1880 vastly expanded the frequency and scope of coverage as national periodicals took up his story. Given the nature of the scandal in which Buchanan and the EMC were caught up—the sale of medical diplomas—the press displayed a surprising lack of critical evaluation concerning Buchanan's personal medical background and qualifications. Once the scandal emerged fully, jibes and epithets rained down upon him from all sides, with writers disparagingly placing his title of Dr. in quotation marks. Yet none of these contemporary writers commented on Buchanan's educational background or the source of his diploma—an especially strange oversight considering the subject of the scandal. The absence of this line of attack suggests that John Buchanan possessed legitimate medical credentials. Several pieces of evidence support this speculation.

A small notice appearing in the *Philadelphia Inquirer* in late 1882 offers perhaps the best evidence. The news item noted that Buchanan had been added to the county registry of physicians in Philadelphia. A prothonotary reluctantly included him under a section of Pennsylvania law allowing physicians without an original diploma in their possession to provide a certified copy of the document or affidavits from the lecturing professors with knowledge of the physician. Whatever documents Buchanan provided were sufficient to satisfy the naturally suspicious official. Furthermore, the newspaper made it clear that the prothonotary knew precisely who he was dealing with—John Buchanan, former head of the EMC and notorious seller of diplomas. The prothonotary undoubtedly scrutinized Buchanan's documentation looking for any flaw he could use as a basis for refusing to list him on Philadelphia's physician registry, but apparently none could be found; thus, the official added Buchanan to the registry, listing his attendance at Glasgow College.[5] It bears noting this claim is consistent with Buchanan's own assertion, in his March 25, 1881, confession in the *Philadelphia Record*, that he held a diploma from Glasgow. This claim by Buchanan was later corroborated (or at least repeated) in a reminiscence penned by Eli G. Jones, one of Buchanan's former students. According to Jones, Buchanan told his students that he studied at, and took an M.D. degree from, the Royal Infirmary at Glasgow.[6]

Buchanan took medical courses in the United States as well. He completed the anatomical course at the Philadelphia School for Anatomy in 1858. A valedictory address given in February 1859 to the graduates of the 1858 course included a John Buchanan from Scotland. That the course was composed of students and physicians from the city's various medical colleges lends additional support to the notion that Buchanan also took a degree from the EMC in the late 1850s, as his former student recalled. The student's memory on this point was supported by a twentieth-century writer's review of the listing of all EMC graduates, which included a John Buchanan in 1858.[7]

A variety of sources confirms Buchanan as a practicing physician in Philadelphia by the mid- to late 1850s. If we accept the chronology of his medical career that he provided in the general remarks section of his 1865 publication, *The Treatment of Venereal Disease*, Buchanan began private practice in Philadelphia sometime around 1858. *McElroy's Philadelphia City Directory* for the years 1859 and 1860, as well as the 1860 federal census, provide contemporary evidence that Buchanan was then a practicing physician.[8] He later commenced a clinical practice from a consultation office at 227 North Twelfth Street that he maintained for many years.[9]

JOHN BUCHANAN, THE AUTHOR

John Buchanan's appointment to the faculty of the EMC in 1860 augured the start of what should have been a promising career. From that point forward, he certainly seemed to be rising rapidly in his profession, assuming an increasingly prominent role at the EMC and, to some extent, within the broader community of eclectic physicians. Although John Buchanan did not replace Joseph Sites as dean of the school until later in the decade, he took on a steadily larger role in the affairs of the school and in eclectic medicine in Pennsylvania. Beginning in 1863, for example, Buchanan served as secretary for the Eclectic Medical Society of Pennsylvania, which routinely met at the EMC building, retaining this position for many years. Buchanan also began serving as the editor for the school journal, the *Eclectic Medical Journal of Pennsylvania*.[10] In fact, his pen flowed in such an impressive fashion that during the 1860s alone he published a half dozen works on medicine.

> *The Treatment of Venereal Disease* (1865)
> *A Practical Treatise on the Diseases of Children* (1866)
> *The Eclectic Practice of Medicine and Surgery: A Text Book for the Student* (1867)
> *The Centennial Practice of Medicine* (1867)
> *A Practical Treatise on Midwifery and Diseases of Women and Children* (1868)
> *The American Practice of Medicine* (1868)
> *The Physiological and Therapeutic Uses of Our New Remedies* (1873)
> *The Dispensary and Pharmacopoeia of North America and Great Britain* (with John J. Siggins, 1878)
> *The Family Physician and Domestic Practice of Medicine* (1884)
> *An Encyclopedia of the Practice of Medicine Based on Bacteriology* (1890)

Buchanan's many works on various aspects of medicine provide another avenue for insight. While the nature of medical works do not generally lend themselves to personal disclosures, it is possible to catch glimpses from these texts into Buchanan's character and mind-set, as well as his professional outlook. At the very least, from these books and his writings in the *Journal*, we can glean a surprising degree of insight into his beliefs and practices as a medical professional under the banner of eclecticism.

A consideration of the entire body of Buchanan's written work suggests a division of his books into three categories. The first consists of his specialized works on specific aspects of medicine, including venereal disease, obstetrics, and diseases of children. All of these texts appeared during the 1860s, a period that represents the apex of his career. The second category of Buchanan's works encompasses those exploring the botanic emphasis common to eclectic medicine, with a close analysis of its *materia medica*. Two of Buchanan's books fall into this category: *The Physiological and Therapeutic Uses of Our New Remedies* and *The Dispensary and Pharmacopoeia of North America and Great Britain*. The third category consists of works giving broad overviews of medicine tailored for various professional and general audiences. Some of these were organized in encyclopedic form (e.g., *The American Practice of Medicine* and *The Practice of Medicine Based on Bacteriology*), but most arranged the content by bodily organ or system (e.g., *Eclectic Practice of Medicine and Surgery; Centennial Practice of Medicine; Family Physician and Domestic Practice of Medicine*).

In considering the entirety of Buchanan's written works, two major characteristics stand out. First, the views he expressed fall squarely in line with the philosophy of most eclectic practitioners of the day. Like most of his eclectic colleagues, Buchanan subscribed to the old adage that *nature heals while doctors collect the fee*. He held that the physician's primary goal was to assist the natural processes, since medicine—at least in the 1860s—could do no more than mitigate the effects of disease. As he asserted, "the cure of disease is not accomplished by medicine—it is aided by it. Nature does her own work."[11] Buchanan's writings also reflected the eclectic *materia medica* of the day. His works often featured appendixes discussing botanic remedial agents (e.g., *Domestic Practice*) or his own formulary (e.g., *Eclectic Practice of Medicine and Surgery*). In keeping with the Thomsonian botanic tradition, Buchanan's writing commonly features lobelia as a treatment. In this regard, his work was consistent with the eclectic predilection for botanic remedies; this had a long medico-religious tradition,[12] holding that indigenous plants represented the best treatment for diseases specific to a geographic area.[13] Buchanan lauded the "liberal spirit" of eclecticism's founder, Wooster Beach, for "emancipat[ing] our predecessors," while castigating the "non-progressive" elements of the profession.[14] His works also contained repeated condemnations of allopathic—and, to a lesser extent, homeopathic—practices. In some instances, these criticisms were veiled, as when he proposed that "enlightened physician[s] . . . aid . . . nature . . . not by stirring up a terrible disorder in an opposite part of the organism . . . or by administering remedies that produce analogous symptoms to the disease." In other instances, he explicitly condemned the allopathic use of toxic minerals, which he labeled "accursed drugs." In Buchanan's view, substances like mercury and arsenic served only to increase patient mortality. He was equally harsh in his criticism of homeopathic notions, rejecting their therapeutic approach as the "imbecility" of passive "do-nothing" medicine.[15]

The second characteristic of Buchanan's writing is that it mirrors in great part the gaps and limitations of the science of his day. Understandably, his writings from the 1860s, in particular, reflect the era's reliance on abstract descriptive concepts, like the notion of a "vital force" animating all life, with human disease arising from a "deficiency or . . . depression of vitality."[16] Another example appears in his work on venereal disease, which he described as the result of sexually transmitted "morbid . . . poisons."[17] Perhaps the best example derives from Buchanan's reliance on "miasmas" as the originating cause for multiple illnesses, from ague to more serious epidemic diseases like cholera (" . . . the effect of a warm atmosphere"), yellow fever ("arising from . . . animal and vegetable miasm"), typhoid ("caused . . . by vitiated air containing emanations from large bodies of [people] crowded together"), and malaria (arising from "decaying organic matter . . . impregnat[ing] the air . . . with a poison[ous] agent").[18]

Because Buchanan intended several of his works for the general reader (rather than for fellow doctors or medical students), he often employed an everyman, commonsense approach in his recommendations for treating illness. His advice to pregnant women included fresh air, tepid baths, outdoor exercise, and loose clothing (no corsets or tight lacing). For young children, he stressed the importance of cleanliness and vaccination. Diet and exercise were common recommendations for all prospective patients. To forestall constipation, Buchanan recommended developing a daily routine, arguing that the best solution was to develop over the long term a daily "habit" of evacuating the bowels at a set time.

Buchanan's general advice to younger physicians echoed this pragmatic note: watch your community for signs of epidemic disease, be careful in administering any purgative to your patients lest it mask or complicate otherwise important symptoms, offer only a "guarded opinion" on "hereditary dispositions," and remain optimistic when treating children as "[they] are extremely tenacious of life and often rally from the most severe disorders."[19]

Buchanan's observations of the human condition in the patients he treated mirrored the biases inherent to the public for whom he sometimes wrote. In his discourses on certain illnesses, he echoed the commonly held racial attitudes one might expect from a white citizen of Philadelphia in the latter half of the nineteenth century. Thus, in his discussion of "cerebral disease," he explained its greater presence or "tendency" in America along racial lines as evidence of a "higher . . . grade of civiliza-tion." Like many of his contemporaries, he diagnosed hysteria as a clinical condition common among middle- and upper-class women of a "nervous or nervo-sanguine temperament." In works intended for a general audi-ence, he shifted his tone from physician-author to physician-moralizer, indulging in long passages on issues he deemed particularly important. In an extended passage on masturbation, for example, he warned physicians and parents alike not to turn a blind eye to the "evils of this practice," calling it "monstrous and unnatural," and asserting that it was a habit conspicuously present among those in insane asylums.[20] Such sentiments were not uncommon during this period. One of Buchanan's faculty col-leagues, John Fondey, offered similar cautions against "self-pollution" and "sexual excess." He even went so far as to propose masturbation as a possible cause for tubercular and scrofulous diseases.[21]

Buchanan's writing grows particularly animated when he draws on his own professional experiences and preferred treatments for patients in his medical discussions. He often used the first person in relating such anecdotes, to stress that the empirical evidence he is sharing with the reader was acquired from firsthand experience. Specific instances of this approach range widely from simple advice regarding preferred *materia medica* ("I have found the oils of pumpkin seed . . .") to recom-mendations for clinical treatments ("I have inserted pledgets of lint, saturated with the solution, to good effect"). In all of these passages, Buchanan adopts a collegial tone, as if speaking casually but directly to another physician. Often the tone is that of an older colleague sharing his professional experiences and tricks of the trade: "The great secret in the use of a bougie is to handle it with the utmost delicacy and twirl it gently. . . ."[22] On occasion, he employs specifics from cases within his own practice as the launching pad for detailed observations. While he shares some cases for their unusual aspects ("I met a peculiar case last summer . . ."), more often his intent is simply to show the outcomes he obtained from a specific treatment: "I will describe the treatment of a case of elephantiasis that occurred in my practice. . . ."[23]

As an author, Buchanan could also be direct, and at times dogmatic, in his admonitions to patients and assertions to fellow physicians. Whether he was recommending what he identified as the "best" treatments for rheumatism, outlining conditional criteria dictating next steps ("My rule is never to operate if . . ."), or even imparting a sense of urgency ("It is a condition that brooks no delay. . . ."), John Buchanan often expressed his views forcefully.[24]

Some of his strongest language appeared in *The Treatment of Venereal Disease*. After more than 125 pages on the nature, causes, and recommended treatments for syphilis and gonorrhea, Buchanan offered "concluding remarks" that were simultaneously predictable and surprisingly radical. He began by establishing his own *bona fides* to weigh in on the subject, citing his large city practice as the only means to appreciate the scope of the problem. He lamented the prevalence of the venereal diseases "contaminat[ing]" so many Americans and "sapping" the nation's "vital[ity]" and stated bluntly, "Syphillis is destroying us. . . ." He also assailed the "antiquated imbecility" of allopaths, claiming that they were further compounding the problem with their toxic mineral treatments. The surprising remedy he put forth was legalized prostitution. "The social evil has reached a point demanding legal enactment for its control . . . [which] can only be effectually exercised by subjecting such houses or individuals, to stringent police regulations . . . only supervision and inspection of the women are adequate to grapple with the spread of the disease."

In making his case, he pointed to historical examples for control of disease, such as the ancients' practice of removing and segregating lepers from the population and more recent European experiments in licensing brothels with "constant inspection" to remove infected individuals.[25] While Buchanan argued from a position of perceived medical necessity to control a transmittable disease, his proposed remedy still surprises, given the tenor of the era in which he made his proposal, less than a decade before the adoption of the Comstock Law, which was designed to suppress the dissemination of pornography and sexual information generally.

More frequently, John Buchanan proved disingenuous in his selection of targets for criticism or praise, as well as in his overall approach to scholarly writing. A cursory glance at the list of Buchanan's published works creates an impression of sustained intellectual labor. However, this portrait withers under scrutiny, as a closer examination of his written work reveals that Buchanan resorted repeatedly to intellectual shortcuts. Portions of his 1868 work, *The American Practice of Medicine*, for example, are taken directly from papers presented by other physicians at the January 1868 meeting of the Pennsylvania Eclectic Medical Society, the proceedings of which were published the very next month in the *Eclectic Medical Journal of Pennsylvania*.[26] In addition to blatant plagiarism, Buchanan routinely resorted to another intellectual shortcut: wholesale repetition. Material dealing with a specific subject in one book often reappeared either verbatim or with relatively minor revisions in later works. His discussion of yellow fever provides one example: he included virtually the same material on the subject in multiple published works between 1867 and 1876.[27]

On the one hand, this is not surprising given the limited advances specific to this disease over such a short time span. While he might refine his text from work to work, Buchanan saw no reason, if his original discussion was well-written and covered the subject adequately, to make substantive changes in his treatment of the topic. On the other hand, this general pattern of recycling content from book to book—some of which had not even originated with Buchanan—might more cynically be explained as a way to enhance book sales in an era of loose copyright laws rather than as an effort to promote or share advances in medical knowledge.

A related criticism might be leveled at the title Buchanan selected for his 1868 work, *The American Practice of Medicine*. At first glance, this title seems reasonable and unobjectionable. However, a very little research reveals that Wooster Beach, the acknowledged founder of eclectic medicine, had produced a three-volume work with the exact same title in the 1830s. Buchanan's adoption of the title might be forgiven and construed as homage to Beach except that the book's dedication page makes no mention of Beach or his earlier work. Once again, a cynical reviewer might see this as a manipulative attempt to derive a financial benefit from readers' confusing his book with the better-known work by Wooster Beach.

A March 1869 editorial by Buchanan in the *Eclectic Medical Journal of Pennsylvania* appears similarly disingenuous today. The topic he addressed was the issue of women enrolling in medical school. He begins by praising women for their competency as nurses, and then first poses and answers (affirmatively) his own question of whether women might not obtain a sufficient "mastery of medical sciences" to become effective physicians. Buchanan asserts that the advantages posed by qualified female physicians were numerous and obvious, including, most notably, the greater frankness that female patients, especially younger ones, would be likely to display in revealing a medical problem or illness to another woman. Rather conveniently, Buchanan timed this pronouncement to coincide with his announcement of a "summer" session for female medical students.[28]

On its face, this pronouncement was not unprecedented. In the Philadelphia community, women had gained admittance to the Female Medical College of Pennsylvania nearly two decades earlier. Moreover, eclectic medical schools at Worcester, Rochester, Syracuse, and Cincinnati were already admitting both male and female students (although the Cincinnati school was vacillating over its commitment to a coeducational model). To an extent, Buchanan's support for a liberal admission policy appeared wholly consistent with the eclectic schools' general policy of challenging orthodox medical practices.[29] However, subsequent events support an alternative explanation for Buchanan's progressive views: that his championing of medical education for women was driven by his pecuniary interest in expanding the EMC's enrollment and thus its financial bottom line.

A series of Buchanan editorials from the period 1869–70 proved even more disingenuous. In a January 1869 editorial appearing in the *Eclectic Medical Journal of Pennsylvania*, John Buchanan blasted the quacks, frauds, and charlatans sullying the reputation of the medical profession. In considering the many "trials of professional life" facing physicians, he lamented the prevalence of "pretenders . . . quacks and imposters" in the profession, whom he claimed had "infest[ed]" the country like a modern twist on a biblical plague.[30] His outrage and indignation at this state of affairs led him, in another editorial published only three months later, to laud the introduction of a bill into the Pennsylvania legislature that would "elevate the standard of our profession." Though eclectic practitioners were often initially skeptical of "medical legislation," seeing it as a ploy by medical regulars to dominate the profession, Buchanan in this instance publicly posed as a progressive champion willing to run that risk so as to reform medicine for the greater good by halting the proliferation of medical charlatans.[31] What is strikingly disingenuous about Buchanan's diatribe is its timing. As will be shown, his call for medical legislation came less than two years after he had secured a charter for the American University of Philadelphia—an institution that existed as little more than a diploma mill churning out the kind of charlatans he decried in his editorials.

The Sale of Diplomas

At some point after John Buchanan became firmly ensconced at the EMC, the sale of diplomas commenced or, if the practice preceded him, accelerated rapidly. Precisely when diploma sales became the EMC's raison d'être is difficult to pinpoint with any degree of certainty. The best marker for when the practice commenced is the charter secured by John Buchanan for the American University of Philadelphia (AUP) in 1867.

According to Buchanan, he and his fellow EMC faculty member William Clark obtained the school charter for benevolent, humanitarian purposes, intending it to provide a vehicle for the "education of the colored man."[32] Buchanan claimed to have received pledges of financial support for the endeavor from Congressman William D. Kelley, a longtime Pennsylvania Republican and staunch abolitionist, and from Matthew Simpson, an influential local Methodist Episcopal minister, whose political friendships extended to President Lincoln and Secretary of War Edwin Stanton. With these promises in hand, Buchanan worked through an unnamed state legislator to secure sponsorship for the necessary bill; together with the legislator, he and Clark claimed to have spent $400 to secure the charter. In a later recap of the AUP's origins, Buchanan described convening an initial class of thirty-six students at a building on Tenth and Chestnut Streets. With the exception of Clark, none of the faculty assembled by Buchanan had any previous connections with the EMC. This lack of prior connection with the EMC, together with Buchanan's later derogatory description of the group as "radical copperhead Democrats," seems to bear out the assertion that they were a new set of players on the local scene. Buchanan's derisive assessment of them may indicate that, at least in this instance, he was working with a different set of contacts within the Democratic Party that had dominated Philadelphia in the prewar years.[33]

If John Buchanan ever truly sought to offer instruction to black Philadelphians at that time, the social and political realities of doing so quickly soured him on the endeavor. In later accounts, he claimed that two full sets of lectures were delivered to AUP students, but not without creating serious disruption at the EMC and in his relationship with longtime colleagues. As Buchanan described it, after a "few months I was compelled to leave the Pine Street College owing to my degradation in lecturing to a negro class." Apparently, EMC veterans Joseph Sites and Henry Hollembaek highly disapproved of the American University endeavor, although Buchanan did not specify their reasons. Buchanan stated that he applied every point of leverage at his disposal to push back against recalcitrant EMC colleagues, including one that struck directly at the EMC's ability to provide cadavers for anatomical dissection. As Buchanan told the story, "I had seventeen dead bodies in the cellar that I had gathered together and owned. I stopped dissections at the college [i.e., the EMC] and that brought Sites and Hollembaek to terms. They sold out to me for $1000." Buchanan's assertions that he and Clark did try to provide legitimate instruction through the AUP, while entirely possible, cannot be accepted uncritically. Buchanan explained that J. T. Goodrich, a former New York and Philadelphia Universalist minister, had held the "books of this colored class"—records that might have provided evidence that lectures had indeed been delivered—but then claimed that the books had perished along with Goodrich during the Great Chicago Fire of October 1871.[34] Why the books were with Goodrich in Chicago rather than in Philadelphia was a point that Buchanan failed to explain. Both the man and the books that might have substantiated the legitimacy and honorable intent behind the AUP's founding were conveniently unavailable.

If Buchanan's rival William Paine is to be believed, the adoption of the name American University of Philadelphia was itself a carefully considered ploy to avert resistance to the idea of issuing degrees to black Philadelphians. He alleged that Buchanan designed the American University diploma to bear a striking resemblance to that issued by Paine's Philadelphia University and, when discussing the AUP, often dropped the word *American* and transposed the remainder of the title. In this way, Buchanan muddied the waters around the similarly named schools, deflecting criticism aimed at his venture by redirecting it toward Paine's school instead.[35]

Whatever the motives of its founders, the American University of Philadelphia soon devolved into a chartered institution existing for no other reason than to act as a second pathway for issuing diplomas. A Pennsylvania senate investigation in 1872 (see chapter 4) provided strong documentary evidence that the school operated almost entirely on paper, functioning only to issue diplomas to individuals in the United States and abroad. Buchanan's lavish distribution of AUP degrees to members of Philadelphia's African American community appears to have been motivated heavily, if not exclusively, by his personal political ambitions. By 1875, he had grown so bold—or perhaps so complacent, considering how easily he was selling diplomas—that the *Eclectic Medical Journal of Pennsylvania* simply conflated its list of the faculty of the two schools into one ("American University of Phila'da and Eclectic Medical College of Penna."), printing a single faculty roster for both.[36] Similarly, advertisements for the two schools in newspapers across the country ran verbatim copy, with only the name of the school changed to differentiate between the two.[37]

Another indicator of the EMC's drift into disreputable practices can be found in the acceleration in faculty turnover that occurred in the 1860s. By the middle of that decade, the EMC's early leaders had either died or left the school. James Buzzell, Marshall Calkins, Thomas Cooke, John Fondey, St. John Mintzer, and Stephen Potter were all no longer with the school.[38] An examination of the faculty rosters spanning the school's entire thirty-year history reveals a steady pattern of attrition and replacement among the EMC faculty beginning after the Civil War. Approximately 105 individuals served on the EMC's faculty over the three decades of its existence. During the school's first fifteen years (1850–65), only twenty-two individuals served as faculty members. This was a marked contrast to the more than eighty individuals serving as faculty at various points in the school's final fifteen years (1866–80).[39]

This steady turnover is relevant for two reasons. First, it signals the EMC's financial instability—a sobering reality shared by many proprietary schools of the era. With a business model dependent on fees from students for matriculation, lectures, books, and other expenses, faculty and administrators of the EMC may have been tempted to resort to unethical practices to create additional revenue streams. Second, the high turnover rate may well indicate that at least some of the individuals listed as faculty members during the EMC's last decade played no role at the school other than as names on a roster. Evidence suggests that names remained on the faculty roster long after the actual individuals had left the school. Thus by the end of the 1860s, the faculty rosters, like so much else characterizing the EMC as an educational institution, had devolved into a mere mask of respectability.

Fixing the origin of the EMC's diploma trade in the early to mid-1860s makes sense for another reason. The Civil War created enormous disruption in educational endeavors across the country. In the listing of medical colleges produced by the 1918 AMA Council on Medical Education, a review of the historical background portion shows more than twenty medical schools that either closed their doors or suspended instruction between 1861 and 1866. While many of these schools were located in contested areas (e.g., Georgia, Missouri, Tennessee, and Virginia), the war's disruption also affected schools in noncombatant areas, such as New York, Pennsylvania, and Vermont.[40] This context makes it easier to imagine how the disruptions of the Civil War offered a convenient screen against closer scrutiny of the EMC's practices.

Enrollment declined significantly in all of Philadelphia's medical schools during the war, though the city soon established a collection of hospitals to treat more than 100,000 wounded soldiers over this period. One school, the Woman's Medical College, suspended operations entirely in 1861 and 1862. One factor in the decline was the fact that students from Southern states had constituted a significant portion of the enrollment in all of Philadelphia's schools. In December 1859 alone, well before the beginning of the Civil War, heightened tensions preceding the 1860 presidential election and an exhortation to return home from at least one Southern governor prompted an estimated two hundred medical students from Penn, Jefferson, and other schools to leave Philadelphia.[41] These larger realities and the looming financial crisis this represented for the Philadelphia schools overshadowed any whispers of the improper issuance of diplomas, although the EMC's 1864 announcement of a recent major endowment raised suspicions in eclectic circles.[42]

Taking these factors and indicators into account, it seems clear that *de facto* diploma sales were occurring at the EMC by the early to mid-1860s. John Buchanan claimed to have become aware of the first questionable transaction involving a diploma sometime after his arrival at the school in 1860. While the question of *when* diploma sales began is important, the more important question—and one even more difficult to answer satisfactorily—is *how* and *why* the practice took hold. Because the best evidence dates the start of the diploma trade to the 1860s, more than a decade after the school's founding, it seems reasonable to infer that the EMC was originally set up as a legitimate school rather than to theorize

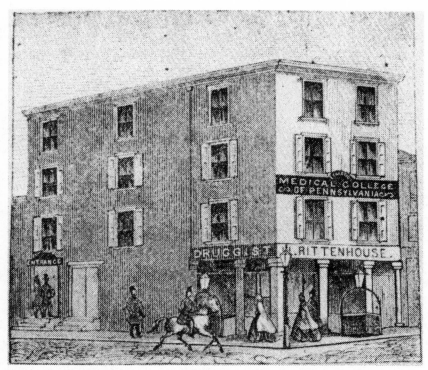

Fig. 5. Eclectic Medical College of Pennsylvania. The EMC operated from this building at Sixth and Callowhill in Philadelphia from 1858 to 1868, before relocating to 514 Pine Street. Image courtesy of the New York Academy of Medicine.

that its later questionable practices had been planned from the beginning. No evidence has surfaced to indicate that the EMC was planned as a criminal enterprise—or as anything other than a legitimate effort at medical education along eclectic lines, in keeping with the reformed medical theories and qualifications of its founders. As to *how* and *why* such legitimate intentions gave way to the barefaced sale of diplomas, the best answers rest with contemporary norms and practices concerning what constituted an acceptable medical education and on what basis diplomas should be issued, not only at the EMC but at medical schools throughout the United States.

In 1860, there existed no single definitive pathway to medical practice in the United States. Aspirants could pursue any of several main routes leading to the role and/or title of physician. Few of these pathways were official and none were exclusive, since there were no legal barriers to the practice of medicine in any state when Buchanan joined the EMC faculty in 1860.[43] At one end of the spectrum, it was possible for individuals to hold themselves out as physicians and practice medicine with little or no knowledge or experience. To set up a practice, an individual had only to acquire the confidence of the local community, often by gaining a reputation and experience through treating friends, family, and neighbors—in essence, by acting as healer for the community. To practitioners of this type, the actual title of physician or doctor was largely irrelevant, since their continuance in that role rested almost entirely on their perceived success in treating patients. At the other end of the spectrum were individuals who had acquired the formal title of physician by obtaining a medical degree issued by one of the approximately 110 medical schools in operation in 1870.[44] On this end of the spectrum, prominent medical educators such as Alfred Stille of the University of Pennsylvania saw a direct correlation between the number of diplomas issued by this burgeoning number of schools and the degradation of the diploma as a credential. As early as 1847, Stille publicly expressed his fear for the credential: "The diploma has lost its value; everyone knows of its prostitution."[45]

Between these two ends of the spectrum, an array of experiences could lead to the practice of medicine. Some individuals became physicians by virtue of their direct working experience with an established practicing physician. This usually involved an apprentice-style relationship of preceptor (the practicing physician) and the preceptee (the aspiring physician). Other individuals completed some portion of a curriculum at a medical school. Still others began practicing after a mixture of these experiences. By the 1860s, it had become more common for aspiring doctors to seek at least a modicum of formalized medical education by attending a course of lectures at a medical school. Understandably, the criteria used by medical schools for issuing diplomas varied from school to school and over time, reflecting the fluid state of affairs in the profession.

One sampling of graduation requirements for many U.S. medical schools in 1861 reflected this fluidity. An examination of the "circulars" for thirty-four medical schools found that twenty-seven schools (nearly 80 percent) usually required students to complete the standard two full courses of lectures to graduate, *but* the schools also were willing to grant exceptions to individuals who either had already completed a course of lectures at another school or had been in practice a sufficient length of time to justify waiving completion of the second course. Sometimes schools required such students to pass an examination before they would waive the second set of lectures; at others they restricted exceptions to students who had previously studied at a "respectable" school or one "in good standing."[46] The range and fluidity of such requirements and restrictions used by many medical schools in the 1860s reflected the less formal standards characterizing the practice of medicine at that time. To further complicate the picture, individual schools routinely tinkered with these standards, frequently altering their requirements for what evidence and documentation constituted appropriate exceptions to their graduation requirements and thus the issuance of their medical degrees.

A second practice that must be addressed involved schools' issuance of nonstandard degrees, such as *ad eundem* and honorary degrees. The Latin term *ad eundem*, meaning "in or of the same rank," signaled a degree completed by someone who had done a portion of the required coursework elsewhere, with the understanding that the completed course was comparable to that offered by the degree-granting school—thus allowing a degree of "M.D. *ad eundem*." This concept and practice dated to colonial America but persisted in all regions of the country in the midnineteenth century. While granting an *ad eundem* degree may not have been the norm, it was certainly not so uncommon as to automatically raise suspicion; such degrees were granted by regular medical schools from California to New York,[47] and by eclectic medical schools other than the EMC (e.g., the Eclectic Medical College of New York).[48] The practice even formed part of the graduation criteria for established Philadelphia schools like Penn and Jefferson.[49] Honorary degrees were equally unremarkable during this period. A search for honorary degrees like that described for *ad eundem* degrees probably would uncover comparable procedures for their issuance by most schools.[50]

In describing medical schools' use of criteria for graduation that recognized education and experiences acquired elsewhere and practices specific to the issuance of a diploma, such as the *ad eundem* degree, one point should be clearly understood. The intent is not to attribute questionable practices to these schools or to imply widespread corruption in the issuance of diplomas; it is instead to point out that the EMC used such practices in common with many other schools. Like many contemporary schools, it issued both *ad eundem* and honorary degrees as a means of recognizing the reality that matriculants arrived at school with an array of medical experiences and education.[51] Further incentive to grant such recognition came from the fierce competition for students among the schools and a business model predicated on student fees. Given these realities, many schools saw the advantages of acknowledging the prior education and experience of prospective students.

The varying nature of medical diplomas and what they represented (or purported to represent) was not lost upon the public. While the story may be apocryphal, a humorous anecdote shared by John Scudder in an 1878 issue of the *Eclectic Medical Journal* reflected physicians' awareness that their patients were not unsuspecting rubes swayed by every certificate, attestation, or diploma waved under their noses. In Scudder's tale, a surviving spouse challenges his late wife's physician in court. When the treating physician points to his diploma as evidence of his medical acumen, the husband explodes in anger and derision, "His diploma! His diploma! Gentlemen, this is a big word for a printed sheepskin and it didn't make no doctor of the sheep as first wore it, nor does it of the man as now carries it."[52] Humor aside, Scudder makes a clear point in this story: in medicine, the Latin most important for any prudent nineteenth-century patient to understand was not the wording of the doctor's diploma but the perennial warning *caveat emptor*—"Let the buyer beware."

In accepting the broad range of paths to medical practice, the EMC was following common contemporary norms, but by the mid-1860s, it made some innovations that began to set it apart from legitimate schools. At this point, the school began advertising "scholarships" as part of its tuition model for students. Rather than requiring a set fee for a single course of lectures (e.g., $60) and the same fee again for the required repeat of the course, the school offered prospective students another option: they could purchase a scholarship before the first course of lectures for a fee ($100) higher than the cost of that course alone but lower than the combined cost of both courses. Moreover, the EMC promised students that by purchasing the scholarship up front, they were entitled to as many lectures sessions as they wanted to attend.[53]

On its surface, the proposal seemed wholly reasonable. This payment structure offered the school higher income up front while presenting any legitimately interested student with unlimited access to the required lectures. What apparently evolved over time, however, was an expectation by the student purchaser of having purchased not simply access to the lectures but the assurance of a diploma at the end of the required courses. A later Pennsylvania senate investigation made clear that as the sale of degrees accelerated, John Buchanan and the EMC altered the intent of the "scholarship" from a guarantee of access to classes to a convenient cover for the direct sale of diplomas. The proposal came to represent a developing *quid pro quo* between the buyer (student) and the seller (the EMC) that a diploma came with the purchase of the "scholarship."

It is important to understand that the EMC took this first step away from legitimacy within the overall context of a business model common to nineteenth-century colleges, including medical schools. For-profit commercial or business colleges proliferated throughout the country, with estimates on their numbers varying from several hundred to several thousand. Like most of its contemporary midcentury medical schools, the EMC was a proprietary endeavor, unaffiliated with a college or university and devoid of any state funding. The impetus for such schools generally arose from a handful of prospective faculty and investors willing to put up sufficient funds to buy or rent a building or lecture hall. Because medical education at that time remained largely a didactic affair based on faculty lectures rather than on clinical and laboratory work, little more was required to establish a school. From a purely financial perspective, such arrangements made sense. In cities housing large numbers of potential students, physicians stood to make more money by banding together and offering instruction as a faculty than they were likely to make by taking on individual preceptors. This proprietary model dates to the 1807 establishment of the College of Medicine of Maryland, which served as the template for all the proprietary medical schools that followed. The Maryland legislature issued a charter establishing the school but granted it no funds. This left the financing and operation of the school to its faculty and/or trustees. Nearly fifty years later, the EMC was founded on such a model and featured both the positive and negative attributes inherent in such schools.[54]

Without question, a "commercial spirit" characterized proprietary schools like the EMC, including significant pressure on faculty to attract and maintain students. Historian Kenneth Ludmerer characterized these schools as more "business . . . than educational enterprises." To be fair, however, one must recognize that the stand-alone character of schools like the EMC was generally not a matter of choice. State funding for higher education proved generally lacking until after the Morrill Land Grant Act of 1862. Moreover, the prospects for affiliation with larger institutions, such as colleges, universities, and hospitals, were small. In many parts of the country, such larger institutions did not yet exist, and where they did (such as Philadelphia's University of Pennsylvania or city hospital), the larger entities had no need for or interest in affiliating with small enterprises, especially medical schools founded by irregular practitioners. This reality led at least one historian to conclude that proprietary schools served the public interest reasonably well through at least the first two-thirds of the nineteen century by producing a cadre of physicians otherwise unavailable to a growing nation.[55]

Still, the financial pressures underlying the proprietary model for medical schools undoubtedly contributed to EMC's drift into unethical practices and diploma sales. The constant pressure to secure incoming students and their fees in order to sustain the EMC was a practical reality never far from John Buchanan's thoughts, and this pressure intensified as the number of medical schools across the country grew; in 1860, there were eight in Philadelphia alone.[56] As the need for funds increased, so did the temptation to lower standards both for matriculation and graduation. In this context, the attraction to Buchanan and colleagues of strategies such as cutting corners in the educational curriculum, withholding funds that might have upgraded instruction and facilities, and rationalizing questionable practices in the issuance of the diplomas becomes more understandable.

When Calvin Newton addressed the 1853 NEMA meeting, he considered the prospects for eclectic schools like the EMC, the EMI, and New York College and saw the future as full of potential but fraught with peril. "If they take [the] high and honorable ground," he explained, " . . . our cause will command the respect of an intelligent community. If, on the other hand, they encourage but a low degree of professional attainments, Eclecticism will lose its hold on the affections of the people, and degenerate till it becomes 'a by-word, a hissing and a reproach among all' classes of society." Newton acknowledged the "unendowed" nature of eclectic schools and urged them to increase their "too modest" tuition. To withstand the inevitable comparison to allopathic schools, he argued that their schools' graduation requirements must be "as high ... or even higher" than those of regular schools, and their faculty among the "ablest of men." In a prescient moment, Newton called for a three-year course of study and firm resistance to any person or institution seeking to entice students with promises of graduation after only a few weeks or months, calling them a "curse to Eclecticism."[57] Clearly, John Buchanan and the EMC failed to heed such advice.

These circumstances represent the broad environment within which we must answer the questions of *how* and *why* John Buchanan and the EMC resorted to the sale of diplomas. The actual answers may be as simple as two words—drift and lapse. Clearly, the school drifted on multiple levels: from its original inspiration to carry the eclectic banner for reformed medicine, from genuine accountability to an independent board of trustees, and from the principle of providing genuine instruction to students. The school also lapsed in its protocols for the issuance of diplomas.

At some point in time, John Buchanan or one of his EMC colleagues first cut a corner in the school's operation, either for convenience or with a premeditated intent to deceive for monetary gain. This may have involved signing a set of blank diplomas in preparation for an upcoming graduating class or signing a diploma on behalf of a faculty colleague temporarily called away. The faculty may have decided to forego a required examination when the examining faculty member was unavailable, or waived the requirement of attending lectures for a student, despite dubious evidence of prior experience practicing medicine. A faculty member may have rationalized overlooking a student's failure to submit a thesis or issuing an *ad eundem* degree despite clear evidence that the student had not completed all the lectures claimed at an earlier school. Perhaps the turning point was issuing an honorary diploma without anything labeling the diploma as such.

However the practice of cutting corners took hold, a financial equation undoubtedly underlay every instance. Every graduating student represented an additional fee going into the school's coffers. Each time a diploma was not issued, that failure represented a corresponding loss of income—money that went uncollected after the labor of instruction. Once John Buchanan reconciled himself and the school to the practice of selling diplomas, the inevitable flow of cash derived from the sales proved too lucrative to abandon. By 1867, if not earlier, Buchanan had committed himself to a practice that reaped a financial windfall in the short term, at least. That he simultaneously was sowing the seeds of his own destruction became apparent soon enough.

Part Two

Crises

"What a wealth of buildings, hospitals, clinics, laboratories, museums, professors . . . we have on paper, and what a paucity we have in fact."

—John Scudder, *Eclectic Medical Journal*, 1877

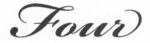

Year of Revelations, 1871

In the spring of 1871, John Buchanan and his EMC colleagues probably had never heard of the *College Courant*. This weekly journal reported on a wide range of topics of interest to American colleges and universities, among them medical education. Though the *Courant* did not specialize in exposé reporting, its publisher, Charles Chatfield, did have some interest in this area. Already in 1871, Chatfield had published *Four Years at Yale*, a revelatory memoir of American college life by Lyman Bagg that was receiving a fair amount of attention for its scandalous depiction of college life and experiences from a student's perspective.[1]

The April 1871 edition of the *College Courant* delivered another sensational revelation by nationally disseminating a news story first published on March 23, 1871, in the *Philadelphia Press*. For the first time, John Buchanan and the EMC drew negative attention from writers, newspapers, and journals far beyond those in the Philadelphia area. Reporter Joseph Reed's article in the *Press* had delivered a devastating critique of Buchanan's activities at the EMC; even worse was the momentum building behind the story as it gathered traction nationally. Journals like the

Courant were always in search of interesting content, and the *Press* article presented a journalistic plum ripe for picking.

The *Courant* article grabbed readers' attention with its provocative title, "A Philadelphia Humbug," and declared its intent to look into that city's "peculiar" but flourishing industry in the "manufacture of academic degrees."[2] What the article then administered was a series of journalistic blows that all but demolished the reputation of Buchanan and the school. The *Courant* revealed how Philadelphia reporters exposed the EMC and its practices along its vulnerable points, using every line of attack open to them. The *Courant* reprinted excerpts of unambiguous correspondence between the school and interested parties seeking to buy diplomas. Accompanying this was an account of several reporters' attempts to purchase diplomas in person from Buchanan. The article also shared the findings of the *Courant*'s close reading of the school's printed materials—much of which supplied further evidence of deliberate deception. The result left little doubt in the reader's mind that naming conventions and much else related to the EMC were secondary to its primary business of cashing in on the issuance of diplomas under the school's legally held charter.

The *Courant*'s detailed description of the EMC facilities alone sufficed to raise the eyebrows of interested readers. The article underscored the profound gap between what the school promoted itself as capable of delivering to its students and the modest reality of its facilities. This section of the article opened with a description of the EMC's three-story building at 514 Pine Street, calling it typical of the "large, old-fashioned" homes that once characterized that area of the city before shifting tastes and city demographics moved the more prosperous residents to other areas of Philadelphia. The structure on Pine Street had stood vacant for many years before the EMC took occupation in 1868, and locals had noted its slow deterioration into an eyesore marred by broken windows and an overall condition aptly described by the press as "decayed . . . dusty, begrimed, and forsaken." When the EMC took over the building, abrupt changes appeared. Masons and carpenters engulfed the building in a flurry of renovation, and multiple signs on its front wall announced its imminent conversion into a medical college. During this interval between the announcement and actual opening of the EMC's new premises, local lore vacillated between two extremes. Nearby boardinghouse owners chattered in anticipation of an infusion of cash from young medical students while others in the neighborhood swapped unnerving tales of the "body-snatchers" sure to accompany occupancy by a medical school, with its need for dissection cadavers.

By 1871, the EMC was fully operational at the Pine Street location, and while the building was substantial, encompassing three stories and an attic, the space it provided came nowhere near that needed for the lecture halls and wards listed in the school's prospectus. The contrast between the lofty descriptions and pictures given by the EMC in many college announcements and the modest realities of the actual premises did not pass unnoticed, especially within the community of eclectic physicians. John Scudder, editor of the EMI's *Eclectic Medical Journal*, wrote scathingly on such deceptive practices. Though his ire in this instance was directed toward a Louisville school, his comments were equally pertinent to the EMC: "What a wealth of buildings, hospitals, clinics, laboratories, museums, professors, brains, etc, we have on paper, and what a paucity we have in fact."[3]

The *Courant*'s description of the EMC noted the many signs on the building advertising various "special diseases" treated by its faculty. Inside the school, John Buchanan presided from two offices spanning the front of the ground floor. Here everything seemed respectable, professional, and entirely proper. The offices were decorated tastefully and filled, as one might expect, with books, pamphlets, and medical literature arranged on tables. The *Courant* focused heavily on the medical "museum" situated behind Buchanan's offices. The museum comprised a single room (50 feet by 18) spanning the back of the entire first floor. Lining each side of the long room, glass cases displayed an array of anatomical models of human organs—most in wax. The focus of many of the displays was male and female anatomy—the sexual organs in particular. In the center of the room stood three large glass displays. Each contained a life-sized wax representation of the nude human form (two male and one female), "true to nature" in every way. The *Courant*'s account made explicit what any reasonably intelligent reader and many citizens of Philadelphia knew firsthand: the museum existed less to nurture scientific pursuits in human anatomy than to lure "lecherous" passersby inside to view what the *Courant* described as its "lascivious" and "shamefully immodest" exhibits. The insinuation was clear. For a small fee, any Philadelphian's prurient interest might be satisfied at the EMC museum.

Despite this contemptuous description, the presence of a medical or anatomical museum in a post–Civil War medical school should not surprise. The existence of such a museum was not sui generis evidence of a school willfully abandoning its educational focus. Since the late eighteenth century, medical schools had been acquiring and cataloging instructive pathological and anatomical specimens for their faculty and students, and occasionally making them available to visitors and the general public. The American antebellum era's "mania for anatomy" and dissection among medical schools reflected physicians' and educators' concerted efforts to establish a scientific basis for medicine. The eclectic medical community, after some initial reluctance, embraced the importance of an understanding of human anatomy and physiology in educating future physicians. As challengers to orthodox medicine, eclectics moved cautiously at first in advocating learned, or more specifically anatomical, medicine. Yet even the father of medical eclectics, Wooster Beach, was sufficiently drawn to this aspect of medicine that in 1847 he acquired anatomical and pathological specimens for the medical museum he had opened in New York.[4]

Over time, however, many museums drifted from the purely pedagogical setting of medical schools to public venues open to virtually any and all paying customers. As this shift occurred, the titillation factor grew more pronounced. Morbid pathology and female reproductive specimens came to dominate their inventory of displays as the competition to draw customers increased. Philadelphia alone had at least two popular anatomical museums in 1871: Charles Kreutzberg's European Anatomical, Pathological and Ethnological Museum and the Museum of Anatomy, Science and Art, both located on Chestnut Street, not too far from the EMC.[5]

That the EMC under Buchanan included anatomical dissection in its proffered curriculum was clear from both the school prospectus (admittedly an unreliable source) and press reports describing the presence of cadavers; that it established a medical museum open to the public meant that the school's interest in anatomy did not preclude it from generating supplementary sources of income. However, the existence of the museum alone did not justify the *Courant*'s depiction of the EMC as an outlier in the world of medical education; instead, it was the *Courant*'s reportage of the nature of that museum in the context of other irregularities by the college that was damning.

The *Courant* next turned its attention to John Buchanan and the faculty, characterizing Buchanan as presiding over a questionable set of instructors. The *Courant* ridiculed the EMC faculty by noting its shifting composition in virtually contemporaneous published rosters. Although several individuals were always included (Buchanan, Joseph Sites, Henry Hollembaek, Edward Down, and James Cochran), the faculty listings seemed amorphous, varying in composition depending on the audience and the publication. Sometimes the faculty roster listed as few as eight members; at other times, it listed as many as seventeen. Had this casual inconsistency in faculty rosters been the only irregularity in the school's printed materials, journalists and readers might have given the EMC the benefit of the doubt, but it was accompanied by Buchanan's odd written transposition and conflation of school names, several iterations of which appeared in both his correspondence and publications. The various school names he used included the American University of Pennsylvania, the American Eclectic University, and the Eclectic Medical College of Philadelphia. This careless—or perhaps deliberately deceptive—treatment of school names implied that the faculty lists were no more sacrosanct. Ultimately, the *Courant* contemptuously dismissed the faculty as a "motley set," "got up . . . for show" to maintain the appearance of a legitimate school. The journal's scathing description went so far as to compare the group to "the figures in the milliner's [shop] window"—a useful but intellectually empty display prop.

The *Courant* assessed Buchanan in similarly sharp terms, describing him as a "short, stout, [and] rather good-looking" Scotsman approaching fifty years of age. The complimentary description ended there. After meeting him in person, the writers characterized Buchanan as a confidence man: "very oily, smooth, and persuasive—apparently perfectly capable of using all the powers which may have been conferred upon the so-called university to put money in his purse."

As proof of the EMC's trafficking in diplomas, the *Courant* published a series of advertisements and circulars posted in European journals. Appearing as discreet advertisements in publications like the *Ecclesiastical Gazette*, the ads outlined a range of degrees (e.g., D.D., M.D.) open to clergymen and gentlemen "qualified by educational attainments and social status." In some instances, the ads listed the diplomas as "honorary degrees," though generally no such limitation was stated or implied. These ads represented all degrees as coming from an institution legally "empowered by charter" to issue such documents, although they omitted the name of the institution. Instead, the ads routed all inquiries to agents of the school through various addresses in London. These ads typically listed prices for diplomas of between £15 and £20, a significant sum roughly equivalent to more than one thousand dollars in 2014 U.S. currency. The details of these diploma sales appeared only in the subsequent written correspondence between the EMC agent and the prospective buyer. Only as the transaction was being completed did the agent reveal the name of the degree-granting institution and its head—for example, the American University of Philadelphia and John Buchanan.

In some instances, the correspondence maintained a pretense of intellectual integrity. In one letter dated October 1870, a Buchanan agent told an English clergyman that obtaining a degree from an established institution in Leipzig or Göttingen would cost £40, but would also require the person seeking the degree to submit several documents, including a "learned dissertation" of at least thirty-two pages. As an aside, however, the agent offered a similar degree from the American University for £25, without any requisite intellectual labor.

The most damning evidence against Buchanan derived from his own handwritten words and from statements attributed to him by reporters who talked with him while posing as prospective students. The reporters obtained a letter written in January 1871 by Buchanan himself to an interested English buyer. In response to an earlier missive, Buchanan all but offered to sell the man one or more degrees with no questions asked.

Dear Sir,

I fully appreciate the contents of your letter. Send me word what honor you do want, and I will have the matter attended to promptly without any parties becoming acquainted with the particulars. Enclose a letter of credit or draft on Brown, Bowen & Co. for £10.

I am very sincerely yours,

John Buchanan

P.S.—If you want more than one D[egree] please inform, and remit in accordance.

The *Courant* reporters' meeting with Buchanan at the EMC culminated in the same overt offer. Their description of the encounter clearly demonstrates how John Buchanan conducted diploma sales. When the reporters arrived, identifying themselves as students considering the EMC, Buchanan welcomed them eagerly, although he turned wary when they hinted that time constraints would make it difficult for them to attend any lectures. They reported that he then closed the door to his office and spoke "confidential[ly]" about the possibility that he might still be able to assist them. When questioned about price, Buchanan deflected the query back to the young men. Already experienced in negotiating diploma sales, he wished to gauge their valuation of the degree they were seeking. "It is customary for us to furnish the degree," Buchanan explained helpfully, "and the gentleman gives us what he thinks proper." The faux students demurred. As reporters they had no intention of setting the price in this exchange. Backed into a negotiating corner by the "students'" refusal to name a price, Buchanan relented, proposing $40 as a reasonable and customary fee.

He also made clear the need for discretion, explaining that "the law is very strict in these matters and the transaction must be perfectly confidential." The faux students agreed to the terms and left with an understanding that they had reached a satisfactory arrangement: they would return with $40 each, and a diploma would immediately be presented to each man. Of course, the reporters did not return; having obtained firsthand confirmation of the allegations raised earlier by the *Philadelphia Press*, they had no need of the degrees themselves.

The articles in the *Press* and the *College Courant* opened the first major breach in the EMC's clandestine sales of diplomas. An exposé by the *New York Herald* followed in early May 1871 under the eye-catching headline, "M.D., $40.—C.O.D." The article spotlighted the multiple similar titles among the Philadelphia schools, characterizing them as holding more "corporate names . . . [than] a Spanish prince . . . has titles."[6] This rapid escalation of the scandal was giving John Buchanan and the EMC a firsthand lesson in the power of the telegraph exchanges to increase the speed and range of news. Telegraph exchanges like the Associated Press were altering virtually everything in newspaper publishing. Any local news story with a sufficiently interesting or unusual angle could be wired telegraphically to a newspaper halfway across the country.[7] The *Philadelphia Press* account about the EMC paled next to the sensational murder stories coming to Philadelphia out of Chicago and New York City and appearing nearly every day in the city papers. However, there is distinct irony in what happened next. A murder case of the high-profile type that Buchanan might otherwise have welcomed as a means of diverting public attention cast an indirect spotlight back on the EMC. This next round of unwanted attention arrived less than four months later.

Death in New York; Repercussions in Philadelphia

On the afternoon of August 26, 1871, Frank Donnigan, a baggage handler at the Hudson River Railroad Depot in New York City, toiled in the muggy heat of the depot's baggage room. Donnigan sorted and arranged baggage for the multitude of trains leaving the station, including a westbound passenger train headed to Chicago at eight o'clock that evening. Among the items set out for loading was a trunk with a lock apparently so suspect that a leather strap had been wrapped around the trunk to secure its contents. As Donnigan grasped the trunk to move it, he detected a strong odor, one so overpowering that he called over the station's bagger master. The two men moved the trunk to another room for closer inspection. After removing the strap, the trunk's flimsy lock gave way under a little pressure. The two men were startled to find that the small trunk, measuring little more than thirty-two inches in length and eighteen inches across, contained the small, slender body of a young blond-haired woman, wedged inside in a grotesque and contorted fashion. There were no visible marks of violence upon the body, but the remains were already beginning to decompose. With this discovery, the New York newspapers launched their extensive coverage of what became known locally and nationally as the "trunk murder."[8]

Two critical aspects of this seemingly unrelated story directed attention back to the EMC. The first was the relatively swift work of the police in tracking down the source of the trunk. The police established the trunk as coming from the home of Dr. Jacob Rosenzweig. As police searches of Rosenzweig's home and office revealed evidence of the botched abortion that had led to the death of the victim in the trunk, Alice Bowlsby, the newspapers simultaneously trumpeted the results of their investigation into the doctor's practice. One aspect of Rosenzweig's background that did not escape notice was his initial evasiveness about his medical training and the source of his medical diploma. It soon became public knowledge that Rosenzweig held a pair of diplomas: one from the EMC and the other from the American University of Philadelphia. Contemporary journalists following the case wrote on the "evil reputation" of the Philadelphia schools, arguing that diplomas from the two colleges were little better than a pathway to "licensed vice and incompetency."[9]

Once the press established the connection between Rosenzweig, the alleged abortionist charged with manslaughter, and the EMC in the public mind, every new article on the case included a reminder of the connection to the attentive reader, who vaguely recalled the doctor's association with dubious Philadelphia schools. Since the case made headlines across the country throughout the fall of 1871, such reminders appeared frequently.

The other aspect of the "trunk murder" story that proved critical for Buchanan and the EMC was the extensive coverage it engendered. The American press and the reading public had demonstrated a fascination with murder stories, especially those featuring beautiful young women victimized by seducers and abortionists in the big city. Since the sensationalized death of New York City's "beautiful cigar girl," Mary Rogers, in 1841, Americans had evinced an insatiable appetite for stories of youth, beauty, and the corruptive influence of the country's burgeoning cities.[10] Edgar Allan Poe, by fictionalizing the Mary Rogers case through his short story "The Death of Marie Roget," was simply among the first to mine a genre that was firmly cemented in the American psyche by 1871. The Bowlsby case possessed not only these elements but an additional sensational touch—her young lover, Walter Conklin, committed suicide out of his grief and shame at the turn of events. Stories around criminal cases like those of Rogers and Bowlsby became staple fodder for the penny press and a spur to the developing nineteenth-century detective or crime story.

One other factor contributed to the press frenzy around this case. Only three days before the discovery of Alice Bowlsby's body, New York Times reporter Augustus St. Clair had published an investigative piece entitled "The Evil of the Age." St. Clair, accompanied by a young woman, had visited several of New York City's abortion providers, including the offices of Jacob Rosenzweig, soliciting information about how to address their "trouble" and how to dispose of the "result." St. Clair even claimed that after viewing Alice Bowlsby's remains at the morgue he recognized and remembered her as a one of the patients he saw waiting at Rosenzweig's office during his undercover visit.[11] The juxtaposition of this exposé in the *Times* to the discovery of the "trunk murder" contributed to the massive response to the Rosenzweig case among the public and the press.

The case dissolved into an unmitigated disaster for Buchanan and the EMC—and part of the public relations damage to the school was self-inflicted. As local newspapers picked up the Rosenzweig case and stressed the doctor's Philadelphia connection, one of Buchanan's faculty colleagues responded with a letter to the editor of the *Philadelphia Morning Post*. In his published letter, Robert H. DeBeust firmly denied any connection between the school and Rosenzweig and claimed a "gross error" by the press resulting in an unfair "stigma to the College." He asserted that no one by the name of *Rozenberg* (italics added) had ever matriculated at

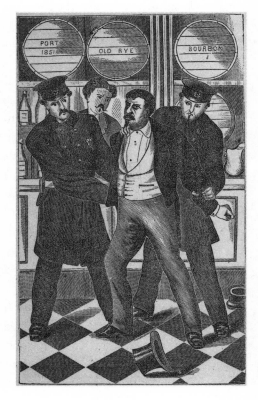

Fig. 6. Illustration showing the arrest of Jacob Rosenzweig. Since Dr. Rosenzweig held a diploma from the EMC, his role in the death of Anna Bowlsby cast a harsh national spotlight on the practices of that school and of Buchanan, as its leader. Print Collection, Miriam and Ira D. Wallach Division of Art, Prints and Photographs, New York Public Library, Astor, Lenox and Tilden Foundations.

YEAR OF REVELATIONS, 1871   77

the school. The *Post* pounced on DeBeust's clumsy attempt at nuanced disavowal and rightfully claimed that DeBeust had misrepresented the graduate in question: his name was Rosenzweig, not Rozenberg. Other critics picked up on DeBeust's assertion that no one named Rozenberg (*sic*) had *matriculated* at the school; that was probably true, they argued, but only because the party in question likely purchased a diploma without ever setting foot in the school or attending a lecture.[12]

The role in the Rosenzweig case of another EMC faculty member and his wife remains perplexing. Within three days after the discovery of Alice Bowlsby's body, police not only arrested Jacob Rosenzweig but identified him as a physician practicing as an abortion provider under the name of "Dr. Asher." As the prosecution collected physical evidence from Rosenzweig's home and Asher's office, a key discovery was a soiled handkerchief with what appeared to be faint monograph that read, "A A Bowlsby." This physical evidence, combined with the autopsy results and the identification of the body made by Bowlsby's personal physician and dentist, gave the prosecution the basis for a strong circumstantial case against Rosenzweig. In light of the tremendous publicity being generated, it is easy to imagine that anyone associated with Rosenzweig, and by extension with the EMC, would have gone to great lengths at this point to distance himself or herself from the case. Inexplicably, however, Cornelia Bowlsby, the wife of EMC faculty member William H. Bowlsby,[13] reached out to Rosenzweig's defense counsel with information she believed pertinent to the case.[14]

The story she told, first at the offices of defense counsel William F. Howe and later under oath at the trial in October, presented a benign explanation for the incriminating handkerchief found at Rosenzweig's home. Mrs. Bowlsby testified that she and her daughter (Anna Martini Bowlsby) had visited Mrs. Rosenzweig at her home several weeks before the events in question. According to Cornelia Bowlsby, her daughter Anna had spilled wine on her gloves, used one of her handkerchiefs to wipe it up, and afterward inadvertently left it behind. Later, from the witness stand, Mrs. Bowlsby examined the handkerchief, asserted that the faded lettering actually said "A M Bowlsby," and proclaimed the item to be her daughter's.[15]

It is impossible to know what motivated Mrs. Bowlsby's testimony. It may have been friendship with the Rosenzweigs or a legitimate desire to see truth prevail if she genuinely believed the handkerchief was her daughter's. A more plausible explanation may stem from her husband's professional relationship with Rosenzweig. According to one reporter, the two men allegedly "exchanged patients," though it is unclear whether this included prospective clients for abortion. John Buchanan offered another connection as well. In his confession, published a decade later, Buchanan claimed that, in early 1871, Dr. Bowlsby brought Rosenzweig to the EMC and procured a diploma for him from Joseph Sites.[16] Taking together these alleged and known connections, Mrs. Bowlsby's testimony may have originated as an ill-advised attempt by the EMC to protect one of its own.

Under cross-examination, the district attorney discredited both husband and wife by forcing her to acknowledge that her husband was the same William Henry Bowlsby who had been "expelled" from the New York Eclectic Medical Society. Even more damning, her testimony piqued the interest of New York journalist Arthur Pember. He launched his own investigation and soon published an exposé featuring Dr. Bowlsby as a faculty member and a local "agent" for the EMC who was only too happy to arrange for the purchase of a diploma—price negotiable.[17]

Rosenzweig's trial culminated with his conviction for manslaughter and a seven-year prison sentence. Mrs. Bowlsby's testimony failed completely, as the judge directed the jury to disregard her testimony. Because her daughter did not testify (allegedly because of illness) and because Mrs. Bowlsby had neither witnessed her daughter monographing the handkerchief nor particularly noticed the handkerchief before seeing it as part of state's evidence, the judge deemed her testimony inadmissible as hearsay. The Bowlsbys' involvement, rather than exonerating the defendant, only heightened public consciousness of Rosenzweig's connection with the EMC.

In the aftermath of this case, John Buchanan and his colleagues adopted a preferred strategy for combating negative publicity in the press—deflection and bribery. Whenever possible, they argued that jealous competitor schools had instigated the stories attributing diploma sales to the EMC. Then Buchanan or a colleague offered to recompense reporters willing to drop that story line and write another, more positive story. The school's November 1871 interactions with a *New York Herald* reporter reflected this tactic.

The *Herald* reporter identified himself to Buchanan and several colleagues at the EMC's Pine Street location. Buchanan and his faculty welcomed the reporter's unannounced visit and took the opportunity to tell their side of a story that had recently appeared with a negative spin in the *New York Tribune*. According to Buchanan, the entire affair had been "instigated" by William Paine, his former EMC colleague, who was now a rival firmly entrenched at Philadelphia University and whose "jealousy," Buchanan claimed, animated his "slander[s]" of the EMC. Buchanan asserted that "he [Paine] has done everything in his power to injure us." The reporter noted Buchanan's assertion that Paine had successfully manipulated individuals at the Eclectic Medical College in New York who had connections to the *Tribune*, playing on the New York school's competition with the EMC for students. After deflecting the accusations against the EMC back toward those who raised them, Buchanan and the reporter entered the next phase of their conversational minuet—the bribe. Buchanan lamented that Paine had successfully "put up a job" against EMC through the *Tribune* article. In fact, he claimed that the *Tribune* correspondent had attempted to blackmail him, demanding $400 to suppress the story he planned to write. Two EMC colleagues (Phillip A. Bissell and J. Dunbar Hylton) affirmed Buchanan's story, claiming that they had been present for the conversation with the *Tribune* reporter. All three men provided the *Herald* reporter with affidavits sworn before a Philadelphia alderman. When the reporter returned the following day to discuss the affidavits, first Bissell and then Buchanan hinted at their desire to "make it worth something" to the newspaperman if he would publish the affidavits as part of a story "in behalf of the institution [EMC]." When the reporter balked at the notion of a "bribe," the two men backpedaled at the injection of the unseemly word into the conversation, saying "Oh no . . . we don't mean . . . anything of that kind." Buchanan agreed that the publication of a good story and the affidavits would be helpful to the school and stressed that his actions were motivated not from personal considerations but from a desire to raise the EMC "out of the mire" of recent negative publicity. When the reporter tried to entice a little evidence of "good faith," a suspicious Buchanan seemingly shut down the conversation by saying, "I can't do it." A few minutes later, however, Buchanan reached into his desk, extracted a pair of five-dollar notes and slipped them discreetly to the reporter, saying, "This goes no further than you and I."[18]

Buchanan or his EMC colleagues undoubtedly employed similar tactics on multiple occasions to circumvent or suppress negative stories destined for the newspapers. In this instance, the tactics failed. The reporter declined the bribe, donating the $10 to charity as the story hit the newsstand on November 30. The entire episode thus became another in the series of metaphorical punches that Buchanan and the EMC absorbed throughout 1871. As the Rosenzweig case moved to trial in late October of that year, John Buchanan turned his attention to political matters.

POLITICAL CONNECTIONS AND CANDIDATE BUCHANAN

During the summer and fall of 1871, John Buchanan must have been alert to rumblings of official or political fallout from the various negative articles about the school that had been appearing regularly since the *Press* article in March. He and his EMC colleagues had enough contacts in local and state government to monitor developments easily. Two of Buchanan's fellow faculty members, Joseph Sites and Joseph Fitler, had served on the Philadelphia Common Council as 16th Ward representatives in the 1850s, while Fitler had also served on the Board of Commissioners for Kensington, a district of Philadelphia. Another colleague, Phillip Bissell, was likewise politically active, as indicated by his run for political office in 1871.[19] It is difficult to say much more about the political connections and influence of Buchanan and the EMC with any degree of certainty. Still, it seems telling that nearly a decade later, a contemporary of Buchanan's in the Philadelphia medical community shared his own take on the man's ability to avoid catastrophic legal or political fallout in the early 1870s.

Dr. Daniel Garrison Brinton, an eminent scientist in the fields of medicine, archaeology, ethnology, and linguistics in Philadelphia, served as co-editor or editor of Philadelphia's premier medical journal, the *Medical and Surgical Reporter*, between 1867 and 1887. In an 1880 editorial reflecting on Buchanan's career, Brinton asserted that "some years ago" he had been "a power in the pot-house politics of this city" and speculated that Buchanan had proven "useful" to one or more local officeholders. Such connections allowed the EMC dean to benefit from what Brinton described as "indirect but efficient" assistance by persons with political influence. Brinton's credibility is bolstered by the fact that he had known

Buchanan since the late 1850s, when both men attended the Philadelphia School of Anatomy. Other contemporary Philadelphia journals struck a similar note but made even more direct assertions. The *Hahnemannian Monthly*, for example, alleged that Buchanan "owned somebody" in the local and/or state political arena.[20] Eclectic colleagues outside Philadelphia probably shared these suspicions. They were more concerned, however, with what modern political operatives would call damage control. On October 5, 1871, the National Eclectic Medical Association passed a resolution ruefully acknowledging the complicity of "Eclectic teachers" in the sale of diplomas and pronouncing their "unqualified condemnation" of such "unlawful and wicked proceedings."[21]

Such charges that Buchanan and the EMC wielded political influence in Philadelphia after the war are entirely plausible. During the 1860s and 1870s, the city's political landscape constituted what one historian described as a "classic study of machine politics on the municipal level." Especially after the Civil War, Philadelphia's political structure included several anomalous features that laid its civic affairs open to manipulation, if not outright exploitation, by unscrupulous individuals. One such feature was the city's blurred lines of accountability, arising from the "overlap" of elected officials' functions created by the prewar consolidation of the Philadelphia county and city political systems. The byzantine network of elective and appointive positions resulting from this consolidation left the average Philadelphian's head swimming as to just *who* was responsible for *what* in governing the city.[22]

A second feature of the city structure at this time was its "saloon politics." This was an era characterized by informal arrangements and backroom deal making. The insider knowledge and connections possessed by Sites, Fitler, Bissell, and Buchanan must have proved invaluable, granting them warning of events to come and periodic access to political advantage.

A third feature of Philadelphia's political structure after the Civil War was its domination by the Republican Party. This created a new entry point into local affairs, though one strongly resisted—both philosophically and at the street level—by the Democratic Party. It was at the street level that Philadelphia politics played out in its most hotly contested form. At this level, both sides employed tactics like the use of "repeaters" (i.e., individuals voting at multiple polling stations in a ward or district) to pack the ballot box for favored candidates or voter intimidation by volunteer fire companies, which had long acted as a political strong arm of machine politicians. These downstream political tactics acted as an additional buffer to that provided by the state's 1869 Registration Act. This law empowered Philadelphia's Republican-dominated Board of Aldermen to appoint specified officials to "certify" rolls of qualified voters and directed any challenge by individual voters to the courts, where they were unlikely to prevail. It also provided for hourly announcements of the running vote total at each polling place—ostensibly to call out voter fraud as it developed but in practice, as one political veteran explained, to alert party bosses of the need to mobilize additional voters.[23]

At the time the Rosenzweig case broke in the press, John Buchanan had turned his thoughts increasingly to politics. He had first tested Philadelphia's political waters in 1869, running unsuccessfully in the Fifth Ward for a seat on the City Council. Despite this setback, he remained active in local affairs by serving as a "watcher" for the Republican 26th Ward in the 1870 elections.[24] Buchanan next set his sights on the October 1871 election for the state legislature, declaring his candidacy as an Independent Republican running in the fourth legislative district. Although Buchanan seems not to have been suspicious by nature, the timing of the earlier *Philadelphia Press* article may not have been coincidental, coming as it did little more than six months before the election. Buchanan apparently did not consider the possibility that political forces may have been behind the timing of the story that loosened an avalanche of negative press. Instead, he devoted his attention to an election day that became memorable for its violence.

Buchanan's experience as a Republican poll watcher in 1870 may have planted the seed for his campaign strategy in the 1871 election, including an erroneous assumption as to how he might safely employ this strategy. Like many fellow residents of Philadelphia, Buchanan had watched the city's black citizens march to the polls in the fall of 1870 and taken note of the potential power of this newly enfranchised voting bloc to ensure long-term Republican political dominance. Buchanan had also witnessed in the 1870 election the violent attempts made by local toughs and city police under the direction of Democratic Party bosses to thwart black voters' access to the polls; the ensuing violence and intimidation on that day had been serious enough to prompt an outraged U.S. marshall to call in fifty Marines from the nearby naval yard to guard polling stations in the contested wards. Despite indignant protests from the Democratic mayor, Daniel Fox, this show of force had quelled the violence and allowed the remainder of the election to pass in relative peace.[25]

That 1870 election also demonstrated to John Buchanan the potential political power of black Philadelphians to swing elections in one direction or the other. Left unencumbered, these voters presented a decisive advantage to Republican candidates. Conversely, if black voters could be driven from the polls by violence and intimidation, their absence could swing local races to Democratic candidates. For his 1871 legislative campaign, therefore, Buchanan planned to reach out to the black community, drawing on their support to win the election outright or to swing the outcome to a political ally. In adopting this strategy, however, Buchanan directly embroiled himself in the violent racial and political turmoil that characterized postwar Philadelphia and the country as a whole.

When John Buchanan had arrived in Philadelphia during the early 1850s, he entered a city in the midst of rapid demographic change and with a history of racial tensions that flared periodically into violent riots. While some of the worst violence had occurred between 1838 and 1844, before Buchanan's arrival, it was recent enough to be remembered by the city's older adults. Rapid changes in Philadelphia's social landscape, notably a period of rapid and sustained population growth fueled by an influx of immigrants, particularly from Ireland, were stimulating fierce economic and political competition, which manifested itself through racial and ethnic conflict.

Despite a more than fourfold increase in the city's population between 1850 and 1870, Philadelphia's black population had remained relatively static. In the wake of the massive inflows of migrants and immigrants to the city, black Philadelphians composed a dwindling proportion of the city's residents. The explicit and *de facto* segregation practices of the era effectively confined most blacks within an area bordered by Walnut and South Streets running roughly east and west and Fifth to Twelfth Streets running roughly north and south.[26] Nestled within this area was John Buchanan's EMC at 514 Pine Street.

While the EMC's location put Buchanan in close proximity to Philadelphia's black citizens, it would be a mistake to infer too much from this. In most ways, black Philadelphians occupied a "separate world" within the city, maintaining their own social, cultural, and economic sphere. This

Table 4: Philadelphia Population, Including Black Residents, 1840–1870

	1840	1850	1860	1870
Total	93,665	121,376	565,529	674,022
Black (#)	19,000	19,000	22,000	22,147
Black (%)	17%	15%	3.8%	3.4%

Source: "Fast Facts," United States Federal Census, www.census.gov; Elizabeth M. Geffen, "Industrial Development and Social Crisis, 1841–1854," in Russell Weigley (ed.), *Philadelphia: A 300 Year History* (New York: W. W. Norton & Co., 1982), 309; "Table III: Population of Civil Divisions less than Counties," *United States Federal Census 1870* (Washington: Government Printing Office, 1872), 254.

degree of separateness and racial tension runs counter to more general perceptions of the city from those outside the area. While retrospective assumptions may associate Philadelphia with abolitionists and the underground railroad, John Buchanan would have recognized the truth in the terse assessment of Philadelphia given in 1854 by black abolitionist William Wells Brown: "Colorphobia is . . . rampant here."[27]

In calculating his chances for Pennsylvania's Fourth Legislative District, a pragmatic Buchanan reflected on the eagerness of black Philadelphians to vote he had observed in 1870, and considered how he might win their support. The EMC's location offered one advantage; the boundaries for the fourth district included the entire 7th Ward, an area near the EMC in which black voters constituted 15 percent of voters. Buchanan also had another advantage. The charter he had obtained in 1867 to establish the American University of Philadelphia gave him a tool for dispensing political largesse. Buchanan was already using that school and its diplomas to forge ties with the city's black community. In 1869, an issue of the *Christian Recorder* advertised an African American physician, Dr. Thomas Kinnard, as an "agent" of the American University with instructions to " . . . travel over the US and visit and invite colored men who are desirous of studying medicine to attend the lectures" at the school "free of cost." Little else is known about this connection other than the fact that Kinnard had presented himself as a physician to the African American community in Philadelphia for more than a decade and had ties to the city's African Methodist Episcopal (AME) Church.[28]

Buchanan's use of an African American agent was hardly surprising, given his constant search for new sources of income and his political ambitions. However, the tactic was disparaged by critics questioning Buchanan's motives in cultivating ties with the black community. Certainly he proved opportunistic and distinctly entrepreneurial, if not exploitive, in his attempt to tap the political potential of Philadelphia's black community. To this end, he cultivated leaders of the AME Church, which had been founded in Philadelphia in 1794 at the church (still in operation) known lovingly as "Mother Bethel." Several AME leaders received degrees (D.D. or M.D.) from either the EMC or the American University, including John Stevenson, Anthony Stanford, and J. P. Campbell. A later investigation by a committee of the Pennsylvania state senate identified other black Philadelphians who had received medical degrees from those colleges and subpoenaed them to testify; these included John Hall, David Parlow, J. W. H. Hack, Joseph Morrong, and Jonathan Davis. The statement of John Hall before the senate committee gives some sense of how freely Buchanan distributed diplomas within the black community. When questioned whether any of his friends also possessed one of these diplomas, John Hall remarked, "I suppose every butcher in the state of Pennsylvania has got one."[29]

By bestowing diplomas on key members of Philadelphia's black community, either for a fee or free of charge, Buchanan prepared the ground for his political campaign. He acknowledged as much in an appeal to "my colored brothers" in the Fourth District, published as an open letter, in which he said, "For a long number of years we have been identified together—your interests have been mine—we know each other, have stood by each other." In his campaign pamphlet *To My Colored Brothers of the Fourth Legislative District*, Buchanan quoted freely from a letter dated September 16, 1871, and signed by two dozen black leaders and "five hundred others," imploring him to run for office and praising him as a "stern and unflinching Republican . . . zealous for the rights" of his constituents. The pamphlet also contained an open letter to Philadelphia's black voters from Willis Richardson (W. R.) Revels, an influential AME minister in Baltimore and the brother of Hiram Revels, who would soon become the first black member of the U.S. Senate. W. R. Revels proved unabashed in his support of "our mutual friend and brother, John Buchanan," telling black Philadelphians, "You have a candidate before you for the legislature in whom you can trust . . . who has been a benefactor to the colored man. On him you can rely; he will not make you promises that he will not fulfill; he will take care of your interests."[30]

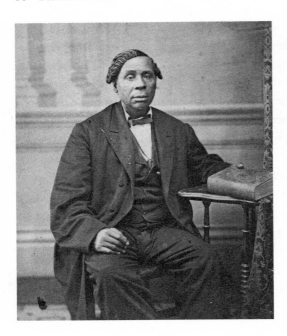

Fig. 7. Willis Revels, a minister of the AME Church in Baltimore. Courted by Buchanan for his 1871 political campaign along with other African American supporters, Revels praised Buchanan as a "mutual friend and brother" to black Philadelphians. Image by permission of the Indiana Historical Society, P0491.

In making his own case for the office, Buchanan offered a mix of broad political platitudes (vowing to "protect the interest of the colored man," for example) and specific promises (such as pledging to secure "colored" appointments to various boards and "fair represent[ation]" on the city's police force). Most telling, however, were his comments targeting the *other* Republican in the race. John Buchanan campaigned as an Independent Republican candidate in a three-man race with Republican William Elliot and Democrat Phillip Bissell. William Elliot was not only the incumbent but a force in local affairs and Pennsylvania politics; he served as a director on the board of the People's Bank of Philadelphia and played a significant role on the city's Gas Trust. Later in 1872, Elliot began a term as speaker of the Pennsylvania House of Representatives. He also appears to have had some familiarity with the EMC and its faculty. An advertisement several years earlier in the *Philadelphia Ledger* promoted Dr. Joseph Fitler's "cure" of Elliot's rheumatism. Despite this connection, however, Buchanan showed no reluctance to castigate Elliot for failing to support the interests of black voters: "I will not, like your present incumbent . . . strike at any favor you ask," Buchanan declared. "You are well aware that Wm Elliott (*sic*) voted against freeing both your Masonic Halls from taxation . . . he has opposed the appointment of colored men in any of the gas works, where he reigns supreme, king of that notorious ring. He has the power to appoint you to positions of importance, which you have the ability to fill, but no!"[31]

Whether John Buchanan genuinely sought to represent Philadelphia's Fourth District in the state legislature when he launched his campaign remains unclear. His earlier political ventures suggest he was truly interested in politics and holding political office, but if we consider the multiple distractions and scandals surrounding Buchanan in the months leading up to the election, it seems impossible that he could have regarded his campaign as anything other than a long shot. Moreover, the campaign presented Buchanan with a financial consideration. In 1871, Philadelphia did not provide voters with a single, uniform ballot. Individual candidates, such as Buchanan, had to purchase and distribute their own "tickets" for voters— two sets if they were courting both Democrats and Republicans.[32] While John Buchanan may have entered the race legitimately intending to win, it seems more plausible that his intent was to siphon sufficient votes from the incumbent Republican, Elliot, to throw the race to the Democrat in the field—his EMC colleague and friend, Phillip Bissell.

In an echo of the urban rioting that had marked Orange Day several months earlier in New York City, the streets surrounding the EMC proved extremely volatile on Election Day, October 10, 1871. The polling site, one block away from the EMC at Sixth and Lombard, became the epicenter for a day of violent confrontations between police and white "roughs" attempting to prevent local black residents of the Fifth Ward from voting. The previous year's election had seen eager black voters waiting en masse at the polling stations when they opened, tickets in hand and already filled out. This strategy had allowed virtually all the eligible black voters to come and go from the polling stations by midmorning, catching the white Democratic bosses off guard so that they failed to mobilize their local toughs and police early enough to block this first wave of black voters. In 1871, however, the Democrats were prepared for an early black presence at the polls; moreover, no federal troops would be forthcoming to protect the black voters. Despite an appearance on the scene by Mayor Fox, full-scale rioting broke out, leaving several dead (including the black educator and activist Octavius Catto) and many dozens more injured.[33] Groups and individuals roamed the area, accosting passersby and voters in an explosion of violence unseen in peacetime Philadelphia since the 1840s. If John Buchanan had expected strong support from black voters in his run for the legislature, the day's violence dashed those hopes, limiting black turnout and dooming his chance either to mount a viable run at the office himself or to swing the race to Bissell. Moreover, Buchanan had other concerns that day—most urgently the distinct possibility that Democratic rioters would target the EMC building because of its policy of accepting black physicians. In the end, the election went decisively to Elliot, with 4,272 votes. Bissell finished a distant second, with 2,300 votes. As for John Buchanan, the newspapers did not even bother to list his vote total.[34]

Five

Senate Inquiry and a Supreme Court Case, 1872

The 1871 election disappointed John Buchanan, but more serious matters soon demanded his attention. In December, the Pennsylvania state legislature announced its intention of convening a special committee to investigate allegations of diploma selling at the EMC. The announcement probably left local Philadelphians puzzled. Why was the legislature acting only now on a matter that had been common knowledge in many quarters for quite some time?

The immediate impetus stemmed from the legislature's adoption of a resolution on May 19, 1871: "It shall not be lawful for any university, college, or other institution incorporated under the laws of this State, with power to grant academic degrees, honorary or otherwise, to confer the same upon any person . . . upon payment or promise of payment by any person in consideration thereof."[1] Subsequent testimony by officials of the University of Pennsylvania, such as Provost Charles J. Stille and Professor Robert E. Rogers, confirmed their role in urging state officials to adopt

89

the law and to make the EMC its primary target. State officials now had a legal basis for challenging the ongoing trade in diplomas. Although this was never explicitly stated, another factor was Buchanan's 1871 legislative campaign, which served as a poorly timed provocation. After the legislature had drawn its line in the sand in May, state officials might have been willing to drop the matter had EMC discontinued its questionable practices and taken immediate steps to return to legitimate educational policies. Instead, John Buchanan's third-party electoral challenge that October to William Elliot, the Republican incumbent for his district in the state legislature and a rising star, proved too much. While speculative, it is logical to link the political maneuverings of Buchanan and his colleagues with the subsequent action of the state legislature: In January 1872, it set up a special investigative committee, charged with finding evidence to support the legislature's ultimate goal of annulling the EMC charter.

THE LEGISLATURE INVESTIGATES

A seven-member committee, chaired by Pennsylvania state senator William M. Randall, convened nine times between February 3 and March 16, 1872, at various settings in Philadelphia and Harrisburg. In total, nearly sixty individuals testified. The deposed witnesses included officials from Pennsylvania University and Jefferson Medical College, as well as faculty and trustees from the EMC and Philadelphia University, reporters from several Philadelphia and New York newspapers, an official with the U.S. Postal Service in Philadelphia, and a parade of current students and graduates from all four schools, who all had varying degrees of firsthand knowledge of—and sometimes conflicting tales of their experiences with—the EMC and Philadelphia University.[2]

The order of appearance for the early witnesses shows that Randall, as committee chair, had a distinct plan in mind. The first few witnesses provided facts and documentary evidence making it clear to the press covering the hearings that the committee had Buchanan, and later William Paine, directly in their crosshairs. The committee hearing opened with testimony from Penn and Jefferson officials, Charles J. Stille, Robert Rogers, and Howard Rand; the editor of the *Medical and Surgical Reporter*, Samuel Worcester Butler; and a postal official, George Fairman. These witnesses introduced an array of letters and documents demonstrating the advertising and sales efforts of the EMC in England, Germany, and elsewhere. The documents included letters from physicians and various officials situated overseas to Philadelphia authorities, particularly those at Penn, seeking to ascertain if that school had any affiliation with John Buchanan and the various agents claiming to represent Philadelphia schools.

The letters and advertisements introduced by Stille and Rogers included inquiries to unnamed local agents overseas that reflected broad foreign confusion surrounding the Philadelphia schools and American higher education in general. One writer from Ireland explained that Europeans found it difficult to "conceive that two universities can exist in the same city."[3] Such misconceptions undoubtedly led some interested overseas parties to respond, under the assumption that they were legitimately exploring the possibility of an "honorary" degree at the city's best-known school, the University of Pennsylvania. Discreet advertisements such as the one following may have led some individuals to respond in good faith: "Degrees, M.D., Ph.D., &c.—The foreign secretary of a 'well-known' university is willing to forward the aspirations of qualified candidates to honorary or other academic degrees. Fees nominal. Address, in confidence, The Foreign Secretary, 10 St. Paul's road, Canonbury, London."[4] However, the documentary evidence also shows that many, if not most, foreigners replying to EMC offers were under no illusion about their nature. They knew that they were embarking on a quid pro quo transaction involving payment for a degree. In most of these exchanges, the names of the Americans offering the degrees, notably Buchanan and Paine, were withheld until later in the correspondence chain.

Testimony from Drs. Butler and Rand showed that the EMC's strategy abroad was also used at home. Just as they did abroad, the Philadelphia schools employed agents and produced a similar pattern of advertisements and inquiries to solicit parties interested in honorary degrees within the United States.

These early witnesses testified cautiously, sticking closely to factual statements and information within their firsthand knowledge. Occasionally their exasperation and sense of indignation at the diploma trade won out. Dr. Rogers, the head of Penn's medical department, pointed out the slipperiness of Buchanan and others by citing their ability to "so successfully cover up their tracks" that implicating them directly proved difficult. Jefferson's Dr. Howard Rand stated bluntly, "The whole thing has been managed very cunningly."[5]

The committee concluded its first day with testimony from a New York reporter, who gave evidence on a pair of well-known but dubious characters allegedly holding EMC diplomas: the notorious Jacob Rosenzweig and a self-proclaimed New York clairvoyant, Madame Cleopatra. These damning revelations came after a postal official with the U.S. Post Office shared information about his investigation of Buchanan and the EMC. His testimony introduced the name of a key, but controversial, future witness: J. Dunbar Hylton, a one-time U.S. postal employee who later joined the EMC faculty.[6]

After laying this groundwork, the hearings followed a methodical course as a long list of individuals testified to their firsthand experiences with or at the EMC and Philadelphia University. Some, such as Cornelius Bates, testified as a graduate and staunch defender of the EMC. Others complained of their experience at the school: "I didn't consider that diploma of any account," said one.[7] A recurring theme raised by many, however, was the sense of urgency they felt to acquire a diploma in a rapidly changing medico-political environment. Many individuals recognized that their less formalized medical knowledge and skills, acquired through mentors or preceptors along with a full or partial course of lectures at a medical school, were quickly becoming insufficient, if not patently unacceptable. Many witnesses seemed to imply a belief that a diploma from a legally chartered institution would soon become the minimum basis for practicing medicine in the United States. Even practitioners with considerable experience, such as the former London physician Idris Davies, testified to their willingness to pay for and sit an examination at an established school in order to qualify for a diploma.[8]

John Buchanan stepped before the committee at a hearing held in Harrisburg on the morning of February 17, 1872. He must have anticipated a torrent of pointed questions and barbed statements.[9] His EMC colleague Phillip Bissell, preceding him as a witness, had faltered badly under the detailed questions posed by the senate committee. The senators opened their questioning of Buchanan with the standard biographical questions posed to every witness: name, residence, occupation, connection to the

EMC. The record of the early portion of this session reveals a tone from Buchanan's questioners that was surprisingly less confrontational than that accorded his colleague Bissell. After the preliminary queries on background and affiliation with the school, committee members began asking Buchanan a series of questions about the EMC faculty: How many members? Who were they? Did all of them lecture? Buchanan responded dutifully to each question, perhaps cognizant of the senators' methods. A dozen witnesses had preceded him. The committee had demonstrated a pattern of opening with easy questions, perhaps consciously designed to settle the witnesses' nerves and lull them into a false sense of comfort and confidence. This made the challenging questions to follow all the more forceful: "Are you in the habit of granting any diplomas from the college when the student has not undergone the full prescribed course?"

John Buchanan had apparently determined his strategy in answering this line of questions. He would explain carefully the categories of diplomas available to, and issued by, the EMC; stressing that these were the same diplomas types issued by most schools.

"No meritorious diplomas."

Apparently confused by the response, the senator queried, "What do you mean meritorious?"

John Buchanan then explained the distinction among the three types of diplomas issued by colleges. "There are three classes of diplomas in medical colleges," he said. "We have what we call an honorary diploma, an *ad eundum* diploma and a degree of merit. The degree of merit is conferred only upon those who attend the prescribed course of study."[10]

Apparently content to follow Buchanan's lead in exploring the various types of diplomas, the senate chairman pressed on. "Do either of these first two classes of diplomas entitle the person receiving them to practice medicine?"

"Not legally."

A senator returned Buchanan's reply as a question. "Not legally?"

"I think not. The *ad eundum* is a degree conferred on top of a degree, a mere honor conferred."

"Do the students procuring that class—"

At that point, Buchanan interjected, cutting off the question. "They are not conferred upon students. The regular degree of merit is conferred on students." He then explained the "prescribed course of study" for the meritorious diploma. He cited the requirements for this degree: three years' study with a preceptor (or eight to nine years in practice), attendance at two courses of lectures, an examination, and a thesis.

The senators next moved to a different line of questioning. John Buchanan listened patiently to their questions about degrees issued to specific individuals. While the transcript of Buchanan's testimony cannot convey the tone or emotions of his testimony, his words at no point reflected exasperation or anger at his interrogators' inferences or skepticism. In each instance, he offered seemingly reasonable explanations to clarify the details behind the individual cases his interrogators put forth. He seemed to have settled upon a strategy for testifying: remain calm, act outwardly friendly, even helpful, and provide detailed answers to every question when possible. By that point in his career, Buchanan had learned that apparent frankness and the verisimilitude afforded by small but telling snippets and incidental details made a statement or story ring true.

At one point in his testimony, however, Buchanan could not resist making an incredible assertion. When a senator asked, "Do you know of any other college or school in Philadelphia that has issued diplomas to students, without requiring the prescribed qualifications?" he answered simply, "They all do it."

When the senators challenged Buchanan to provide examples supporting this statement, he brought up the case of a Dr. Idris Davies and claimed to have a copy of a letter to Davies from Dr. Rand of the Jefferson Medical College offering to sell him a diploma for a fee of $150. When asked if Rand's letter required Davies to sit an examination, Buchanan stated, "The copy I got didn't say anything about the examination," but asserted that Rand had told Davies "he would have to write a thesis." This account differs from earlier direct testimony to the committee by Davies himself, supported by several letters from Rand, stating that Jefferson Medical College would confer a degree on Davies without requiring him to attend classes, as long as he provided proof of practicing as a doctor for seventeen years, sat an examination, and paid a fee. Whatever the specifics of the requirements Jefferson asked of Davies, the college clearly sought evidence that Davies was a qualified and experienced medical practitioner, and required proof of this fact before it would issue him a diploma. Such a process, if executed as described, was wholly legal and not inappropriate, but in the context of the senate hearings, it seemed uncomfortably close to the more dubious practices alleged of the EMC and Philadelphia University.[11]

The committee then shifted its line of questioning to another EMC diploma holder, Dr. A. R. McCarthy. This time John Buchanan struggled in his attempt to implicate other schools' practices. The specific circumstances of McCarthy's experience with the EMC did not lend themselves to shifting the spotlight. Undoubtedly experiencing some nervousness at this point, Buchanan's answers became increasingly brief responses to questions. "Yes, sir" and "No, sir" answers filled this portion of the transcript. The closed-ended questions posed by the senators made it awkward for Buchanan to expand upon his answers. As Buchanan's testimony drew to a close, Senator Strang interjected with a request that harkened to the earlier portion of Buchanan's testimony.

"Will you, at your leisure, give us a little statement in writing, of the character of the degrees and the names you give them at your institution?"

Buchanan agreed to do so. This request gave him the opportunity to play the role of a cooperative witness with nothing to hide. He even offered to supply the committee with the EMC's register of degrees and cash books for its review. After this exchange, the committee chairman dismissed Buchanan from the stand. Whether he ever provided the requested written statement or the school's register and cashbooks is unclear; no mention is made of any of them in the committee's final report.

Senator Strang's request for a written statement seems odd considering a transcriptionist sat with them in the room, capturing all the testimony. Strang may have hoped that a written statement might contradict Buchanan's oral testimony in some way, or he may have intended the opposite: to give Buchanan a chance to finesse his written response in a way that offset his oral testimony. Another possibility is that Senator Strang had no ulterior motive and was simply struggling to follow Buchanan's explanation of diploma types and felt that the transcription would not clarify matters. Whatever Strang's motives, John Buchanan was the only witness to receive this type of request.

If John Buchanan acquitted himself capably in his testimony, his colleagues' statements undercut his position. Even in the dead letters on the printed page of the transcript, these colleagues come across as hedging and deceptive in their responses. EMC faculty member Phillip Bissell testified the same day as Buchanan, though with far less confidence and a greater degree of caution. Simple questions by the senators about the sale of diplomas or asking for his firsthand knowledge drew vague, noncommittal responses: "I have heard some stories. . . . I have seen diplomas of some colleges. . . . I have no recollection. . . . I never inquired about the gentleman's business."[12] On several occasions, he demurred or declined outright to answer on the basis that his response might violate his constitutional right against self-incrimination. When questioned on his current employment status with the school, Bissell tried to disassociate himself from the EMC completely. When asked if he was presently "connected" with the EMC, his muddled answer exasperated the committee. "I suppose I am," Bissell answered. "I do not know anything to the contrary, although I have not been there. I tendered my resignation some time since, and whether it is accepted or not I do not know." Even worse was the testimony from William C. Harbison, a homeopathic doctor and acquaintance of Buchanan's, who was forced to acknowledge that the city of Philadelphia had him under indictment for perjury.[13]

Little better for Buchanan was the parade of African American witnesses called to testify on the basis of the degrees issued to them. The testimony of some of these witnesses evinced their awareness that Buchanan's offer of diplomas was motivated by his desire to gain "political influence" within their community, particularly through members of the African Methodist Episcopal Church, such as A. L. Stanford, John Stevenson, and David Parlow.[14] The latter two men, along with two others called to testify, Joseph Morrong and Jonathan Davis, had been signatories of the letter endorsing Buchanan's run for a seat representing the Fourth Legislative District in the state senate the previous fall, which he had reprinted in *To My Colored Brothers of the Fourth Legislative District*.[15] This fact was not likely to have been missed by William Elliot, who had beaten Buchanan in that race and was now the speaker of the Pennsylvania House of Representatives. Buchanan's challenge to Elliot, and the city's tense racial politics during that era, meant there was nothing accidental or arbitrary about the decision to call so many African Americans to testify. This parade of witnesses served as a reminder to both Democrats and Republicans on the seven-member committee of

Philadelphia's racial politics. For Democrats, it signaled a new political era, in which they could expect a tactic they perceived as pandering for the black vote to become political business as usual. For Republicans, it served as a powerful reminder of Buchanan's cynical ploy to split their party vote and throw the race to his Democratic colleague, Bissell.

The testimony of two reporters, Howard Hanmore of the *New York Herald* and Joseph Reed of the *Philadelphia Press* proved equally damning for Buchanan. Both described personal encounters with Buchanan in which he attempted to bribe them to avoid negative press. Hanmore had visited Buchanan several months earlier, in November 1871. He identified himself as a reporter and found Buchanan and Bissell cordial enough ("They treated me very kindly") but clearly anxious to avoid more negative press. During his visit, Hanmore feigned a willingness to write a positive story on EMC; Buchanan, initially "wary," came around after a series of conversations and proffered $10 to Hanmore, with the possibility of more to follow. Reed recapped his March 1871 story, which had first brought Buchanan and the EMC to public attention. His narrative culminated with Buchanan's agreement to grant him a medical diploma for $25.[16]

The testimony of a large number of the remaining witnesses shifted the committee's focus to William Paine and Philadelphia University. An undercurrent of animus against Paine flowed from many of those who testified. One witness contemptuously described Paine as "more corrupt even . . . than Buchanan," While another characterized him as poisonous ("I condemn him as the deadly upas") and contemptible ("I think little of him"). Perhaps not surprisingly, faculty members and trustees at Philadelphia University either distanced themselves from Paine or rejected him outright. A fellow faculty member of Paine's recounted how a major disagreement among faculty had resulted in a reorganization and prompted his own decision to serve as dean of the school solely for the purpose of "keep[ing] Dr. Paine out." One school trustee, seeking to shift blame away from himself and his fellows, emphasized how they had broadly "empowered" Paine to act on behalf of the school.[17]

If Paine's testimony was any indication, the man possessed a combative nature and wielded a sufficiently acid pen to make him a formidable adversary. In his testimony, Paine decried the injustices and plots against him and Philadelphia University by the city's long-established schools

(Penn and Jefferson), as well as what he felt were libelous allegations made in the *Medical and Surgical Reporter.* His written rebuttals to accusers spared few targets: he called homeopaths "ignorant, bigoted sectarian quacks" and used race-baiting language to label Buchanan's school a "darkey concern." To show his possession of the moral high ground, he even called for the establishment of a "central medical board" to examine the graduates of all Philadelphia medical schools.[18]

Both in his testimony and in a later publication, *Pennsylvania Frauds* (ca. 1873), Paine denied allegations of diploma selling and recalled his own failed attempts to interest the state legislature into opening an investigation of this same matter in the 1860s. However, the biased content of *Pennsylvania Frauds* is difficult to reconcile with his testimony before the senate committee and undercuts many of Paine's forceful denials of corruption, since it is highly selective in its account of the senate investigation, giving considerable attention to favorable witnesses and very little to those critical of Paine and Philadelphia University (e.g., Smith, Murphy, Fleming, McShane, and Harvey). Even stranger was the pamphlet's detailed narrative of how state officials, including Governor John W. Geary, attempted to discredit Paine through a plot implicating him in the corruption case of George O. Evans, a special agent empowered by the governor to secure federal reimbursement for specific expenses incurred by Pennsylvania during the Civil War.[19]

One of the most damning witnesses to testify—and one implicating both Buchanan and Paine—was John Dunbar Hylton.[20] His testimony ostensibly provided the committee with an insider account of the diploma trade. Hylton had joined the EMC faculty in 1870, and he claimed that soon thereafter, when he realized that "things did not seem to be going on right," he dedicated himself to breaking up the operation. Hylton related his attempt to recruit Penn and Jefferson officials in a sting of the EMC and Philadelphia University, an effort that ultimately came to naught. He also described the practices of Buchanan and Paine in detail, including the former's largesse in distributing diplomas to black voters ("I believe almost every colored gentleman [in] the district was presented with [one]")[21] and the latter's insistence on framing the diploma trade as a scheme selling *scholarships*, rather than *diplomas*, to individuals. Emphasizing this point, Hylton stated baldly, "They sell the scholarships," explaining that these sales came with an implied understanding to the purchasers that they were buying the diploma as well. This method seemed an ideal way to "cover up the legal technicalities" arising from the state legislature's May 1871 law prohibiting the sale of diplomas.[22] The technique presented a clever mechanism for thwarting both the intent and the spirit of the law. Hylton's explanation of this tactic exposed how Paine and Buchanan could forcefully deny selling diplomas without necessarily perjuring themselves. As Hylton told the story, Buchanan and Paine posed as innocents bewildered by the presumption of students who assumed that a diploma came with the scholarship.

At the same time, Hylton's testimony occasionally rings hollow, even self-serving, in its tones of moral indignation at the blatancy of the diploma trade. Several witnesses testified that Hylton had personally assured them that he could secure a diploma if they were so interested. Presenting himself as an outraged educator and professional acting disinterestedly, Hylton claimed such incidents were attempts to gain direct evidence against Buchanan and Paine. His coy, somewhat guarded, denial of one witness's testimony, however, seemed more akin to the action of a cooperating witness hoping to avoid prosecution than to the disinterested actions of an outraged educator and professional.

The hearings concluded on March 16, 1872. The committee hurriedly finalized its report, reading it into the legislative record only four days later. The final report proved unequivocal in its tone and damning in its conclusions. The committee dismissed any charges of wrongdoing by Jefferson Medical College and the University of Pennsylvania, but cited ample evidence that Drs. John Buchanan, head of the EMC and American University of Philadelphia, and William Paine, leader of Philadelphia University, had "openly engaged in the sale of diplomas." Perhaps thinking particularly of the origins of Philadelphia University, the committee also raised, but did not answer, the question of the "complicated and mysterious legislat[ive]" actions that brought these schools into existence. The report hinted that these schools had operated within a culture of impropriety in place since their founding, but it included no evidence to support this intimation.[23]

From the testimony of dozens of witnesses offering an array of "astounding facts," the committee concluded correctly that the two schools had engaged in an "open and systematic" sale of diplomas. The report expressed outrage at practices so blatantly designed for monetary gain that not only were degrees issued to individuals who had failed to attend even a partial course but individual recipients often lacked "any medical or scientific attainment whatever." In this manner, the "nefarious business" of Buchanan, Paine, and their schools had become so "notorious" that it cast a shadow upon even the city's premier legitimate institutions for medical education, Penn and Jefferson. The committee recommended that the legislature repeal the statutes incorporating the two schools.[24]

THE PENNSYLVANIA SUPREME COURT

On March 22, 1872, the Pennsylvania legislature delivered what should have been a fatal blow by repealing the charters of Buchanan's and Paine's medical schools. Local newspapers delighted in the demise of the diploma mills and applauded the legislature for doing "exactly what was right." At the same time, John Buchanan and his attorney turned a careful eye to Pennsylvania's state constitution and the exact verbiage of the repeal. One thing immediately obvious was a legislative oversight. The legislature had repealed the charters for the EMC and Philadelphia University but there was no mention of Buchanan's other institution, the American University of Philadelphia. Legally chartered in 1867, the American University served as a second conduit for diploma sales. In essence, the legislature closed two doors of the diploma trade but inexplicably left open a third. The mystery behind this oversight disappears if one accepts John Buchanan's 1881 confession. In a lengthy interview with the *Philadelphia Record*, Buchanan claimed to have disbursed $3,000 among some or all seven members of the senate investigative committee.[25] If true, this may account for the otherwise inexplicable omission of the American University from the bill repealing the school charters.

Buchanan displayed a cunning shrewdness in refusing to accept the repeal of the EMC charter as a fait accompli. He and his attorney scrutinized Pennsylvania's 1857 constitution, the legal basis for the legislature's decision to repeal the EMC charter, and came to the conclusion that the 1857 constitution did not grant the legislature authority to repeal charters issued by a previous legislature predating the current (1857) constitution. This would mean it lacked the power to repeal the EMC's charter, which had been issued in 1850. Buchanan then used an indirect method to get this matter into the court system. He directed his EMC colleague, Henry Stickney, to seek out a local attorney, Kinley J. Tener. He also gave Stickney a signed diploma for an EMC graduate named Chilton Allen, an individual who John Buchanan knew had long since left the country. Stickney was to present Tener with a "made up" story alleging lost time, damages, and other injuries supposedly suffered by Allen because of the repeal of the EMC charter. Buchanan directed Stickney to have Tener secure a second attorney, who would "sue" Buchanan and the EMC on Allen's behalf while he (Tener) defended them against the suit. By raising the issue through proxies, Buchanan could argue a critical point of law without directly confronting the court with a legal contest between the EMC and the state. The lawsuit brought against Buchanan by "Allen" reached the state supreme court quite quickly, and on March 1, 1873, the court handed down its decision. Ruling in favor of the defendant, John Buchanan, Pennsylvania Supreme Court Justice Agnew held that the amended 1857 constitution did not grant the legislature the "power of repeal" for entities—in this case, the EMC—established under the prior constitution. Thus, the state had acted without proper authority in repealing the school's charter. According to the ruling, any "forfeiture" of the charter could come only through judicial proceedings—and the operations of the senate investigative committee did not qualify.[26] In a surprising turn of affairs, less than one year after the legislature had extinguished the EMC as a legal entity, the school rose from the ashes to resume operation.

MORE LEGAL TROUBLES

Though the EMC emerged from the potentially disastrous events of 1871–73 with its operations largely intact, significant damage had been done. While whispers and occasional questions about practices at the EMC may already have been current by the late 1860s, the school had remained largely in good standing within the eclectic community. After the revelations of 1871–72, however, eclectic critics considered Buchanan and the EMC beyond the pale. The period immediately after winning *Allen v. Buchanan* offered Buchanan perhaps the last opportunity to reestablish the EMC as a legitimate institution by ending its questionable or outright fraudulent practices and working to rebuild the school's relationships within the eclectic community. Buchanan did neither.

Faced with condemnation from within the eclectic community, Buchanan instead unleashed a torrent of abuse at his detractors, characterizing them as "mongrel, chaotic and brainless." He called out specific eclectic schools for their "burlesque on medical teaching," calling the American Medical College of St. Louis a "slaughterhouse," describing the charter obtained by the Bennett College of Eclectic Medicine as worth no more than that obtained by "a tobacconist," and labeling the Eclectic Medical College of New York as nothing more than "a grand burlesque upon the profession." He even went so far as to attack the mother of eclectic medical schools, the Eclectic Medical Institute of Cincinnati, describing it as little better than "a common school."[27] Buchanan's writing degenerated into unseemly name-calling. Those drawing his ire included eclectic stalwarts like Drs. Robert S. Newton and John Scudder, whom he disparaged as "lardaceous" and a "dead beat," respectively.[28] If Buchanan had retained the faith of any eclectic colleagues following the senate investigation, they all abandoned him after his vitriolic writings of 1874.

During the thirteen-month interregnum in the EMC's legal operations (from March 1872 through March 1873), Buchanan leaned heavily on the valid charter he still held for the American University of Philadelphia. With business as usual under the auspices of the EMC temporarily suspended, Buchanan resumed the offensive through a retitled version of the EMC's journal (the *Journal of Progressive Medicine*), in which he offered a revisionist and self-serving history of the EMC that omitted inconvenient facts.

In this account, Buchanan claimed the school had been undermined by the "corrupt influences" of former faculty members who sought to hide their own misdeeds by adopting a name for their new college—Paine's Eclectic Medical College of Philadelphia—so closely mirroring that of the EMC as to inevitably confuse the two schools. Buchanan stated that in this way Paine and his new colleagues had dragged the original EMC into the tainted mud of their "parasite" school's disreputable activities. He then reassured EMC graduates that "all the living graduates" of the school would receive an *ad eundem* degree from the American University. The piece ended in a barrage of platitudes ("truth can never be obliterated") and a call for action: to resist allopathic persecution by securing pledged support from local elected officials. Buchanan rallied his supporters using the language of dissent and reform, reminding his readers of his colleague Joseph Sites's admonition that "freedom . . . in medicine, as in religion and politics, is as essential as . . . the air you breathe."[29]

These personal attacks and diatribes garnered attention by themselves. Yet Buchanan may have drawn just as much attention through the extravagant claims and advertisements printed in the *Journal of Progressive Medicine*. In its pages, Buchanan touted his "cure" for cancer, offering to sell the "formulae" for preparing and applying his "Great Cancer Antidote" for $10.[30] The *Journal of Progressive Medicine* carried a similar cure for consumption. Despite the implausible nature of these pronouncements, Buchanan was not alone in making such claims. During this same period, his EMC colleague Joseph P. Fitler widely advertised "Rheumatic syrup," as well as curatives for gout, lumbago, and other diseases. EMC faculty members had indulged in such extravagant advertising for some years, starting at the college's foundation in 1850 with John Fondey's electromagnetic treatment for tubercular disease.[31]

The publicity created by Buchanan's revisionist history and attacks on other doctors and medical schools, and by the inflated claims made by him and his colleagues for their patent medicines and cures, took a new slant in light of the notoriety surrounding Buchanan and the EMC. Episodes that might once have passed unnoticed were now potential grist for the reporters' mill. For the rest of the 1870s, most of Buchanan's activities took place in the unwelcome glare of a politico-legal scrutiny that he had not experienced previously. Six months after *Allen v. Buchanan*, a reporter visited Buchanan to inquire about the Cuban consulate's questioning of a physician with credentials from the American University. The reporter's account of the interview showed Buchanan once again presenting an implacable demeanor. When the reporter handed him a story from the previous day's *Philadelphia Inquirer*, Buchanan read the article, sighed heavily, and commented, "They are again at the same work." He then carefully answered the reporter's queries about the physician in question, explaining that the man had been issued a diploma only after completing a three-month "private course" and providing evidence of course work completed abroad together with and "some years" of experience in private practice.[32] This interview demonstrated another of Buchanan's favored tactics in dealing with the press—playing the role of victim. Affecting the tone of a persecuted party, he patiently delivered detailed, seemingly reasonable answers to specific questions.

The best example of the heightened scrutiny directed at Buchanan concerns the publicity aroused by his treatment of a patient, Emily Vandergrift, in 1874. Despite public preoccupation that year, both locally and nationally, with the kidnapping and disappearance in July of four-year-old Charley Ross, the local press remained eager to pursue any story concerning John Buchanan and the EMC. This story began when Vandergrift wrote to Buchanan in response to an advertisement for his medical practice, and later traveled to Philadelphia, on or around September 10, 1874, for a consultation. According to testimony at the coroner's inquest, Buchanan examined Vandergrift, told her that she had a "serious rupture" that might require surgery, and placed her at the home of a professional nurse in preparation for the surgery and postoperative care. Vandergrift paid Buchanan $75 in advance for his services. Nothing more occurred until September 13, when she became seriously ill with "chills . . . fever and vomiting." Buchanan did not treat her until two days later, when he limited his treatment to "dry cupping"—a practice he cited in his published works as a preferred alternative to the incisions and skin scarifications of the "wet cupping" once commonly used by allopathic physicians. Buchanan never operated, as Vandergrift died later that same evening. In filling out her death certificate, he listed "fever" as the cause of death.[33]

Whether Buchanan's signature on a death certificate sufficed to raise suspicion or whether the newly widowed Mr. Vandergrift raised the cry of medical malpractice is unclear. A coroner's inquest convened the following afternoon, although Buchanan did not attend. A detective testified that he had initially sought Buchanan at No. 225 North Twelfth Street, the address he provided on the death certificate, only to find that he had not lived there for several years. He soon tracked Buchanan down at 514 Pine Street (the EMC building) and arrested him. Damning evidence came from the physicians who had conducted the postmortem examination of the body. Their findings showed no evidence of disease or a rupture, although the woman's "bowels were congested all through." They cited the cause of death as exhaustion resulting from pain and vomiting. The coroner's jury deliberated briefly and returned its verdict: "That . . . Emily J. Vandergrift came to her death from exhaustion, the result of disease of the bowels, caused by criminal malpractice . . . at the hands of Dr.

John B. Buchanan." In a confession later published in the *Philadelphia Record*, Buchanan claimed that he disposed of this legal matter after paying $1,250 to "the lawyers."[34]

In one regard, this accusation of medical malpractice against Buchanan does not surprise and may have had little to do with his skills as a physician or his standing within Philadelphia's medical community. Beginning in the mid-nineteenth century, medical malpractice, once a rare allegation, became an increasingly common charge brought against physicians by patients or their families reacting to real or perceived negative outcomes. One historian tracking malpractice cases reaching state appellate courts noted a 450 percent increase in such cases between 1860 and 1890. Physicians lamented the increase of these "vexatious" civil suits. That Vandergrift's family pressed the matter against Buchanan may have reflected evolving patient perceptions of what constituted acceptable care and outcomes and the potential vulnerability of even established physicians possessing assets sufficient to warrant a legal effort to secure damages.[35]

Despite the serious nature of the charge against Buchanan and his being held over for arraignment, no trial took place. As for several other legal matters that followed in 1876 and 1877, Buchanan's arrest was reported in the newspapers only to disappear soon thereafter as a veil of silence descended. In each case, the legal problem seemed to quietly disappear. In the 1960s, one medical historian searched the court records for this period as part of his broader research into Philadelphia's extinct medical schools. Finding no bills of indictment or bond-related documents, he speculated that Buchanan had a "confederate" in the offices of Philadelphia's Quarter Sessions Court.[36] One might propose a similar explanation for the lack of follow-through on Vandergrift's death in 1874: perhaps Buchanan or a friend had contacts among the city aldermen. These officials held an amorphous portfolio of extensive *de facto* functions and powers that often included handling court cases. The alderman system offered an ideal platform for "delay and favoritism" in legal matters,[37] characteristics that appear to have benefited Buchanan in this case.

John Buchanan faced more legal troubles in 1876. In mid-April, an elderly man approached a young woman near Sixth and Chestnut Streets. He handed her a pamphlet that she deemed sufficiently "improper" that she passed it along to her brother, a reporter with the *Philadelphia Record*. He alerted the police to what the newspapers later termed "obscene materials." Under police questioning, the old man admitted that he was employed by Dr. John Buchanan, the printer and publisher of the materials, who was soon arrested.[38]

Not surprisingly, the newspaper accounts fail to give precise information on the contents of the pamphlet. While American newspapers titillated their readers with sensational stories, they usually refrained from publishing explicit details on sexual matters. The *Philadelphia Record* did, however, hint at the nature of the contents in reporting that Buchanan was charged with "issuing certain books and cards in the form of advertisements conflicting with the law relating to obscene publications."[39]

This description of the pamphlet as an "advertisement" allows the reader to surmise two distinct possibilities. First, it may have contained promotional material for the EMC's museum, which, as noted earlier, prominently featured male and female nudes and anatomical displays of sexual organs. Beginning around this time, a growing social ambivalence about the suitability of such displays, together with the growing number of obscenity laws, was causing a steady decline in the popularity of medical museums open to the public. Second, the "obscene materials" may have dealt with female hygiene and/or contraception. This seems a reasonable explanation, considering the various accusations over the years linking John Buchanan to abortion and the 1873 passage of the Comstock Law for the suppression of obscene literature, which provided a legal basis for such prosecutions.[40] Whatever the contents of the paper, at least some local officials seemed eager to take this opportunity to make life difficult for Buchanan.

This case proved more difficult for Buchanan to dispose of than most of the legal matters he had faced during this period. He posted $1,000 bail and then quietly disappeared, amid press speculation that he had fled to Europe. This rumor may well have been true. Years later, a friend of Buchanan's talked of accompanying him on a transatlantic journey at a time of considerable personal trouble for the doctor. Buchanan may have journeyed to London, intending to remain. One piece of evidence for this concerned a promissory note that Buchanan left with a Philadelphia stable man, Dan McCaulley. The note came due during the doctor's alleged absence, and when Buchanan failed to appear, the local court issued a judgment in the stable man's favor. Consequently, in early June, a constable assigned to secure the EMC property against creditors' liens arrived to find workmen emptying the premises. Little remained inside, although what did included some human remains and dissecting instruments in the third floor dissection room.[41]

The constable followed the wagon, loaded with a portion of the school property, into Camden. There Philadelphia authorities found a larger cache of EMC property. All the materials were brought back to the EMC, but only after the Philadelphians fended off individuals claiming to be New Jersey authorities seeking to secure the property for creditors on their side of the Delaware River.[42] It seems likely that the people claiming to be authorities from New Jersey were actually employees of Buchanan; D. B. Brinton, editor of Philadelphia's *Medical and Surgical Reporter*, noted that during this period Buchanan relocated his operations to Haddonfield, New Jersey.[43] The removal of the EMC property may actually have been an attempt by Buchanan to secure his assets against seizure. In any case, by the summer of 1876, Buchanan and the EMC appear to have closed up shop. Soon thereafter, though, circumstances changed yet again.

In September 1876, cooler temperatures finally encouraged Philadelphians to brave the crowds and venture over to Fairmount Park, a 285-acre tract just west of the Schuylkill River that had become home to America's Centennial Exposition. In mid-September, while the exposition enjoyed booming business, John Buchanan resurfaced in Philadelphia. A sharp-eyed customs official had identified a shipment consigned to Buchanan that contained blank diplomas. Acting on this tip, the police placed the EMC property under watch and soon arrested Buchanan near the school premises under the 1871 state law prohibiting the sale of diplomas. Once again, Buchanan posted $1,000 bail to secure his release.[44] Buchanan now had two outstanding legal matters to resolve.

As it turned out, though, neither case ever came to trial. His earlier arrest on obscenity charges had a trial date set for February 16, 1877. When it finally arrived, the matter was delayed, not once but twice. The whole affair then quietly disappeared, with no further mention in the press.[45] As for the charge of selling diplomas, it did not even progress that far. This case, too, quietly disappeared, with no further publicity or apparent impact on Buchanan.

John Buchanan's string of legal challenges present an interesting question: how did he wriggle out of these cases? At this late date, a lack of information renders the question unanswerable. These cases may have been an indication that Buchanan had grown careless in conducting his and the school's affairs. Alternatively, Buchanan's arrests may testify to the determination of local authorities to make it untenable for Buchanan to continue his operations in Philadelphia. However the cases arose, the apparent failure to convict in each instance is even more interesting, making it seem likely that Buchanan still retained sufficient connections and influence among Philadelphia's politico-legal authorities to protect him from successful prosecution. There is some evidence for this.

In his later confession, Buchanan described the bribes he paid at various points in his career. In the death of Emily Vandergrift, he admitted to paying a bribe of $1,250 to dispose of that case; he also described paying $250 to a "prominent lawyer" to dispose of the 1876–77 cases. A sympathetic alderman or a bribed clerk, working discreetly at some nondescript city desk, may have helped him avert conviction in some of these judicial matters. The bail money paid in the diploma sales case of 1876 went to a Philadelphia alderman, and, as noted earlier, the aldermanic system seemed especially vulnerable to the granting of favors. The combination of a well-paid attorney and Buchanan's connections inside the aldermanic system of justice in Philadelphia probably played a key role in dispensing with these cases.[46]

CONTINUED DEFIANCE

Given the events overtaking Buchanan and the EMC in the 1870s, it seems surprising that both were in a reasonably good position as the decade drew to a close. Despite the near misses arising from legislative investigations and multiple arrests, John Buchanan emerged relatively unscathed in several critical ways. None of the mid-1870s legal matters culminated in a conviction or any jail time longer than that needed to secure the funds to post bail. The *Allen v. Buchanan* decision should have been nothing more than a temporary reprieve—a wake-up call spurring state and local authorities to definitive legal action and a brief window of opportunity for John Buchanan to reestablish EMC as a legitimate institution. Instead, neither the leadership in Philadelphia nor that in Harrisburg took the necessary judicial steps to terminate the EMC charter.

John Buchanan failed to recognize this period as one of the last opportunities for him and his school to change course. While he somehow escaped from the multiple legal entanglements that should have derailed his career permanently, his behavior shows them to have had some impact. By the end of the 1870s, Buchanan was acting carelessly, if not recklessly or desperately. The economic depression in the United States that followed the Panic of 1873 undoubtedly aggravated the situation for Buchanan and the EMC. His increasingly aggressive outbursts and indiscreet business operations may well have reflected a growing financial pressure.

The strongest evidence for this appeared in the July 1877 issue of the *Eclectic Medical Journal of Pennsylvania*, of which Buchanan was still editor. That issue carried questionable pronouncements, and exhibited odd editorial decisions. After listing nearly fifty EMC graduates, along with their thesis titles and precepting physician, Buchanan boasted that the school expected a "large class" of matriculants from Europe in the fall and planned an expansion of its hospital. In language that shifted oddly between present and future verb tenses, he described the hospital as a "chiefly private" enterprise and made the exaggerated claim that it could accommodate nearly one hundred patients. He also announced plans for a "permanent endowment" that would secure and retain "eminent" lecturing faculty. In a linguistic irony, he described the endowment as a "*scheme . . .* receiving the earnest attention of our graduates [italics added]."[47]

While advertisements for legitimate and quasi-medical products had long appeared in the the journal's back pages, they had not often been prominent in the editorial section. Now that section openly championed products like the "Electro-Voltaic belt" and the merits of ozone as a therapeutic agent. In fact, Buchanan offered to "furnish [the] apparatus" and "give instruction how to make and apply" ozone. This open huckstering continued as the journal touted both an "eclectic pharmacy" and a steam printing press, operating at the EMC's 514 Pine Street address.[48]

Most striking of all was the brash, defiant tone that Buchanan struck in his editorializing. In a short piece entitled "We Still Live," he offered a backhanded acknowledgement of the struggles afflicting himself and his school over the preceding decade, asserting "We still live! Surviv[ing] the assaults of external and internal foes; . . . like the firm oak which has withstood the tempest, stands more erect when the storm has passed. . . ." Then, in a tone of blustering resolve, he declared, "We are determined to maintain the reputation of the Eclectic Medical College . . . and we will do it."[49] The very next page, however, carried his most brazen pronouncement yet, one that undermined any pretense of respectability and further cemented the reputation of the EMC as a diploma mill. It appeared as an "important notice" to fellow physicians and prospective students, offering his services for private instruction leading to a degree.

> Possessing unusual facilities for educating students, we have made arrangements to receive into our private offices a limited number of students of both sexes, enabling them to become thoroughly acquainted with the Practice and Science of Medicine *in the shortest possible time.* . . . [I] make these arrangements, though at considerable personal inconvenience, because of the deplorable ignorance in which most medical students are found on leaving the Colleges . . . the country is full of physicians who know all about cell structure, &c., but who cannot diagnose a fever. . . . *Diplomas from a Chartered University will be granted as soon as the student is competent.* [italics added]

Buchanan further promised his private students access to school facilities and the opportunity to gain extensive clinical interactions. Students would move from his lectures and tutelage directly to the "bed-side," where they could apply what they had learned. Buchanan claimed that the extensive clinical opportunities he could provide would allow them to "treat more cases than many practitioners do in a year." Female students were promised "all the Obstetrical cases and Diseases of women they can attend to." Buchanan set the price for all of this ("Instruction, including diploma fee") at $300. Interested parties were directed to send all questions and "further particulars" to John Buchanan, M.D., 514 Pine Street, Philadelphia.[50]

Buchanan's offer was stunning in its explicitness. Coming from any quarter, the quid pro quo intimated by phrases like "in the shortest possible time" and "as soon as the student is competent" would be sufficiently eye-catching to raise questions, if not outright suspicion. Coming from a physician and an institution already linked to the illegal sale of diplomas, the offer seems a foolhardy act of self-incrimination. This same journal issue carried advertisements for a dental department of the American University and a "University College of Pharmacy." These paper institutions seem to signal that Buchanan and his EMC colleagues

were anxious to squeeze every drop of possible revenue from the charters in their possession.

The cast of characters now surrounding John Buchanan at the EMC
were likewise dubious—wholly different than the stalwart early founders of the school. Even longtime colleagues like Joseph Sites and Henry
Hollembaek had departed. Instead, Buchanan's faculty included family
members (e.g., his brother-in-law, Martin V. Chapman), political friends
(e.g., Philip Bissell), and an assortment of nondescript colleagues, most
of whom were EMC graduates. The evidence suggests that by the late
1870s, the EMC delivered little or no real instruction; the faculty members were cronies and opportunists rather than legitimate physicians.

By the close of the decade, the EMC was far removed from its earliest days, when the school carried the eclectic banner of reformed medicine in the East and its legitimacy was unquestioned. John Buchanan
appeared to understand that times were changing as consensus grew in
favor of medical registration laws, boards of medical examiners to issue
licenses, and the formation of a national association of American medical
schools. Although this awareness was admittedly unstated and perhaps
even unconscious, the pages of the *Eclectic Medical Journal of Pennsylvania*
reflected a growing sense that time was running out for the EMC and
its diploma sales.

" . . . when [he] undertakes to sell the right to
practice medicine to any Tom, Dick or Harry in
Philadelphia who can raise $100, it is coming too close
to home . . . to be any longer suffered to exist."

—*Philadelphia Record*, March 1, 1880

Six

The Return of Medical Licensing Laws

When John Buchanan joined the faculty of the EMC in 1860, there were
no legal constraints on the practice of medicine in the state of Pennsylvania. Indeed, with the exception of North Carolina, there were no legal
constraints on the practice of medicine anywhere in the United States.
From a socioeconomic perspective, America's medical marketplace remained "open" and highly competitive.[1] At that time, the notion that
an elected official or some designated officer of the state should be empowered to restrict a citizen's ability to engage in his or her chosen trade
struck many Americans, and perhaps most physicians, as an infringement
of fundamental rights and an unwarranted governmental intrusion. In any
case, such governmental action was not yet possible, since large portions
of the country, especially west of the Missouri River, lacked sufficiently
developed state or territorial governments to enforce such powers.

When John Buchanan's career at the EMC came to a halt only twenty
years later, however, the country's social and political environment had
changed so markedly that nineteen states and the District of Columbia
had already enacted legislation establishing a state's right to do precisely

that—to regulate the practice of medicine, ostensibly in the interests of public health and safety. An obvious question arises. What happened to change so profoundly the medical and sociopolitical climate of the United States in fewer than twenty years?

Any account of the rebirth of medical licensing laws in America during the mid- to late 1800s might reasonably discuss a range of factors contributing to this shift. Successful lobbying for such laws by physicians, both individually and collectively, tops that list of factors. Medical historians and sociologists agree on the key role played by physicians in lobbying for the adoption of legislation codifying medicine as a profession and setting legal constraints around its practice after the Civil War. Where historians differ in describing the emergence of these post–Civil War medical licensing laws tends to be in the nuances each chooses to emphasize in describing the role of physicians. Many point to the impact of physicians' professional aspirations—a desire for greater prestige and socioeconomic influence—as the driving force behind the advent of medical licensing laws. Others have shaded the story to show how competing philosophies of medicine (allopathic, homeopathic, and eclectic) waged internecine battle around medical licensure as if the outcome were a zero-sum game permitting only a single survivor. Still other historians have pursued a parallel path by tracing the burgeoning number of nineteenth-century medical schools and their graduates as an economic imperative to control entry into the medical marketplace through licensing. However, an assertion common to almost all these accounts is the suggestion that steady advances in nineteenth-century medical science provided a key impetus to licensure. This explanation carries an appealing measure of intuitive logic—specifically, that the standards for medical professionals, their education, and licensing, all rose in response to the insights gained from bacteriology and therapeutic advances. As one historian has recently pointed out, however, this narrative thread does not hold up well under scrutiny, since the establishment of medical licensing laws predated most of the medical advances associated with the late nineteenth century.[2]

The rise of medical licensing stemmed from more than simply the lobbying efforts of physicians and the growing pains associated with a nascent medical profession and educational system. Important factors outside medicine were also at work. A growing public awareness of, and perhaps impatience with, the effects of America's laissez-faire economic system on individual consumers began developing in the last quarter of the nineteenth century. According to one legal scholar, the tremendous volume of laws passed in the areas of public health and sanitation between 1850 and 1900 represented a failure of pure free-enterprise theory, which holds, after all, that quality goods or services should ultimately drive bad ones out of the market or force lower prices.[3]

Some people, including physicians, however, were not willing to wait for the hidden hand of the marketplace to sweep away medicine's detritus. The dangers of tainted food and water (which now could be sterilized, processed, or treated to avoid most contaminants) and the later validation and understanding of germ theory provided an almost moral impetus for the enactment or refinement of laws designed to protect the public health. It might be argued that a *belief* in beneficent scientific and medical advancements meant that the public and legislators were not content to wait for good doctors to drive out the bad ones in the competitive marketplace.

Another factor relevant to this discussion is the general reassessment taking place as to the purpose of such government regulation through licensing laws. In the 1830s, most people condemned physician licensing as an attempt to protect power and privilege. After the Civil War, however, many people had come to view the concept of licensing as a mechanism to protect the general public as well as the interests of independent educated professionals, who seemed vulnerable in the emerging age of industrial titans and financiers. The post–Civil War years witnessed the birth of large corporations that seemed to threaten the idealized vision of America as a nation driven by the economic engines of the yeoman farmer, the artisan, and the small businessman. The steady demographic shift toward urbanization meant that a growing number of Americans now had less firsthand knowledge than they once had of the skills of the physician, attorney, or other professional they might occasionally need to consult. The sheer size of growing metropolitan areas like New York City, Philadelphia, St. Louis, and Chicago created a vastly different environment for interpersonal and business relationships compared to those in less populous rural settings.[4]

At the same time, there emerged a sense of intrinsic value delivered to society through the labors of qualified professionals, be they physicians, lawyers, engineers, or architects. Admittedly, some of the impetus for this change of view derived from the assertions of value made by professionals themselves through their associations and societies—for example, the American Medical Association (1847), American Bar Association (1878), American Institute of Architects (1857), and American Society of Civil Engineers (1852). Some scholars have argued that this post–Civil War "professionalizing trend" bestowed authority and confidence on individuals at a time when deference to authority seemed otherwise weakened in the early Darwinian era.[5] For many urban Americans they could simply look at their surrounding city environment to gain some appreciation for the value of expertise. The professions of architecture and engineering provide clear examples. With multistory buildings rising ever higher and more and more steel bridges spanning American waterways, the work of such professionals was visible and tangible to all. Moreover, the compressed space and crowding of cities meant that poor design and its resulting structural failures posed risks to all, creating a powerful impetus to ensure quality construction by legislating the training and conduct of these professionals. Creating a regulatory framework ensured adequately trained and knowledgeable architects and engineers capable of carrying through large-scale construction projects that served a readily apparent public good.

While the work outcomes of physicians might lack the visibility of bridges or buildings, they involved the same balance of risk to benefit. Effective medical treatments and sanitation supported a community's overall public health and well-being, while ineffective or unsafe treatments and neglect of public health issues by ignorant and unqualified practitioners threatened them. This was especially true during the periodic outbreaks of epidemic diseases (notably yellow fever, typhoid, and cholera) that plagued America's increasingly crowded urban centers and port cities. Such outbreaks had already compelled local and state authorities to protect public health by imposing quarantines and moving to pass other sanitary and public health measures. Half a dozen states established boards of health in the immediate postwar years, and all but a handful had followed suit by 1900.[6] The establishment of individual state boards of health and of a short-lived National Board of Health further normalized the concept of local or state intervention in matters of health.[7]

These public health efforts aligned with the reintroduction of occupational licensing in the United States, including medical licensing after the Civil War. Authority for this governmental role derives from the Tenth Amendment: "The powers not delegated to the United States by the Constitution, nor prohibited by it to the States, are reserved to the States respectively, or to the people." This amendment remains the bedrock of federalism. The Constitution enumerated a wide range of powers explicitly to the federal government, but those not specifically ascribed to the federal government or falling within its implied powers rest with the states and/or the people by virtue of the Tenth Amendment.

One of the key concepts to derive from this is that of the police powers of the individual states. The United States Supreme Court later identified these as the authority of each state to impose "reasonable regulations" to protect the broad interests of the citizenry, including their "public health and safety."[8] Occupational licensing, including that for medicine, falls under the heading of the police powers of the individual states, as recognized under the Tenth Amendment.

Occupational licensing gained steady momentum after the Civil War. The basic idea, of course, was hardly new. During the pre-Revolutionary War era, colonies had licensed tradesmen such as auctioneers and peddlers, ostensibly with some notion that this served a public benefit, even if simply by limiting a potential public nuisance. While the same justification (i.e., protecting the public) can be applied to almost all occupations, its obvious pertinence to the medical profession was advocated vigorously by members of that profession themselves.[9] Consequently, many colonies, and later states, imposed actual or de facto licensing of physicians until the Jacksonian era rejection of licensing in the 1830s. The growth of alternative schools of thought in medicine and the widespread view that licensing laws were by their very nature anti-democratic led to the wholesale dismantling of these laws nationally.

REGISTRATION LAWS AND LICENSING BOARDS

North Carolina was the first state to emerge from this interlude in American medical regulation. The shift occurred in incremental steps, beginning when the state's long-dormant medical society reconstituted itself in 1849. Ten years later, legislation created the North Carolina Medical Board. Several features of the North Carolina law presaged what was to come in other states. This law did not make graduation from medical school a blanket requirement for a medical license there. North Carolina had too many practitioners with no formal education or training for such a requirement to be practical. The law also exempted some prospective licensees from the board's examination requirement, most notably through a pragmatic "grandfather" clause exempting doctors already actively practicing medicine in North Carolina. However, the law did empower the board to examine physicians entering the state without a medical degree. Once the board issued a license, state law required the insertion of a public notice giving the names of licensees in at least two newspapers within thirty days of license issuance.[10]

North Carolina's grandfather clause represented a concession to the realities of the mid-nineteenth-century medical landscape. While some physicians would have preferred laws that precluded a fair number of their colleagues by imposing minimum credentials for licensure, many understood (or soon learned) that legislative realities made it impossible to secure support for overly exclusionary laws—particularly those clearly targeting colleagues along sectarian lines. There were simply too many physicians lacking formal credentials whose situations deserved genuine consideration. A wholesale rejection of physicians with many years' practical experience represented a politically infeasible approach.

These practicing physicians cannot be dismissed collectively as charlatans or quacks. They were caught up in a transition from a long-established system featuring informal or "on acceptance" criteria for those practicing medicine to a new system requiring formal qualifications (e.g., a medical degree) and licensure under the auspices of a state medical board. The advent of this new system posed a legitimate challenge to these individuals' vocation and livelihood.

Several generations of physicians in post–Civil War America had been practicing medicine for years, with varying degrees of success in the eyes of their patients and communities. They often possessed no formal medical degree. Their education may have been a full or partial course of lectures from what modestly passed as a medical college. Often it may have involved self-study and working for a period of time with a practicing physician—a kind of a mentor/teacher relationship that may even have been sufficiently formalized as to call it a preceptorship.

While the physicians who later purchased one of John Buchanan's medical degrees undoubtedly included a proportion of outright frauds and charlatans, many of them were in fact legitimate practitioners trying to adapt to changing socio-legal expectations for the profession. This latter group comprised individuals with a genuine interest in medicine, who had been practicing for years without formal credentials. They saw the acquisition of a diploma as a formality, now required to bring them into conformity with the emerging era of state regulation of medicine.

In one aspect, North Carolina's legislation proved atypical compared to that introduced in other states in the 1860s and 1870s—North Carolina established a medical licensing board empowered to examine and issue licenses. More common were simple registration laws, requiring only that a physician register with a state or local office, usually that of the local county clerk. In some states, the physician had to produce a medical school diploma in order to qualify and get his name added to the register. In other states, no such requirement existed; individuals entered the registry simply by presenting themselves before the county clerk and self-identifying as a physician.[11] In the 1870s, multiple states and territories enacted comparable medical registration laws. In places like Arizona, the Dakotas, Texas, Kansas, Montana, and Wyoming, these laws had little or no immediate impact. They probably served more as statutory window dressing heralding a hoped-for future state of settlement.

In more settled regions of the country, however, this was not the case. In large states settled much earlier, like Illinois, New York, Ohio, and Pennsylvania, the enactment of medical registration laws prompted considerable discussion and debate. In the federal census of 1870, more than 62,000 individuals identified themselves as physicians. The physicians in the four states just mentioned accounted for one-third of this national total of physicians.[12] These individuals exhibited a wide range of education and training. On one end of the spectrum stood a relatively small number of physicians with formal medical education and a degree from an established medical school affiliated with a university. Some of these doctors even had educational and clinical experience acquired in European centers for medicine, like Paris. At the other end of the spectrum stood a much larger number of physicians who were largely self-taught or who had learned through apprentice or preceptor-style experiences in cobbling together a modest body of what might pass reasonably for medical knowledge.

Physicians practicing in states settled earlier, like Pennsylvania and New York, sensed that registration laws were a modest first step in what

Table 5: Jurisdictions Enacting Medical Licensing Laws after the Civil War

Jurisdiction	Registration Law Enacted	Examining Board Established	Eclectic (E) and (H) Homeopathic Boards Established
North Carolina	1859	1859	
Ohio	1868	1896	
South Dakota	1869	1893	
North Dakota	1869	1890	
Arizona	1873	1881	
Texas	1873	1876	1901–1907
District of Columbia	1874	1896	1896–1929
Kentucky	1874	1874	
New York	1874	1890	1890–1907
Nevada	1875	1899	
New Hampshire	1875	1897	
Wyoming	1875	1899	
California	1876	1876	1878–1901
Montana	1876	1889	
Vermont	1876	1898	
Alabama, Illinois	1877	1877	
Missouri	1877	1883	
Pennsylvania	1877	1893	
Kansas	1879	1879	1879–?
New Jersey	1880	1890	
Arkansas*, Colorado, Florida**	1881	1881	1903–1955* 1899–1921**
South Carolina	1881	1888	1904–1908 (H)
Washington	1881	1890	
Nebraska	1881	1891	
Connecticut	1881	1893	1893–1935 (E) 1893–1979 (H)
Georgia	1881	1894	1894–1913
Wisconsin	1881	1897	
Mississippi, New Mexico, West Virginia	1882	1882	
Louisiana	1882	1894	1894–1979 (H)
Rhode Island	1882	1895	
Minnesota	1883	1883	
Delaware	1883	1895	
Michigan	1883	1899	
Virginia	1884	1884	
Indiana	1885	1897	
Iowa	1886	1886	

Table 5 (cont.)

Jurisdiction	Registration Law Enacted	Examining Board Established	Eclectic (E) and (H) Homeopathic Boards Established
Idaho	1887	1899	
Maryland	1888	1888	1892–1957 (H)
Oregon, Tennessee	1889	1889	
Oklahoma	1890	1903	
Utah	1892	1892	
Massachusetts	1894	1894	
Maine	1895	1895	
Alaska	1913	1913	

Sources: *Polk's Medical and Surgical Register of the United States* (Detroit: R.L. Polk), editions for 1890, 1896, 1913–14, 1914–15; *Revised Statutes of Arizona Territory* (Columbia, Missouri: E. W. Stephens, 1901); *First Annual Report of State Board of Health of Illinois, 1878* (Springfield: Weber, Magie & Co., State Printer, 1879); *Compiled Laws of Kansas, 1879* (St. Louis: W. J. Gilbert, 1879); *General Statutes of Kentucky* (Frankfort: Major, Johnson & Barrett, 1879); *Changes in General Statutes of 1878, State of Minnesota* (St. Paul: West Publishing Co., 1883); *Laws, Memorials and Resolutions Territory of Montana* (Helena: Robert E. Fisk, 1876); *Revised Statutes State of Missouri, 1879* (Jefferson: Carter & Regan, 1879); *Revised Statutes State of Missouri, 1919* (Jefferson: Hugh Stephens Co., 1920); *Statutes of State of Nevada, 1899* (Carson City: State Printing Office, 1899); *Public Statutes State of New Hampshire* (Concord: Edson Eastman, 1900); *Documents of 123rd Legislature State of New Jersey* (Trenton: John L. Murphy, 1899); *Statutes at Large State of New York, 1871–74, Vol. IX* (Albany: Weed, Parson & Co., 1875); *General Statutes State of New York, 1890* (Albany: Weed, Parsons & Co., 1890); *First Annual Report State Board of Medical Registration and Examination of Ohio* (1897); *Statutes of State of Ohio, Vol. II 1866–68* (Cincinnati: Robert Clarke & Co., 1876); *Digest of the Laws of Pennsylvania, Vol. II* (Philadelphia: T and J. W. Johnson & Co., 1896); *Digest of the Statute Law of State of Pennsylvania* (Philadelphia: George Bisel Co., 1912); *Revised Civil Statutes State of Texas Sixteenth Legislature* (Austin: State Printing Office, 1887); *Acts and Resolves Passed by General Assembly State of Vermont* (Burlington: Free Press Association, 1898); *Revised Statutes of Wyoming* (Laramie: Chaplin, Spafford, Mathison, 1899); Ronald Hamowy, "The Early Development of Medical Licensing Laws in the United States, 1875–1900," *Journal of Libertarian Studies* 3, No. 1 (1979).

would likely be a series of measures creating a system for medical licensure. Even if a given state did not initially require the registering physician to present a medical degree, the addition of such a requirement represented an obvious next step toward more rigorous regulation. But by itself, that small first step seemed likely to accomplish very little. The tremendous variance among the approximately 110 medical schools operating in the United States in 1870 meant that medical degrees failed to confer anything close to a common level of educational and clinical experience.[13] It was clear to many people that even registration laws requiring a medical degree did little more than create a roster naming those who had self-identified as practicing medicine in the state and giving the location where they were doing so. As these laws generally did not distinguish among diplomas, those issued by lesser institutions were just as effective in putting physicians in compliance with the law as were those from more legitimate and rigorous schools.

Registration laws may have achieved some success in driving itinerant physicians from these states, but at what price? These laws posed no serious hurdle to individuals holding diplomas from schools such as the EMC, and, in fact, they introduced a negative consideration. In states like Pennsylvania that initially limited their medical legislation to a registration law, practical experience demonstrated what critics of such legislation had predicted: in treating every diploma the same and making no attempt to delineate the minimum educational basis that the diploma should represent, these laws added an economic value to the diploma that it had not previously possessed.

An editorial in the *Philadelphia Medical Times* criticized Pennsylvania's registration law along these lines, complaining that it had "degraded" the profession by placing "irregulars and charlatans" on the same plane as mainstream practitioners.[14] Such dissatisfaction was echoed elsewhere. A contemporary Michigan physician claimed, for example, that his state's registration law drove those practitioners who lacked a written credential to obtain one by whatever means necessary, including "buy[ing] diplomas."[15] In practice, therefore, poorly crafted registration laws actually benefited schools like Buchanan's, which held legally issued state charters.

Over time, the inherent flaws in registration laws helped to spur further legislation, intended to create legally constituted bodies of medical examiners at the state level, empowered to assess and pass judgment on the qualifications of all individuals presenting themselves as physicians entitled to legally practice medicine—to establish, in essence, state boards of medical examiners to determine a physician's qualifications and fitness before issuing a medical license to practice. The fortunes for medical licensing in America had turned and turned again in rapid fashion. After being dismantled in the 1830s as anti-democratic and of little value in an era of limited therapeutic benefits coming from any physician, medical licensing laws revived little more than a generation later, reappearing with greater vigor as proponents argued that such laws protected the interests of the very public who had earlier dismissed them.

It should be emphasized that not everyone accepted public protection as the real motive behind these laws. Many argued that the laws were really designed to protect the emerging professional standing of the physicians themselves. In fact, the scorn poured by physicians who saw themselves as skilled professionals on peers whom they labeled frauds and "quacks" led one later writer to define *quacks* as "practitioners who continue to please their customers but not their colleagues."[16] This witticism hints at the skepticism felt by many during the last quarter of the nineteenth century as medical licensing laws took hold in state after state.

Dr. John Rauch and the Illinois State Board of Health

Not surprisingly, the reestablishment of medical licensure unfolded differently from state to state. In some states (as in North Carolina), medical legislation was enacted piecemeal. In others, such as California and Illinois, a single stroke of the pen enacted sweeping legislation establishing an entire system of medical licensure, including a board of medical examiners. California's 1876 Medical Practice Act might have served as a template for laws in other states,[17] but did not; California's geographical isolation from much of the rest of the country and the lack of a galvanizing figure on its new board prevented the state's experiment in medical regulation from gaining greater national attention. It fell to Illinois instead to lead the way, influencing legislation across the country and incidentally having a profound effect on the fortunes of John Buchanan and the EMC.

The driving force behind Illinois's medical licensing system was John Rauch, a former Civil War surgeon and passionate crusader for sanitation and public health. Like a growing number of physicians, Rauch understood that simple registration laws were inadequate to guard patients from those practitioners whom he and many others deemed insufficiently trained at best and medical frauds and charlatans at worst. He supported taking the important next step: replacing simple registration laws with broader legislation establishing a state medical board possessing the power not only to require each physician to produce a medical diploma but also empowering the regulatory board to evaluate the quality and underlying educational basis for that diploma. The American Medical Association embraced this position in 1875, though the organization enjoyed far less influence in the nineteenth century than in the early decades of the twentieth century.[18] Despite the AMA support, this next step in medical regu-

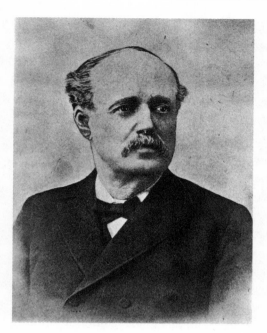

Fig. 8. John Rauch, M.D. Rauch and the Illinois State Board of Health championed licensing laws and vigorous medical regulation. The board placed the EMC on its list of disapproved medical schools. Image courtesy of U.S. National Library of Medicine, Digital Collections.

lation developed slowly. By the summer of 1880, when John Buchanan and the EMC reached their dramatic crossroads, only seven states and territories required doctors to produce any demonstrable proof of fitness to practice, such as passing a licensing examination, beyond merely presenting a medical diploma.[19]

In the meantime, however, John Rauch emerged as the most significant public proponent of medical licensure, influencing states first to establish systems for the evaluation of credentials and later to require higher educational standards among medical schools. With Rauch's support, Illinois established its state board of health in 1877, and both the board and the law underpinning it became models for those adopted in other states. The impetus for the Illinois law had several sources. Public health matters posed an increasing challenge to state and local authorities in Illinois during the early 1870s. Major problems included the profound contamination to the Chicago River, the virulence of endemic and epidemic diseases such as yellow fever, and the generally poor sanitation existing in the state's major cities. Illinois's response to these local and regional realities reflected an emerging national trend as many states were adopting health boards to address public health and sanitation issues.[20]

Rauch, a graduate of the University of Pennsylvania medical school, emerged as the region's greatest advocate of public health, first on Chicago's board of health and later as president of the American Public Health Association.[21] His desire for a state board of health meshed with the political goals of the Illinois Medical Society, which was pushing legislators not only to create such a body to address health and sanitation issues but also to limit the practice of medicine to "well-educated men," irrespective of their particular philosophy of medicine. This latter aspiration was particularly striking in the mid-1870s, when so many physicians aligned themselves with specific philosophies or schools of medicine, shunning interaction with, much less recognition of, practitioners from other schools of medical thought. In leading the Illinois State Board of Health, first as its president and then its executive secretary, Rauch demonstrated a personal aversion to sectarian issues and a commitment to fairness. Determined to circumvent internecine squabbles and require higher standards for all medical practitioners, he worked to include homeopathic and eclectic physicians on the Illinois board along with orthodox physicians.[22]

Within its first year, the board confronted and resolved a potentially damaging situation stemming from inquiries it had made regarding the educational experience of graduates from Hahnemann Medical College in Philadelphia and the Eclectic Medical Institute (EMI) of Cincinnati who were seeking to practice in Illinois. Critics of the board latched onto these inquiries as evidence of bias against eclectic- and homeopathic-trained practitioners. In both cases, however, Rauch and the board demonstrated a willingness to consider new evidence and, despite some initial reservations, chose to license graduates of both schools.[23]

Rauch visited the EMI in 1877, probably at the request of the school. Faculty member John Scudder described Rauch as diligent in his fact-finding and in "earnest" about executing the board's authority to the "full intent and meaning" of Illinois law. The two men found common ground in their shared belief that a medical degree should not shield the "disreputable or unprofessional" individuals within the profession. Within the pages of the school's periodical, the *Eclectic Medical Journal*, Scudder praised Rauch's efforts to remove "traveling humbugs" and "charlatan[s]" from Illinois's list of prospective licensees. Satisfied by what he saw during his on-site inspection of the EMI, Rauch eased school officials' fears before leaving Cincinnati. He told Scudder he would report to the board that the EMI diploma should be deemed satisfactory in the hands of any "legitimate holder" of the degree.[24] The judicious handling of these schools by Rauch and the Illinois board paid dividends later, when other states began taking closer notice of Illinois's list of recognized medical schools.

Illinois's 1877 Act to Regulate the Practice of Medicine contained two critical features. The first was statutory language creating a state agency empowered to issue a license based on either submission of a diploma or successfully passing an examination administered by the board. The second key feature stemmed from the law's provision for licensure by examination, which allowed the board to verify the "genuineness" of a diploma. The critical phrase in the act spoke of the board verifying diplomas from "legally chartered medical institutions *in good standing* [italics added]."[25] Supported by the state's attorney general, John Rauch and the Illinois board drew a broad interpretation of this clause, giving the board considerable latitude in determining which schools' diplomas it would recognize.

With this legal coverage behind it, the board exercised wide-ranging authority that culminated in a list of recognized medical schools whose graduates were eligible for a license in Illinois.[26] This meant the board was not satisfied merely to uncover individuals seeking to obtain a license under fraudulent conditions—by presenting a forged or stolen diploma, for example. The board would go further, seeking to identify individuals presenting legitimate diplomas from legally chartered schools but with no reasonable underlying educational basis for the issuance of the diploma. In essence, the board was targeting diploma mills.

Rauch pointed with pride to the large number of Illinois's physicians who left the state or "quit practice" within the first year of the board's activities—a number he estimated at 38 percent of the total. The board took specific aim at "spurious" diplomas and identified nine schools whose diplomas they refused to recognize. Rauch believed that several more schools were suspect but the board lacked firm evidence of dubious practice, or those too would have seen their graduates denied licensure. In its first year, the board denied an estimated four hundred individuals medical licenses, deeming their diplomas to have been either purchased or obtained upon "nominal" examination.[27]

Rauch and the board also made clear that their work would go beyond denying licenses to the graduates of such schools; they also intended to curb dubious institutional practices by "regulating" medical schools. The first step came on July 1, 1878, when the board adopted resolutions mandating a specified length of education as a requirement for licensure. In this case, they defined "actual attendance" as including "two full courses of lectures" of sixteen weeks each and separated by at least six months between each course.[28] This was the opening salvo in a protracted battle by first the Illinois State Board of Health and later state medical boards collectively to establish ever-higher standards for medical education as a condition for medical licensure.

It would be difficult to overstate the efforts and activities of John Rauch and the Illinois board. At the time of Rauch's efforts in the late 1870s, state medical boards were emerging as the sole legal entities with the authority to set and administer standards for medical licensure, including minimally acceptable standards for medical education. This was an important consideration, since Rauch's efforts predated the later establishment of voluntary efforts to reform medical education, such as the reestablishment of the Association of American Medical Colleges in 1890 and early efforts at national accreditation of medical schools through the work of the AMA Council on Medical Education in 1904.

Historians such as Kenneth Ludmerer have pointed out the impressive work of progressive medical schools like Harvard, Michigan, and Johns Hopkins in the last quarter of the nineteenth century, specifically, their role in promulgating a model for medical education built around university and hospital affiliations. Irrespective of state medical board initiatives, many medical schools like these voluntarily committed themselves to pursuing a model of academic medicine, building on the rapid expansion of medical knowledge, especially in bacteriology.[29]

John Rauch and the Illinois board were not concerned with these schools and their graduates. Their efforts focused on the schools not affiliated with a university, proprietary endeavors like the EMC, with business models that depended primarily, if not solely, on students' tuition and fees for their funding. Rauch viewed these schools with suspicion, seeing them as particularly vulnerable to exploitive practices, such as the sale of diplomas already occurring at the EMC. Over the decades that followed, the medical licensing boards of other states, like Illinois's, provided the necessary leverage to force substandard proprietary schools to either raise standards or close their doors. By 1932, only a few schools categorized as Class C or "nondescript" schools were still operating. Included in this group was a handful of virtual diploma mills, whose graduates were all but unlicensable in the vast majority of states. In this manner, medical licensing boards became the regulatory hammer pulling the few remaining rusty nails from the wooden foundation of medical education.[30]

By the time the Illinois State Board of Health issued its annual report for 1880, John Rauch was prepared to publish the detailed results of its extensive investigations into the quality and conditions of American medical schools. The report emerged from the board's extensive information-gathering on medical schools throughout the country. In conducting this research, the board had queried schools on a range of issues, including their standards for preliminary education or entrance requirements, the specific branches of medicine being taught, the length and interval of lectures, examinations, student access to clinical and dissection opportunities, and their practices regarding advance standing for students with prior experience with preceptors. Rauch admitted to applying greater "scrutiny" to more recently established schools but the Illinois board showed remarkable objectivity in its licensure of graduates considering the tenor of the times and the often vitriolic sectarian exchanges occurring within the profession.[31]

The 1880 report included a directory of medical schools meeting the Illinois board's requirements for recognition of their diplomas, which included detailed information about each school. The report also listed eighteen schools whose graduates would not be licensed by the state of Illinois. While the board included six irregular schools (i.e., those with nontraditional approaches such as homeopathy and eclecticism) in this group, it listed twenty irregular schools in its directory of approved schools, with nine more awaiting a final decision by the board.[32] Fear among eclectic physicians that sectarian considerations would dictate the board's decisions proved unfounded.[33] This objectivity by the Illinois board did not benefit John Buchanan, however. Among the Philadelphia schools it identified as inadequate were Buchanan's EMC and American University, as well as William Paine's Philadelphia University.

In one way, individuals like John Buchanan, rather than being the sole or even primary targets of legal and regulatory authorities like the Illinois board, were simply the most *convenient* targets. They served as the means to a greater end, a mechanism for bringing to heel the larger group of practitioners whose education and training (however sparse or informal it may have been) had once sufficed at the dawn of medical regulation in America. John Rauch revealed as much in his board's first annual report when he reveled in the estimated one-third of practitioners who left Illinois within the first year of the board's activities.[34] In essence, those, like Rauch, determined to raise the standard of medical practice took aim at diploma mills like Buchanan's as a way of indirectly striking at the practitioners *buying* these diplomas. In his board's third annual report, Rauch, with "great pleasure," reported Buchanan's recent arrest, noting with satisfaction that since its inception, the board had routinely denied licenses to graduates of Buchanan's institutions.[35]

Without question, when the state of Pennsylvania joined forces with the *Philadelphia Record* in 1880 to shut down John Buchanan and the EMC, they were acting from the belief that they were removing a public menace. By exposing Buchanan and his diploma mill, they were alerting the public to the danger posed by unscrupulous doctors using purchased degrees to practice without legitimate medical education or training in order to profit from the desperation of patients seeking relief wherever they could find it. Few people then or now sympathize with the medical charlatan. For John Buchanan, however, his arrest in June 1880 was the culmination of a series of disastrous events that had begun, unbeknownst to him, with a clandestine meeting several months earlier in January.

Part Three

Fall

"The diploma selling business has
reached such proportions that the
public is getting aroused."
—*Cincinnati Medical Gazette*,
October 1880

Seven

John Norris and the *Philadelphia Record*

The date and place of the meeting that sealed the fate of John Buchanan and the EMC went unrecorded. Even the identity of all the individuals present that day is uncertain. The allusions to this meeting that were published afterward provide some insight into what transpired, however, and allow for reasonable speculation on much that must have occurred. We know the identities of two of the participants: John Norris, the city editor for the *Philadelphia Record*, and Henry W. Palmer, Pennsylvania's attorney general. Moreover, based upon the agreement reached during this meeting and the events that transpired later, two other likely participants can be named: William M. Singerly, owner and publisher of the *Record*, and J. Howard Gendell, a prominent Philadelphia lawyer.[1]

The subsequent vigor with which John Norris pursued the case against John Buchanan suggests that he and Singerly requested the meeting with the attorney general. The *Record*'s owner and his city editor knew of the resolution passed in December 1879 by the state legislature calling on Palmer to break up the diploma trade centered in Philadelphia. They also knew that, despite repeated previous calls for action along these lines, few signs of activity or vigorous prosecution of the matter had followed. Singerly and Norris brought a surprising offer to the meeting that day. Singerly expressed his willingness not only to commit the financial resources of the *Philadelphia Record* to exposing the work of John Buchanan but also to strongly pursue sufficient evidence to allow for a successful prosecution of Buchanan and others engaged in the sale of diplomas. Under the plan they proposed, the *Philadelphia Record* would "advance" the funds necessary to pursue the case and "trust" that the state legislature would later reimburse the newspaper. In essence, the *Record* agreed to underwrite the costs of the investigation in a demonstration of "public spirit" for the greater good of the city and the state.[2]

Palmer had no reason to refuse the offer, so Norris and Gendell laid out their plan. As they had studied the matter, there were two issues to be addressed: First, what legal basis could be used to challenge the schools in question? And second, how could they acquire the necessary evidence to secure individual convictions as well as the annulment of the charters of the diploma mills? Based on the stories they had heard and information gleaned from reliable sources, they had no doubt that the activities of John Buchanan at the EMC and Thomas Miller, now head of the faculty at Philadelphia University, violated the Pennsylvania state law that banned the conferral of degrees based upon payment or promise of payment. Since the crime was only a misdemeanor, however, state prosecution on this basis would have minimal effect. The penalties involved (a $500 fine and six months in jail) seemed inadequate when compared with the damage inflicted by the diploma trade on the city's reputation and the injuries likely suffered by patients at the hands of graduates from these schools. The discussions that day must have drifted into the actual operations of the EMC. How were Buchanan and the EMC conducting the trade? How were the sales of diplomas being carried out?

The information they had gathered so far indicated that Buchanan conducted much of his business by mail, rather than through personal transactions on-site at the EMC. With this understanding in mind, the group planned their preferred course of legal action. Their primary goal would be to prosecute the schools and their leaders for mail fraud under a federal law (Title 18 U.S.C., Section 1341) passed by the U.S. Congress in 1872, with the state misdemeanor charge serving as an added bonus. The federal law in question made it a crime "to scheme or artifice

Fig. 9. Henry W. Palmer. As Pennsylvania's attorney general, Palmer expressed the state's gratitude to John Norris and William Singerly for their critical role in bringing Buchanan to justice. Image LC-DIG-hec-16236 courtesy of the Library of Congress, Print and Photographs Division, Washington, D.C.

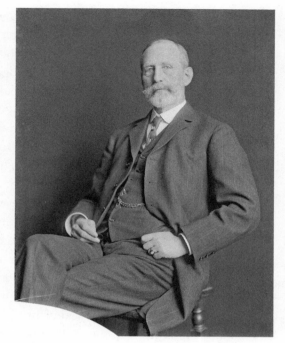

to defraud . . . by means of the post office."[3] Norris and the others felt that a potential conviction on this charge carried sufficient teeth to either scare Buchanan and his cohorts into abandoning the diploma trade permanently or, as they would have preferred, send them to prison for eighteen months.

At some point, those at the meeting turned to the practical matter of acquiring the evidence necessary to secure an indictment and conviction. The four men determined that John Norris would take on the role of a diploma seeker attempting to secure a medical degree through correspondence with Buchanan. In fact, Norris would assume multiple guises, writing to the school as different individuals, each seeking a degree. The group would arrange for Norris's letters to be crafted and sent from various locales across the country. This was an important tactical detail. It would not only preserve Norris's identity but prevent complications, since if the various inquiries were mailed locally, bearing a Philadelphia area postmark, Buchanan might eventually request personal meetings with his "correspondents." The strategy also ensured that the transactions were conducted solely through the U.S. mail—the key to pursuing multiple counts of mail fraud. Norris collaborated with Gendell in crafting each letter in the chain of correspondence that later ensued.

At trial it would be critical that the correspondence showed a genuine and explicit quid pro quo of payment for a diploma. Ideally, the correspondence should also show that John Buchanan neither expected the diploma seeker to demonstrate medical knowledge as a condition of sale nor cared whether or not he had such knowledge. Finally, Norris and Gendell tried to craft the letters so as to prevent all avenues for Buchanan to evade, rationalize, or explain away the transaction to a judge or jury; after all, he had done this in the 1872 state senate inquiry by claiming that the degrees granted by the EMC were honorary ones to established physicians. This approach would help insure a clear demonstration of Buchanan's intent to "defraud" both the public and medical licensing boards concerning the true medical expertise of those granted one of his diplomas.

In building their case, Norris, Singerly, Palmer, and Gendell chose John Buchanan and his schools, the EMC and the American University, as their primary targets. However, they also identified Philadelphia University as an additional target. A group of Methodist ministers now controlled William Paine's former school, one of whom, Thomas Miller, seemed to be stepping up the questionable issuance of diplomas. Since Miller was showing a startling lack of discretion in conducting this trade, the group determined that an on-site sting operation against Miller might be an effective strategy, with the twenty-three-year-old John Norris posing as an erstwhile medical student hoping to reduce or eliminate the time needed to acquire a medical degree. The group decided to begin this operation immediately to secure evidence against Miller and Philadelphia University, while Norris also began the slower process of crafting letters and corresponding with Buchanan to secure the documentary evidence needed for mail fraud charges.

A WARNING SHOT

On February 27, 1880, John Norris and a colleague at the *Record*, Lucius Maynard, spent the portion of a day meeting with the Rev. Thomas Miller, dean of Philadelphia University, which was located at 209 North Tenth Street. The two men portrayed themselves as prospective medical students, short on funds but long on ambition and anxious to turn a modi-cum of instruction into a medical degree and a paying patient clientele. Norris's subsequent written account of this meeting with Miller sounded a seriocomic tone. In a series of vignettes reporting their encounter, Nor-ris juxtaposed a word picture of the earnest but obtuse Miller, narrating from a chalkboard as part of an impromptu lesson on prescription writing, with descriptions of conditions in the building, almost laughable in their lack of any real capacity to provide instruction. Norris created a devas-tating portrait, reproducing Miller's recitation of how to mix a solution for teething children as he chattered on in a shabby room surrounded by life-sized demonstration aids, including a human skeleton and a human figure crudely made of cloth stuffed with sawdust. Norris also described in disparaging terms the floor-to-ceiling glass cases lining three walls, which contained what would be generously characterized as a "slim" anatomical collection.[4] By providing an almost verbatim transcription of portions of his encounter with Miller, Norris offered a damning portrait not only of the man and his university but of an array of broader issues: diploma sales, the uneven standards for medical education, and the lack of any meaning-ful oversight for these schools.

Norris proved an ideal choice for this role. Though he was young enough to pass for an aspiring medical student, he was actually a veteran Philadelphia newspaperman. The son of a Pennsylvania Civil War veteran killed at the Battle of Gettysburg, Norris graduated from Girard Col-lege in 1871 at the age of fifteen. After beginning to train as an engineer, he abandoned that field to redirect his energies toward Philadelphia's newspaper business—possibly at the suggestion, or with the assistance, of his cousin Samuel Hudson, another Philadelphia newspaperman. Af-ter three years with the *Philadelphia Press* followed by a successful run at the *Philadelphia Times*, Norris joined the *Philadelphia Record* in 1877.[5]

The timing proved auspicious, as the *Record* was enjoying impressive growth and an expansion of its circulation under its new owner, William M. Singerly. The newspaper had first appeared in 1870 as the *Philadel-phia Public Record*, later dropping *Public* from its title. Its first publisher, William Swain, had been determined to challenge the dominant role of the *Philadelphia Public Ledger*, but after a noteworthy launch and a failed marketing ploy in 1873, the *Record* settled back into a more modest pres-ence and circulation within the city.[6]

Singerly's purchase of the *Record* in 1877 changed not only the paper's fortunes but the landscape of newspaper publishing in Philadelphia and across the country. At that time, the *Record* carried a circulation of about 6,000 copies daily—a limited but respectable presence in what was an extremely competitive market. Roughly a dozen newspapers were in circulation in Philadelphia during this period. The *Record* was a morning daily, competing with several strong challengers for the morning circulation market, notably the *Philadelphia Inquirer*, the *Public Ledger*, and the *North American*. Several other papers put out evening editions, including the *Philadelphia Herald*, the *Philadelphia Telegraph*, and the *Philadelphia Evening Bulletin*. From modest offices at Third and Chestnut, Singerly redesigned the *Record* as a penny paper by leveraging his wood and paper pulp factories to hold down costs. By the 1880s, the *Record*'s daily circulation topped 100,000, and by the 1890s was approaching 170,000.[7] This rapid rise in circulation testified to Singerly's business acumen, especially since the paper leaned heavily Democratic in a city that had gone decisively Republican in the years after the Civil War. Even the *New York Times* lauded the *Record* as "one of the best" newspapers in the country.[8]

The *Record*'s massive growth meant that opportunities abounded at the paper for talented and ambitious young men like Norris, who soon became the paper's city editor. He possessed the qualities Singerly claimed to desire in a reporter: ambition, drive, and education. But Singerly claimed to want even more—reporters with presence—an ability to interact effectively with people spanning all walks of life in a major American city. He wanted a reporter to be "fundamentally a gentleman"—not in style, dress, or manners but in displaying integrity and purpose in seeking the factual truth behind a story. Years later, an interviewer queried Singerly on the secret to the *Record*'s success. In his reply, he stressed the paper's commitment to "truthfulness" and shared an anecdote from his earliest days at the paper. The foreman of the composing room had approached Singerly with a reporter's story fresh from the field, concerned that it touched on a potentially sensitive subject. Singerly replied with a question of his own—"Do you know the right and the wrong of this?" When the foreman responded that he thought they did know the facts, Singerly declared, "Print the right! And let that be the rule from this day on."[9]

Singerly surely had this anecdote polished and perfected through multiple retellings; it was perhaps even apocryphal. It would be easy to

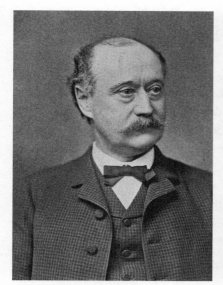 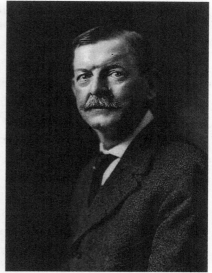

Above left: Fig. 10. William Singerly. As owner and publisher of the *Philadelphia Record,* Singerly brought significant financial resources to bear in pursuing Buchanan and shutting down the EMC. William M. Singerly portrait courtesy of the *Philadelphia Record* Photograph Morgue [V07], Historical Society of Pennsylvania *Above right:* Fig. 11. John Norris, city editor of the *Philadelphia Record.* Norris's persistence in coordinating investigative and legal operations culminated in Buchanan's arrest on multiple charges in June 1880. Image LC-USZ62-75445 courtesy of the Library of Congress, Prints and Photographs Division, Washington, D.C.

cynically dismiss the story today as self-serving pontification. In considering the track record of the newspaper and the arc of John Norris's subsequent career, however, this anecdote may be more revealing than we might assume. The sentiment it expresses does seem in line with the culture cultivated at the *Record* under Singerly, one that encouraged aggressive, hands-on reporting and investigation, not simply because it resulted in stories that built circulation but as a means of holding elected officials and those in power accountable for events occurring on their watch. In essence, what took hold at the *Record,* and what drove John Norris personally, was a reportorial philosophy arising from outrage at the effrontery of human avarice in all its guises and impelled by a strong desire to see justice served and the guilty punished. This approach was one that John Norris had already been acquiring through his experiences at the *Times* and the *Press;* he had learned the reporter's trade there on criminal cases like the nationally infamous Charley Ross kidnapping in 1874, when he had doggedly chased leads well after the case had grown cold, abandoned by most others.[10]

Norris's exposé of Miller simultaneously conveyed pity and scorn for a man who blithely acknowledged having bestowed upon himself both M.D. and D.D. degrees under the seal of the school. Miller proved laughably naïve in his interactions with the two reporters. He agreed to take them on as his "private students," and, after accepting their $25 first installment toward the total tuition fee of $100, added them to the roster of students who had ostensibly completed the prior class beginning five months earlier, in October 1879. Not content with this postdated record keeping, Miller presented Norris with a series of admission cards for various lectures on such subjects as anatomy, surgery, physiology, chemistry, obstetrics, and materia medica, all of which carried dates showing that the classes had commenced months earlier, in October. Miller even filled out a certificate for the reporter, identifying him as a student of the school who was "entitled to practice Medicine from this date, February 27, 1880."

Miller's casual willingness to incriminate himself and the school, both verbally and through documents, seemed almost comical, but had serious implications. After Miller showed Norris a daunting set of medical texts, he reassured him that practicing medicine was "easy." He then reached for several bottles arranged next to the inkstand on his desk and held up each one in turn for a closer inspection. The bottles contained aconite (i.e., wolfsbane or monkshood), belladonna (i.e., deadly nightshade), and nux vomica (i.e., "poison nut" from the strychnine tree). Pointing at the bottles, Miller declared, "I always carry [these] about with me . . . they will cure every disease man ever had." Then he reached into his coat pocket to show Norris and Maynard a small case with a dozen small vials containing the three poisons and an array of other solutions.

Miller's pride in exhibiting his traveling pharmacopeia and his breezy self-confidence about using them stunned Norris. It was not the mere presence of these drugs in Miller's medicinal arsenal that was so alarming; diluted forms of these botanicals were standard treatments among allopathic, homeopathic, and eclectic physicians in the mid-nineteenth century.[11] What troubled Norris was his sense that Miller had no real understanding of the underlying properties of these drugs and their potential to inflict harm. For Miller, the dilution or mixture of these toxic substances into an ostensibly safe solution was nothing more than an exercise in following the printed instructions given in whatever pharmacopeia he happened to be consulting.

At one point, Norris interviewed the parishioners at Eden Methodist Church at Lehigh and Fifth Streets, where Miller served as a pastor. Few there understood what had motivated their minister to take up medicine so suddenly. They were genuinely perplexed that a man of Miller's seemingly good character had become associated with "that college," as one parishioner termed the school. This same man confided to Norris that the school's "bad reputation" was known to everyone but that Miller had staunchly defended the school and William Paine when they had pressed the point with him, claiming that Paine had been "maligned" unfairly. Norris's investigation uncovered the presence of several Methodist ministers on Philadelphia University's board of trustees, which probably accounted for Miller's new role in medicine and defense of the school's former dean.

Miller concluded that day's meeting with Norris and Maynard by telling the two men that if they would follow his guidance, " . . . I will make good doctors of you." By the time Miller walked them to the door, Norris was running through a mental catalogue of the diploma trade in Philadelphia. Allegations of dubious practices at the EMC and Philadelphia University dated back more than a decade. During Norris's career as a journalist, he had witnessed the senate investigation of the EMC and Philadelphia University, which had thoroughly discredited both John Buchanan and William Paine, but he had also witnessed its curious aftermath: the legislators' strange oversight in annulling the EMC charter but failing to annul that of Buchanan's paper institution, the American University of Philadelphia, and the rumors that omission prompted; the surprising reversal of Buchanan's fortunes when the Pennsylvania state supreme court later overturned the legislative annulments; and then the strange silence that followed *Allen v. Buchanan,* when no one appeared interested in pursuing the matter into the judiciary, the only means for legally addressing the matter. When Norris and Maynard left Philadelphia University that day, Miller offered a heartfelt good day and a final salutation, "Now, gentlemen, don't fail to let me hear from you!"

Norris responded with a seemingly good-natured, "Oh, no, Doctor, you will hear from us tomorrow." Norris's reply to Miller arrived via the next morning's edition of the *Philadelphia Record*. The front page trumpeted the "Doctor Factory" operating in the city's midst and explained how one of their reporters had become a "sawbones in two minutes." The bulk of the article provided a detailed description of the *Record* reporters' interactions with Miller, culminating in their postdated status as students at Philadelphia University and receipt of a certificate attesting to their status with the school and their preparedness "to practice Medicine" immediately. The article succeeded as an effective and damning portrait of Miller and the school.

On March 1, 1880, an editorial in the *Philadelphia Record* laid out that paper's motives in the matter of the diploma trade. Pointing to the medical licensing laws that had begun taking hold among the states over the previous decade, the *Record* asserted that they were changing the medical environment, and urged immediate action to deal with the sale of diplomas, arguing that the licensing laws raised the stakes and the legal implications of issuing the M.D. degree. As the *Record* asserted, the appellation "M.D." was not an inconsequential honorific akin to "Colonel." If that had once been the case, it was no longer true. Now, a person granted an M.D. degree would gain a legal status and authority not previously associated with physicians. The *Record* also asserted, rather disingenuously, that the medical diploma traders had raised the stakes themselves by seeking new buyers in the United States, instead of confining their trade to an international market. That assertion had no basis in fact, since the Pennsylvania senate investigation of 1872 had clearly demonstrated that diploma sales in the United States were already common a decade earlier. Nevertheless, having raised the battle, the *Record* offered no quarter, laying out a moral imperative for action: "The medical quack is an enemy of the human race . . . a factory of bogus medical practitioners is a public nuisance of the worst sort . . . There is no end to the murderous mischief it may perpetrate. Making counterfeit doctors is infinitely more dangerous than the coinage of spurious dollars."[12]

John Buchanan did not feel the full implications of the *Record*'s crusade until several months later, but the repercussions for Miller and Philadelphia University came quickly. By mid-March, a Methodist conference had removed Miller as minister at his church. In June, the state of Pennsylvania began quo warranto proceedings against the school to examine its alleged abuse of those powers granted it under its charter.

Two months later, authorities arraigned Miller on forgery charges for signing the names of several Philadelphia University trustees on the certificate he had issued John Norris during the latter's February 27 visit. By the following spring, March 1881, proceedings against Philadelphia University had culminated in a legal ruling that included a "decree of ouster." Miller and the school trustees agreed to a decree that allowed the state to "[in]validate all past acts" under the school's charter.[13] With that decision, Philadelphia University—established in 1853—no longer had any official, legal existence.

The *Record*'s exposure of Miller and Philadelphia University could hardly have escaped the attention of John Buchanan. The story probably brought to mind the resolution passed by the Pennsylvania state legislature just a few months earlier, in December 1879, which had requested that the state attorney general's office initiate legal action against the EMC, the American University, and Philadelphia University for "abuse of its franchises."[14]

From Buchanan's perspective, weeks had passed with no legal proceedings commencing or even seeming imminent. Was the resolution a toothless measure designed to placate an ambitious councilman, a disgruntled faculty member at Penn or Jefferson, or some other unknown party? After all, John Buchanan had come to expect periodic flare-ups of scrutiny and targeting in recent years, and without definitive evidence against him and the EMC, some critics were content to level accusations through the newspapers, such as those appearing only weeks earlier.

In January 1880, the *Philadelphia Inquirer* and the *Philadelphia Times* had expressed indignation over the "mysterious disappearance" of a young woman, Mary Ash. Both newspapers pointed an accusing finger at Buchanan, insinuating that Ash had been "decoyed" into Philadelphia by a man named Goff and "last seen . . . in the neighborhood" of Buchanan's offices. They also stated that Buchanan could not be located for questioning. The girl's father had sworn an affidavit before a local magistrate claiming Ash was either dead or dying after "criminal malpractice" at the hands of John Buchanan. The local press seemed surprised when the girl returned safely home a week later, though the article carrying this information did not garner a headline of its own. Editorial staff buried it as just one more item in the "Police Intelligence" section of the *Inquirer.* The young woman told reporters she was "much annoyed . . . [by] the notoriety" stemming from the erroneous reports of her absence when she had simply been visiting a friend in Philadelphia.[15]

John Buchanan probably reassured himself that the newspapers were a nuisance but not a source of concern and that any real threat would come from the politicians and the courts, not reporters. He may even have resolved to begin making discreet inquiries to see what was afoot in Philadelphia and Harrisburg. If he did follow this line of thinking, he would soon be surprised to realize just how wrong he was. John Norris and the *Philadelphia Record* already had him in their crosshairs.

A STING OPERATION

John Norris's plans received a jolt several weeks later with a round of unanticipated publicity regarding John Buchanan and the EMC. Unknown to Norris, a chain of correspondence begun in early February 1880 by the United States ambassador in Berlin had been making its way to the Philadelphia mayor and the public in late March. On February 2, the American ambassador to Germany, Andrew White, wrote to inform the U.S. secretary of state of the anger of German authorities over questionable diplomas originating in the United States.[16] White had long been irritated by the antiquated pedagogy of many American institutions of higher learning, but he regarded the Philadelphia-based trade in diplomas as being on a different plane. It was a national "disgrace" marring American education. White's letter described his own experiences in Berlin where he had personally examined several "sham" diplomas, in particular one made out to a Paul Volland and signed by John Buchanan, M.D.[17]

The U.S. secretary of state, William Everts, forwarded White's missive to the Interior Department's Bureau of Education, along with his own letter seeking assistance in ferreting out the "status and general reputation" of the schools and persons mentioned. Bureau Commissioner John

Facing page: Fig. 12. This cartoon, entitled "The Philadelphia Physician Factory," appeared in April 1880 in the humor magazine *Puck.* The renewed national interest in diploma mills nearly unraveled Norris's carefully laid plans. Image courtesy of the U.S. National Library of Medicine, Digital Collections.

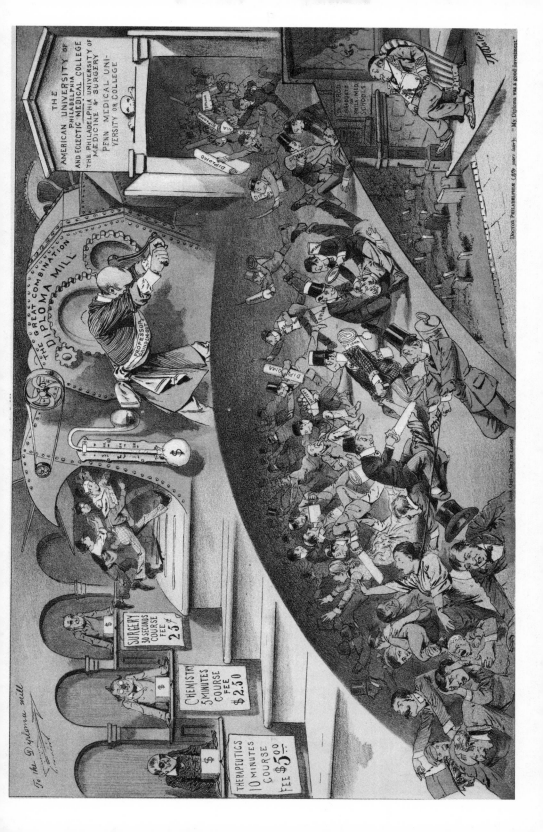

Eaton then forwarded a copy of all the correspondence to Philadelphia's mayor, William Stokley. By 1880, inquiries of this nature concerning the EMC were nothing new to the mayor's office. Stokley shared this latest inquiry with the local newspapers.

When the story broke in late March 1880, Norris must have winced at its timing. While Buchanan had been used to scrutiny in the past, it had never come from such high-level officials. For Norris, this turn of affairs threatened to precipitate a worst-case scenario in which Buchanan closed up shop, liquidated his assets, and bolted the scene. While such an outcome might put an end to the EMC and leave Buchanan, the major player in the diploma trade, out in the cold, a resolution that never brought Buchanan to justice in a court of law hardly seemed satisfactory. Buchanan might even be able to remain in the area and continue operating with a lower profile, in which case he would be extremely cautious in his actions and guarded in responding to inquiries from diploma seekers. Given such a scenario, Norris feared that it might prove impossible to ensnare him in even the most carefully plotted sting.

This round of publicity threatened to undermine the trap that Norris and his colleagues were setting with their correspondence. Norris had already written to Buchanan using several false identities. He had sent letters posing as Dr. John William Fanning of Tippecanoe City, Ohio, and as George Austin Dawson of Chester Court House, South Carolina, among others. To accomplish this, Norris had secured critical help from Thomas Barrett, a U.S. postal agent, who provided him with the various postmarks he needed to carry out this sting, such as those from Tippecanoe City and Chester Court House. In the guise of Fanning and for a negotiated price of $100, Norris was attempting to obtain two diplomas showing an M.D. (one in English from the EMC and the other in Latin from American University of Philadelphia), as well as a certificate showing membership in the National Eclectic Medical Association. All of these documents were to be postdated to April 1878 at the request of "Fanning," who claimed in his correspondence that April 1878 was the date he had arrived in Ohio and assumed the practice of medicine. As George Dawson, Norris secured a law degree from the American University. He sought a second law degree under the name Henry Dawson from the American University and a diploma under the name John McLean for a "master in electrotherapeutics" from the Philadelphia Electropathic Institution.

This last school was a wholly nonexistent enterprise, although one that apparently required Norris or a surrogate to attend several lectures on the "medical virtues of electricity" before obtaining a diploma.[18]

Norris demonstrated a deft touch in framing his letters. On the back of the stationery he used for the imaginary Dr. Fanning's letters to Buchanan, Norris placed preprinted text touting Fanning's medical acumen:

"DR. FANNING's GREAT REMEDIES
DR. J. WILLIAM FANNING's LUNG MIXTURE AND BLOOD PURIFIER.
FANNING's FEVER AND AGUE REMEDY. . . .
Thousands testify to its wonderful effects and life-sustaining powers.
Read a few of the many remarkable cures from the doctor's case book."[19]

Writing as Fanning, Norris began with a straightforward query regarding the possibility of securing a medical diploma. Then, playing on Buchanan's vanity, "Fanning" alluded to a copy of Buchanan's 1868 *Practical Treatise of Midwifery* in his (Fanning's) possession and enclosed $1.25 in the letter in case a newer edition was available. By citing the price list from an older edition of the EMC's *Eclectic Medical Journal of Pennsylvania* and offering to journey to Philadelphia to close their deal should they come to agreeable terms, Norris signaled that Fanning may not have been fully aware of all the circumstances surrounding the school in recent years. Even here, however, Norris included a subtle mix of messages, commenting, for example, "I saw in the *Dayton Journal* about Minister White and the Latin diplomas—I want one in English." In this single sentence, Norris/Fanning signaled some knowledge of the brewing scandal while hinting at a willingness to avoid looking too closely into the matter. These touches, together with Fanning's sometimes deferential tone ("As to the dip[loma], I will be guided by your advice"), established what Norris hoped would be a "mutual confidence" between the two correspondents.[20]

Buchanan's May 1880 reply offered reassurance of its own: "Minister White is quite wrong on the matter. The plan was in all cases to sell a *scholarship*" [italics added]. Buchanan's reply also featured a blunt tone: " . . . if you mean business . . . send in your full name, date, a very short thesis, and if you can spare it $100, at least no less than $65." Fanning responded in kind, saying "I do mean business; business of the most serious nature." Further negotiation led Fanning to provide the requested thesis, a short paper entitled "Electricity as a Curative Agent." Norris's later characterization of the paper in the *Record* left little doubt as to its dubious quality. As he described it, the paper opened with general assertions about the virtues of eclectic medicine, followed with material copied from various schools of medical treatment, and then included another stroke to Buchanan's ego by lifting entire sections from, and then citing, his *American Practice of Medicine*. Accompanying the thesis was a final letter from Fanning, asking how they should conclude the "other matter"—that is, the transaction for the diploma. Fanning wished to know whether payment and shipment should be made through the Adams Express Company.[21]

Norris's correspondence is described in some detail to illustrate how he approached his letter writing with Buchanan. Viewed collectively, the correspondence unfolded at the pace one might expect. Fanning was supposed to be an interested but cautious physician, practicing far from Philadelphia. In order to sound the appropriate note of authenticity, his letters had to contain an element of courtship ritual. An unquestioning willingness to immediately send money for a diploma would have been suspicious. Fanning's letters needed to reflect more than a desire to close the deal and secure the diploma; they needed to betray a hint of anxiety and some trepidation. They needed to reflect enough awareness of the attention generated nationally by White's letter to convey a tacit understanding that the deal being brokered was best alluded to through indirect language ("the other matter"). The two parties needed to establish an understanding without spelling out too clearly its exact terms. Fanning needed to be just enough of a scoundrel for Buchanan to feel comfortable that he was interacting with one of his own.

In the meantime, the fallout from the *Record*'s exposure of Philadelphia University, as well as from Ambassador White's correspondence, reverberated in the Philadelphia press throughout the spring of 1880. Reporters monitored the accelerating repercussions for Miller and his Philadelphia University colleagues as they were called to account by the Methodist Episcopal Judicial Council and the local Methodist Preachers Association.[22] Criminal cases with any hint of a connection to the EMC or Philadelphia University, like one in which an alleged diploma holder was accused of poisoning his wife, garnered front-page attention.[23]

All the while, questions about the Philadelphia schools continued to be asked. In early April, the Texas Board of Medical Examiners contacted Mayor Stokley's office to inquire about the EMC, explaining that it had been investigating individuals holding EMC diplomas who demonstrated "no evidence of study or fitness for medical practice." Similar inquiries reached the mayor from Germany, England, France, and the Channel Islands. At the same time, the Massachusetts Medical Society reported to their state's legislature that they possessed "proof positive" of the sale of diplomas in Philadelphia. Meanwhile, local Philadelphia reporters delved into the story behind Ambassador White's letter. They scrutinized the details of the specific diploma and its holder cited in White's letter and gave particular attention to an accompanying certificate signed by Phillip A. Cregar, a Philadelphia notary. Cregar had certified the document as a "regular diploma" of the EMC, that the school was "regularly incorporated" and "in good standing," and that the affixed signatures, including that of John Buchanan, were "genuine."[24]

Astute reporters also noticed that Cregar's certificate included the signature of the Philadelphia County prothonotary, William B. Mann—the same William Mann who had served as John Buchanan's attorney during his legal troubles of 1876–77. The coincidence proved too much for curious reporters. They descended upon Cregar, who sought to minimize his connections with the school. He defended himself by claiming to have seen the school's charter firsthand and to have notarized only a handful of EMC diplomas. As Cregar explained to the press, he had no reason to believe the signatures affixed to the diploma were anything but genuine.[25]

During this flurry of newspaper scrutiny, a brief silence hovered over Buchanan and the EMC in late spring 1880. Despite the twin blasts of publicity stemming from the Miller exposé and Ambassador White's letter, Buchanan, for a brief period, became a figure on the margin of these stories rather than their focal point as the broader, fundamental issues embedded in these stories became explicit: What is the basis for the issuance of any diploma? And how can flagrant abuses in their issuance be corrected?

It would be helpful to have some insight into Buchanan's thoughts during this period. Unfortunately, the obvious sources for such insights are nonexistent. If Buchanan kept a personal journal or diary, none has survived or resurfaced. Similarly, no statements by Buchanan appeared in the press during this period. No letters, official papers, or records from the EMC remain to offer even an indirect glimpse into Buchanan's state of mind or his planning as events accelerated in 1880. We are left with speculation.

One assumption that might be drawn is that Buchanan now spent less time at the EMC. Much of the silence in the press may be attributable to the simple fact that Buchanan was staying away from the school to the extent possible as a means of avoiding ambush interviews by reporters; the offices of the *Philadelphia Record* and the *Philadelphia Inquirer* were both conveniently situated for reporters near Third and Chestnut, only blocks away from the EMC. At the same time, based upon Buchanan's timely replies to Norris's Fanning/Dawson letters, it is clear that he either remained near the school or was using an intermediary to pick up letters addressed to him there.

What may have occupied his thoughts even more than unwelcome publicity in the late spring of 1880 were prospects for establishing a new eclectic medical college in Michigan. It is difficult to say how far such plans had progressed at this point, though several months later John Buchanan would be apprehended with sixty shares of stock in the Detroit Eclectic Medical College on his person.[26] It is possible that he, either alone or in concert with others, had been mulling over the possibility of a school in Michigan for some time, only to have the publication of the White letter accelerate discussions and planning along these lines. With Buchanan's subsequent arrest in June, these plans gained an added impetus.

A RAID AND AN ARREST

At 5:00 P.M. on the afternoon of June 9, 1880, a letter carrier stepped up to the front door of the EMC.[27] He knocked and waited for an answer. When the door opened, the man stated that he had a certified letter for Dr. John Buchanan. A brief conversation ensued and the letter carrier entered the building. The man who answered the door had turned and begun walking away, only to look back and see the letter carrier standing with his back braced firmly against the door. The scuffling of footsteps sounded briefly outside before a group of men pushed their way into the EMC. Special Agent Thomas Barrett of the U.S. Postal Service; a federal deputy marshall named Reuter; Philadelphia's police chief, Samuel Givin; and two reserve police officers had pressed inside. Joining them was John Norris.

The group found John Buchanan upstairs, hunched over a female dental patient that he had placed near a window for added light. The postal agent, Barrett, introduced himself and then asked whether Buchanan had received letters from parties in Tippecanoe City, Ohio, and Chester Court House, South Carolina. Buchanan acknowledged as much. Then U.S. Marshall Reuter began reading an affidavit from John Gibbons, the U.S. commissioner for education: "On or about June 5, 1880, John Buchanan did devise a scheme and artifice to demand and to be effected by means of the post office establishment of the United States, and did in and for the purpose of executing said scheme and artifice take a certain letter out of the Post office of the United States at Philadelphia."

John Buchanan watched as police then searched the premises while Norris and Barrett pored over every document turned up in their search—the matriculation book, the roster of graduates, sixteen express-receipt books, and stacks of correspondence, including more than fifty letters to and from diploma seekers, as well as registers documenting the financial transactions. The correspondence proved particularly damning. Despite Buchanan's characterization of the financial transactions as those for purchasing a scholarship, the letters revealed the truth in an unequivocal fashion. These transactions were a quid pro quo submission of money (ranging from $30 to $150) in exchange for a diploma.[28]

At one point, Norris and Barrett attempted to count the number of diplomas issued before settling on an approximation. They placed the estimated number at 3,000 diplomas. Later, after an analysis of all the paperwork confiscated at the EMC, Norris and the *Record* revised the estimated number of EMC and American University diplomas in circulation as being closer to 11,000. The official school registers accounted for only 1,500 diplomas. The vast majority were issued through sales, either brokered directly, through the mail or in person, by Buchanan and colleagues, or through agents for the school situated elsewhere in the United States and Europe. In their final analysis of the documentary evidence, Norris and the *Record* claimed that only a "very small" portion of the diploma holders were "legitimate doctors." As one example, the paper compared the thirty students apparently in attendance in 1880 to a listing showing slightly more than 100 graduates expected that year.[29]

In addition to its publication of the EMC's questionable "graduates," the *Record* provided its readers with a helpful guide for determining which diplomas were wholly bogus. The *Record* detailed how to assess these based on the date of issue and the faculty listed on the diploma. "Any diploma bearing the name of R. A. Simpson since 1878 is fraudulent," the *Record* declared, adding, " . . . any diploma bearing the name of C. H. Kehnroth prior to 1879 must be looked upon with grave suspicion."[30] The *Record*'s publication of several thousand diploma holders' names garnered interest from newspapers and journals throughout the country, some of which were eager to republish the names of any EMC and American University degree holders ostensibly residing in their states. A physiomedical publication, the *Cincinnati Medical Gazette*, lamented the damage to the cause of reformed medicine inflicted by Buchanan and the EMC. Twice the *Gazette* published lists of physicians holding Buchanan-issued diplomas, lamenting, "Heaven save us from such!"[31]

As the search of the offices progressed that day, authorities began to believe that they had some sense for the materials on hand. Then someone pointed out the one item they had not yet located in any great volume— the actual diplomas being sold. The records made clear that Buchanan's office at 514 Pine Street served as the base for the operations. Yet they had found no cache of blank diplomas or even evidence of periodic deliveries of such documents. With a renewed sense of purpose, the group began checking desks for false drawers, tapping on the walls to sound for hidden compartments, looking behind pictures on the wall. Finally, someone kicked away a carpet lying in a corner of the room. Under it was revealed a trapdoor and a steep set of stairs leading to the basement. John Buchanan tried to minimize the find by claiming it to be the way into his personal laboratory. The *Philadelphia Inquirer* later gave it a more ominous description, labeling it a "drug shop." More importantly, once they secured adequate lighting, Norris and the others found the additional physical evidence of the diploma mill they had been seeking. In a far corner of the basement was an entire printing operation—a composing room and three-quarter Gordon press; electrotype plates for the EMC and the American University; and a half-ton cache of blank diplomas, some signed by the EMC faculty, others not.[32]

Also scattered about were flawed versions of a recent circular. Dated June 1, 1880, the circular carried a generic salutation ("To the Editor—

Dear Sir") and a proposal that if the editor printed the enclosed advertisement once a week for eighteen months, John Buchanan would remit a signed "scholarship" for the American University of Philadelphia, fully executed with signatures, seal, and so on. The editor could "sell or dispose of [the scholarship] in any way you deem best." Local newspapers subsequently highlighted this last piece of evidence as a recent and particularly damning tactic, although in reality Buchanan had been advertising the American University in American newspapers for close to a decade.[33]

The scope and volume of the materials seized that day were remarkable. They were so extensive that it took the *Record* until mid-July to publish a complete description of all the contents. Not only did the materials document the extent of the diploma trade under the legal charters of the EMC and the American University, they also revealed the blatant criminality of an enterprise that had grown so large that it was issuing diplomas and certificates for nonexistent entities (e.g., the Liverpool Anthropological Society), paper institutions (e.g., Livingston University), and legitimate institutions wholly unaffiliated with the EMC (e.g., the Eclectic Medical Institute).[34] The scope and volume of materials seized that day suggest that Norris and his fellows had caught Buchanan wholly unawares. Apparently he and his colleagues had made no effort to remove documents to a safer location, despite the massive attention focused on the diploma trade in the months prior to the raid. In June 1880, Buchanan and the school seemed to have been operating through a stunning combination of greed, hubris, and carelessness.

The search of the EMC premises provided an additional humiliation for Buchanan. One of the reserve officers came down from the fourth floor attic to report an "overpowering stench" of human remains. A cursory look at the fourth floor dissecting room found the partially dissected remains of human corpses in an advanced state of decomposition. The stench was so strong that even a copious layer of lime had failed to mask the smell. The next day, the city Health Department removed the remains of four or five corpses for burial in a pauper's field. Conditions in the room were characterized by "filth, disorder, [and] vermin." An examination of the hospital ward two floors below found comparably "filthy" conditions. The Health Department ordered the immediate closure of the building as a "nuisance . . . to public health" until the hospital and dissecting quarters could be adequately cleaned and disinfected.[35]

The Legal Noose Tightens

Police arrested John Buchanan that day on multiple charges: violation of federal law by using the U.S. mail with intent to defraud, violation of Pennsylvania state law regarding the sale of diplomas, and forgery. This last charge stemmed from assertions by several EMC faculty members that they had neither signed certain diplomas nor given Buchanan authority to do so on their behalf. Warrants had been issued against the entire EMC faculty, and two members, Charles G. Polk and John J. Siggins, were arrested with Buchanan during the initial raid on June 9.[36] Newspapers across the country picked up the story of Buchanan's arrest. The main elements of the story did not vary, although some newspapers, such as the *Wheeling Register*, labeled Buchanan an "abortionist" and heavily stressed this earlier allegation as a way of damning him doubly.[37]

At noon the following day, while the Health Department labored to clean the second and fourth floors of the EMC, John Buchanan appeared before Commissioner Gibbons in a hearing on the charges of mail fraud. He must have been shaken by the hearing's outcome. After listening to detailed testimony from John Norris and Thomas Barrett, including cross-examination by Buchanan's attorney, William Mann, Gibbons ordered that Buchanan be held in custody and set his bail at the staggering sum of $10,000. This drew an immediate protest from Mann, who claimed the amount "excessive" but noted that Buchanan was prepared to offer funds to meet bail set at half that amount. Gibbons declined, whereupon authorities next hauled Buchanan to a nearby magistrate court to face charges for the illegal sale of diplomas and forgery. Evidence provided at the time by EMC faculty member Charles Polk indicated that most of the signatures on the diplomas offered in evidence were forged. He pointed to several names—specifically, those of James Cochran and David Diller—and testified that Cochran had been dead for several years and Diller had left the EMC four years earlier. On this basis, the magistrate ordered Buchanan held for the illegal sale of diplomas and set his bail at $2,000, with another $1,000 for each forged signature. The events of that afternoon brought his total bail to approximately $20,000.

If Buchanan had not fully appreciated the gravity of his personal and financial situation at the time of his arrest, he understood it now. The totality of his ruin crashed down on him during these initial hearings.

His prior court experiences had been nothing like this. They had always culminated with, at the worst, an overnight stay in jail while he worked through family, friends, and his attorney to secure the necessary modest funds for his release. The bail amounts had always ranged between $500 and $1,000, of which only a portion had to be presented in cash, with the rest in the form of a bond pledging security for the remainder.

Even if Buchanan could get the collective $20,000 bail reduced substantially, it would still take time to raise such a sum. For apparently the first time in his life, John Buchanan spent more than a night in jail. Over the next ten days, he and his attorneys labored to obtain a bail reduction that would give him some chance for release while awaiting trial. The first opportunity did not arrive until June 17, when the U.S. district court heard Buchanan's request for a reduced bail. This hearing marked a small victory, accompanied by a setback. Judge Butler did reduce Buchanan's bail on the federal charges from $10,000 to $5,000, but he refused the surety offered by Buchanan's daughter based upon property she owned in New Jersey.

Buchanan and his attorney, William Mann, then tried a different tack. Obtaining another hearing before Commissioner Gibbons regarding the $5,000 bail amount, Mann offered surety for the bail from Buchanan's brother-in-law, Martin Chapman, and from one of Buchanan's friends, Daniel Cleary. Gibbons expressed satisfaction with the $5,000 amount and the surety from Cleary and Chapman. Having obtained Gibbons's agreement, Mann returned Buchanan to Judge Butler's court. Over the objections of the district attorney's office, Butler claimed that if Gibbons was satisfied with the amount and the parties providing surety, then he was too.

Mann then had his client taken to the Court of Quarter Sessions for a separate bail hearing on the state and forgery charges. This session included heated wrangling back and forth between Mann and a lawyer from the district attorney's office. The latter described Buchanan as "a man of some means" and intimated that he presented a flight risk. He also put forward the interesting argument that since the other court had set a $5,000 bail on a mail fraud charge that carried a penalty of only eighteen months, then the bail for the diploma sale and forgery charges should be far higher, since conviction for forgery could result in a sentence of up to ten years. The judge considered this point, but since John Norris had been unavailable on short notice to answer the judge's questions regarding the prosecution's case, he agreed to a reduced bail of $5,000. Having obtained the reduction, Mann asked for and obtained a thirty-minute recess, after which he returned with Joseph Koecker, a local Philadelphia architect, who agreed to provide surety for Buchanan. The judge allowed the lawyer from the district attorney's office to pose a few questions to Koecker, who admitted that he expected Dr. Buchanan to "indemnif[y]" him "against possible loss." In prescient fashion, the attorney finished with a warning to Koecker should Buchanan fail to appear, " . . . If I have to get the money from you, I shall have no compunction in doing so."

The workings behind a series of nineteenth-century bail hearings would not usually warrant this degree of attention. Given what later transpired on August 17, 1880, however, these details provide insight. The prosecution's vigorous defense of the significant dollar amounts set in the original hearings and their determined efforts to thwart any reduction were unsurprising. They were familiar with Buchanan's prior history in Philadelphia courts—a history in which he had posted much smaller sums for bail and then somehow managed to mysteriously delay the appearance of the original charges in the court docket before they ultimately disappeared. It stood to reason that Buchanan would find it more difficult to tap into any remaining political connections from within the confines of a jail cell. Furthermore, in describing him as someone possessing financial "means," the prosecution was signaling their concern that Buchanan might employ these means to flee the state.

For Buchanan, these bail hearings reinforced just how much more serious his legal position was this time. He faced state and federal charges that could put him in prison for a significant period if convicted. The national interest in the case meant that, even if he could manage to arrange intervention on his behalf, it would be impossible to do so discreetly. For all intents and purposes, the publicity had nullified the legal and political influence of Buchanan's friends and contacts. The level of scrutiny directed toward the EMC and the interest of federal officials meant that Buchanan's contacts could no longer work for him behind the scenes as they had in the past.

Authorities set Buchanan's arraignment in U.S. district court for mid-August. This provided ample time for meetings with his attorney, William

Mann, as they planned how to address the pending charges. While the forgery charges were troubling because of the lengthy sentence the judge could impose if Buchanan was found guilty, the evidence was actually weak. Buchanan knew that the diplomas seized in evidence featured a confusing mix of authentic and spurious signatures. Evidence for the prosecution from a handwriting expert could be negated by contradictory evidence for the defense from another expert. The forgery charges most likely had a different purpose: to help those determined to convict Buchanan to raise his bail to the highest amount possible and to help convince several EMC faculty members into becoming witnesses for the prosecution.

The mail fraud charges were more worrisome. The evidence collected through Norris's efforts was damning and unequivocal in proving a pattern of payment for diplomas. Mann might argue, correctly as it turned out, that there was no intent to deceive or defraud, since the purchaser of the diploma understood the quid pro quo nature of the transaction and was himself attempting to deceive others (i.e., prospective patients) about his medical expertise and qualifications as a physician. In the cold light of reason and logic, this defense might prevail. However, this point of law would be argued in an environment tainted by the heavy publicity surrounding the case, where such nuances might not carry the day.

Buchanan's confidence about gaining a courtroom victory probably weakened and collapsed in July and early August. Friends and colleagues that he had counted upon for support were becoming harder to find and sometimes less than sympathetic. Days after his arrest, Buchanan received a short letter from Phillip Bissell, his longtime EMC colleague. Bissell's edged humor seemed to indicate a falling-out between the two men.

> Dear Buck: I see you have a free advertisement again in the papers. It will bring a fresh grist to your mill. 514 Pine Street will be advertised all over the world. Buy a new steam press to print diplomas on—the sale will be unprecedented, not withstanding the hard times.
>
> Yours Bissell

Bissell's letter arrived in a large yellow envelope at the offices of the *Philadelphia Record*. Bissell addressed the letter to Buchanan, although he directed it to be delivered by Barrett, the postal agent who took part in the sting operation. On the outside of the envelope, Bissell had scrawled, "Open Letter." The *Record* interpreted this literally and obliged by publishing the letter on June 15, 1880.[38]

It is probable that Bissell later regretted drawing attention to himself. Once authorities had more closely analyzed the mountain of documents seized at the EMC, Bissell felt compelled to write the *Record* disavowing any connection with the EMC by claiming a case of mistaken identity. Bissell asserted that he was being confused with a "relative of mine," Augustus Post (A. P.) Bissell. The documents seized on June 9 undercut this strained explanation.[39]

Even EMC colleagues of Buchanan's who had remained in the fold soon fell by the wayside. Faced with warrants for their arrests on charges of signing diplomas for the purposes of illegal sale, most of the faculty had scattered, although not all escaped successfully. One of these was Charles H. Kehnroth, EMC professor of chemistry and toxicology. A friend of Buchanan's, whose son lodged in Buchanan's home, Kehnroth was arrested on July 6. Before a magistrate the following day, the state produced a receipt, issued by the Adams Express Company and signed by Kehnroth, which attested to his delivery of the box containing the diplomas sent to Fanning and Dawson as part of Norris's sting operation. Authorities had another EMC faculty member, John J. Fulmer, standing by for the hearing. He testified that the signature on the receipt was Kehnroth's. Kehnroth remained in jail for some time, unable to raise the $4,000 bail.[40]

Another setback came the following week. Phillip Cregar, a former principal of the Philadelphia Girls Normal School, had served as the notary for the Volland diploma prompting Ambassador White's outraged letter. On July 12, he appeared in court to answer misdemeanor charges of "uttering a forged document." The prosecutor's questions were pointed and specific. Cregar acknowledged notarizing some of the Buchanan diplomas but insisted, despite newspaper accounts of thousands of diplomas issued by the EMC and American University, that he had personally notarized fewer than ten. The prosecutor pressed Cregar to explain why he would notarize even one EMC diploma when the school was so notorious for selling diplomas. Cregar admitted having "heard in a general way of the abuses" at the EMC but stressed his understanding that the abuses had occurred previously, under William Paine.[41]

More importantly, Cregar asserted that he had exercised due diligence as a notary. He related a conversation he had had with John Buchanan earlier that year, in which Buchanan had shown Cregar the school charter and denied that any payments for diplomas had been sought or accepted. In fact, Cregar testified, Buchanan had adamantly stressed that "the university is honorable" in its methods and explained that the school issued some honorary diplomas but "nothing more than what is done by every reputable medical institution." Buchanan and his EMC colleague Henry Hollembaek offered to write out sworn statements to allay Cregar's concerns. Cregar claimed that Buchanan had been "so earnest" in their conversations that he had felt no reason to doubt him or the school.[42]

Cregar seems to have conducted himself well under questioning. His answers seemed reasonable and his manner neither evasive nor overly defensive. However, this façade soon crumbled. Cregar failed to reappear in court the following day, and the *Record* briefly reported him as a "fugitive" from justice. Once again, someone with connections to John Buchanan and the EMC had broken publicly under the intense scrutiny of the case.

A series of separate but related incidents in early August underscored the gravity of Buchanan's situation and the extensive resources that John Norris, the *Record*, and local authorities were dedicating to their goal of obtaining a conviction.[43] After Buchanan's arrest, authorities and reporters remained alert to the general activities at the EMC. In due course, they obtained a copy of correspondence between Kehnroth, writing on behalf of American University of Philadelphia, and W. J. Fletcher, a diploma seeker in Ohio. The letter exchange demonstrated that even after the raid on the EMC building and Buchanan's arrest, diploma sales had not ended completely. Consequently, police and reporters kept Buchanan, his associates, and the EMC under a "close watch." Their vigilance paid off on July 27 when authorities tracked a man leaving 514 Pine Street carrying "two large bundles" to a steel-plate print shop. They suspected that the bundles contained blank diplomas and perhaps a steel-plate seal for either EMC or the American University.

Meanwhile, in another development, *Record* reporters learned that Buchanan's son-in-law, John Fitzpatrick of 432 Pine Street, had sent a $30 package COD to a man in Ohio, only to quickly change his mind and ask for its return. It was rerouted back to Philadelphia, but was accidentally sent to a different express office than the one from which it originated. There it sat, unbeknownst to Fitzpatrick.

John Norris believed that this package probably contained diplomas or other evidence pertinent to the case against Buchanan and saw an opportunity to possibly secure further evidence. Lacking a warrant, he used a ruse to gain access to the package. Consulting the city directory, he found another man named John Fitzpatrick, who agreed to claim the package after Norris explained the situation to him. Norris accompanied this second Fitzpatrick when he claimed the package and witnessed it being opened. The package contained two diplomas, one from the EMC and another from the American University, along with a certificate of membership in the National Eclectic Medical Association. All of the documents carried John Buchanan's signature and were backdated to 1877.

Then, as prearranged with Norris, the second Mr. Fitzpatrick exclaimed in surprise that he "had never sent such a bundle" and suggested that it must have originated from the John Fitzpatrick at 432 Pine Street. The express company sent word of the package to the correct Fitzpatrick, who appeared later that afternoon to retrieve it. Meanwhile, Norris swore out an affidavit as to the contents he had seen, and a local magistrate issued arrest warrants for both Buchanan and Fitzpatrick. Neither man had any idea that their activities had been discovered. Thus, they were completely caught off guard by what happened next.

Around the same time that Norris worked his ruse to access materials at the express office, events came to a head back at the print shop, where authorities had witnessed two bundles from the EMC delivered in July. Either through a tip or active monitoring of the print shop, authorities were alerted when someone picked up the two bundles and delivered them to a corset shop at 212 South Eighth Street. A vigil on this shop paid off soon after dark when John Buchanan's son, George, arrived. He took up a casual but watchful position in front of the store for twenty minutes before Fitzpatrick emerged.

The two men then hurried toward 514 Pine Street, carrying the package from the print shop and a steel plate for printing American University diplomas. Police arrested Fitzpatrick en route; another officer confronted George Buchanan at the entrance to 514 Pine Street. The district attorney's office now had more evidence of ongoing attempts to sell diplomas, including the steel plate used to print the American University diplomas, and John Norris had another sensational headline for the August 5, 1880, edition of the *Record:* "Buchanan's Audacity—the Dean Again Trapped—Conspirators Caught Red Handed."

Having been caught with the steel plate and blank diplomas, George Buchanan confessed to several facts: that he resided at 432 Pine Street, where the returned express package had been delivered; that he was a professor of dentistry at American University; and (pertaining to the intercepted correspondence between Kehnroth and the diploma seeker W. J. Fletcher) that no one named Fletcher had attended that school at any point during the past three years.

In relating all this to his father, George probably also told John Buchanan of an exchange that took place in court between Buchanan's attorney, Mann, and John Norris. Mann asserted that Fletcher had been a student at the EMC and offered to bring him from Ohio to attend a subsequent hearing. Norris brushed aside the bluff. "We will save you the trouble and have him here ourselves."

Norris's defiant tone and threat are noteworthy. He would neither be bluffed nor intimidated. He had proved doggedly persistent in pursuing this story, far beyond what any reporter had previously done. There had been newspaper investigations of the EMC in the past, but none of those reporters had ever taken such an active role in the story, or in efforts to gather evidence for the legal authorities. Earlier reporters had been content to print their stories and move on to the next assignment, satisfied with striking a blow through words and nothing more. Not so with Norris. He seemed committed to living this story in multiple capacities—as investigator, reporter, witness, and prosecutor. From John Buchanan's vantage point, the most disconcerting element of the situation was that Norris seemed to have access to unlimited resources in pursuing his story. In early August 1880, John Buchanan had good reason to be worried.

Eight
The "Death" of John Buchanan

FLIGHT

When did the idea first occur to John Buchanan? When did he decide that a single dramatic act of deception—faking his own death—was the answer to his mounting problems? The ruse had two advantages. First, it would resolve his legal problems: dead men do not stand trial or serve jail sentences. Second, it would eliminate the financial consequences of simply fleeing. If Buchanan were dead, the bail funds supplied by friends and colleagues would simply be returned to them. The same would hold true for any money Buchanan himself had put toward his bail: it would be returned to his estate.

The notion of faking one's death and starting life anew was far from original in 1880. Fictional variations abound in Western literature. However, John Buchanan did not need to have read such accounts to hatch a similar scheme. He had firsthand knowledge of two such episodes. The ploy was known to journalists too, well enough that one newspaper, seeing it as a popular method of escape, labeled it the "drowning dodge."[1]

According to one press report, a former Buchanan pupil at the EMC, named "Foster," plied a similar maneuver a decade earlier. Apparently Foster had pursued and married a wealthy widow living near the EMC. Months after the wedding, Foster disappeared from Philadelphia along with the woman's funds. Soon thereafter, word arrived from upstate New York that a small skiff, containing a hat, coat, and papers identified as Foster's, had been found on the St. Lawrence River. This evidence convinced both the widow and the local authorities that Foster had drowned. Later, Buchanan received word from his former student, very much alive and well and now in California, enjoying the windfall he had stolen during his brief but lucrative marriage.[2] Whether this story is true in all aspects is impossible to say. However, it bears noting that the list of the EMC graduates for the class of 1870 includes a "W. H. Foster," and in June 1870, the *Philadelphia Inquirer* published an account of a local physician, Walter H. Foster, who disappeared during a fishing trip.[3] This evidence weighs heavily in favor of John Buchanan possessing firsthand knowledge of at least one faked suicide.

There is also evidence that another man, supposedly an "intimate acquaintance" of Buchanan's, considered the same exploit as a way of extricating himself from legal trouble. According to the same journalist who had reported Foster's tale, a Dr. William C. Harbison made detailed preparations to carry out a similar ruse in the mid-1870s, plans that included an impersonator who would jump from a ferryboat as part of a feigned suicide. While this particular faked suicide never came off, it seems plausible that Harbison did contemplate such a plan and was acquainted with Buchanan. Newspaper accounts of Harbison's misadventures in Philadelphia during the 1870s reveal a pattern of behavior that routinely crossed professional and legal lines. Harbison was among the witnesses called by the 1872 Senate committee investigating alleged diploma sales. Questioning before the committee revealed that Harbison was under indictment for perjury at that time and was well aware of his legal right against self-incrimination.[4] Harbison's legal troubles only increased. Between 1875 and 1879, he ran afoul of local authorities on at least four occasions: in 1875, he was charged with the "indecent disposal" of a corpse; in 1876, he was charged with two crimes, malpractice and conspiracy; and and in 1879, he faced multiple charges, including that of being accessory after the fact to an assault, arising from the murder of a young woman.[5] If we are judged by the company we keep, Buchanan's links to Foster and Harbison speak volumes about the man's moral compass.

While Buchanan's knowledge of these episodes may have inspired his "jump" from the ferryboat *Philadelphia* in the early hours of August 17, 1880, his recognition of the need for such a drastic measure probably dated no earlier than the week before. On August 9, Buchanan's brother-in-law, Martin Chapman, allegedly sought out John Norris, proposing a bargain in which Buchanan would relinquish the charter for the EMC and transfer title of the school's property to Norris.[6] In approaching Norris with such a blatant offer, Buchanan and Chapman misjudged their antagonist. Norris had no interest in abandoning his journalistic ambitions for some dubious property. Far from wanting to rest on his professional laurels, Norris's previous exposé of Philadelphia University was merely an early example of his career-long commitment to hands-on investigative journalism, and he was eager to apply and refine the same tactics of methodical evidence gathering he used for that story earlier in 1880 to other stories of skullduggery. Indeed, Norris's tactics against Miller and Philadelphia University, while extremely effective, were little more than a trial run for his campaign against Buchanan and later against even more powerful foes, such as the Philadelphia stockbrokers William and Louis Ladner.[7]

Norris's ambitions, so alien to Buchanan, and his consequent refusal to let go his hold on the EMC story, may have been the proverbial last straw for Buchanan. It left him with few options for derailing his case from tracks now leading inexorably toward conviction and prison. In the two days following Norris's rebuff of Chapman's overture, Buchanan accelerated preparations to stage a faked suicide. Two different press accounts alleged that in the days preceding the August 17 leap from the *Philadelphia*, Buchanan and a young woman believed to be his daughter made inquiries around the wharf of the Market Street ferry in Philadelphia. In each instance, witnesses claimed that the pair asked questions about the ferry schedules and tidal currents on the Delaware River, and in one account, the ship's engineer, John Holton, was said to have calculated the running of the ebb tide for the inquiring couple.[8]

Neither press report explained how Buchanan and the woman with him justified posing such questions without raising undue suspicion, and Holton later denied calculating the ebb tide for them. Moreover, after his initial testimony confirming his belief that it was Buchanan who jumped from the ferry, Holton recanted that part of his statement. The threat of perjury charges may have contributed to the vehemence of Holton's denial concerning the alleged conversation.

Setting aside Holton's denial, identifying the specific ferry from which to stage the jump was one of the first practical tasks Buchanan had to complete to move the plan forward. Despite some potential drawbacks, the *Philadelphia* was a natural choice, since Buchanan had routinely used this ferry over the years in traveling between the city and his residence in New Jersey. His presence on the *Philadelphia*, therefore, would hardly appear suspicious, as it mirrored his prior routine. Moreover, Holton was well-acquainted with Buchanan from years earlier, when he had been a student of the dean at the EMC.[9]

Regardless of whether Holton had prior knowledge of the scheme or simply participated in its execution, he could play the critical role of corroborating witness, testifying to Buchanan's presence. As long as Holton had observed the doctor's impersonator boarding the boat, and provided that the lighting conditions and impersonator's disguise were adequate, he might testify in good faith that he believed Buchanan to have been onboard, whether he observed the actual jump or not. As events transpired, the presence on board of crew member Joseph Middleton the night of the jump offered a second corroborating witness. Middleton knew Buchanan by sight from long years when his work on the ferry coincided with the doctor's frequent trips across the Delaware River.[10]

The drawbacks to using the *Philadelphia* derived from two critical elements. First, the press might uncover Holton's past association with Buchanan and seize upon this connection to raise doubts. Second, alert readers familiar with the *Philadelphia*'s daily route might find their suspicions aroused by the fact that the ferry ran between Smith and Windmill Islands, both landmarks potentially reachable by a swimmer. Such drawbacks could not compete with the urgency of Buchanan's need, however. With his August 17 hearing fast approaching, he must have decided that the *Philadelphia* would have to be the site of the faked suicide, since an even more pressing problem awaited resolution—securing an imposter for the leap.

On the evening of August 11, a closed carriage with several passengers pulled up to the home of Thomas Coyle in nearby Linwood, Pennsylvania. Coyle, a former U.S. marine now working in the shipyard at

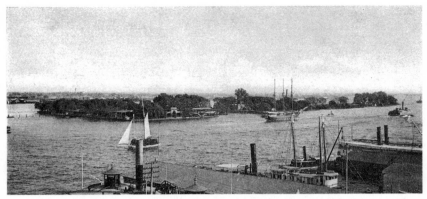

Fig. 13. Smith and Windmill Islands. In 1880, a Buchanan imposter jumped over-board as the ferryboat *Philadelphia* approached these islands in the middle of the Delaware River. For a brief period, many believed the drowning suicide. Image courtesy of Adam Levine Collection/PhillyH2o.org.

Chester, had won local celebrity as a sportsman. In 1875, for a $1,000 prize, he had waged a highly publicized long-distance swimming match against J. B. Johnson, an English swimmer widely renowned as the first man to attempt swimming the English Channel. Although Coyle failed to defeat Johnson in their thirteen-mile swim down the Delaware (he surrendered the effort after ten miles), the feat established him as a swimming champion on the Eastern Seaboard. For several years before 1880, Coyle's name periodically appeared in local newspaper reports of his latest distance swimming challenges.[11]

One of the passengers in the carriage, James Longbotham, stepped down from the rig and knocked on the door, asking for Coyle. Hearing that he was away that evening, Longbotham left a message with Coyle's son, claiming he worked with a newspaper interested in writing a story on his father. He urged the boy to have his father contact him at his saloon near the train depot in Chester, Pennsylvania. Intrigued by the prospect of further press coverage Coyle did visit Longbotham at the saloon several nights later, on August 14. After some preliminary conversation, Longbotham broached the critical question. Could Coyle jump from a moving ferry on the Delaware River and swim to safety? When Coyle answered that he could, Longbotham took the plunge. Telling Coyle "I've got a job for you, then," Longbotham offered to pay Coyle $50 to jump from a moving ferry into the Delaware and swim toward a waiting skiff. He then added the kicker: Coyle would have to make the jump in disguise, sporting a pair of false side-whiskers and wearing padding under his shirt to make him appear heavyset. Longbotham declined to elaborate further. He assured Coyle that he would contact him later with details of the exact time and place for the jump.[12]

By the time the two men separated that evening, they appeared to have reached an understanding. As it turned out, each man had read the other well enough that both were soon making alternative plans. Coyle left that night initially pleased with the prospect of easy money. As time went on, however, he became increasingly concerned about the nature of the job—specifically, the vague circumstances surrounding the jump and the deferral of its details until later. Finally, Coyle reached the un-settling conclusion that the job might be a ploy to cover up a murder. Sufficiently alarmed by the conversation, he alerted the Chester police.[13] Meanwhile, Longbotham must have sensed Coyle's suspicion, despite his acceptance of the job. He raised his concerns with Martin Chapman, who had accompanied him to Coyle's residence several nights earlier, and one or both men decided to secure someone else for the job. A man known only by the last name of Shepard finally accepted the offer.[14]

Whether at the urging of the police or prompted by his own curiosity, Coyle called on Longbotham at the latter's home several days later, on Monday, August 16. The saloon keeper was absent, but in a conversation with his mother, Coyle was led to believe that the matter requiring his services had been "dropped" after a long discussion by Longbotham and several men who had visited her son the day before.[15] Coyle departed, believing that the scheme—whatever its true nature—had been aban-doned. He had no way of knowing that Buchanan or his friends had se-cured another swimmer for the jump planned for later that same night.

Earlier that day, the U.S. district court judge had called up Buchan-an's case for mail fraud. The grand jury delivered a true bill, and an ir-ritated Judge Butler asked the lawyer William Mann why his client was not present. Explaining that ill health had confined Buchanan to bed at his New Jersey home, Mann assured the judge that the doctor would be present in court the following day. Despite the prosecutor's protests that Buchanan should forfeit his bail for his failure to appear, Butler agreed to hold the matter over until the following day, August 17.[16] Meanwhile,

John Buchanan had already slipped quietly out of the area, making his way toward New York City and from there farther west.

Later that night, events unfolded aboard the *Philadelphia* much as they had been planned. Thomas Vanduser accompanied a disguised Shepard onto the boat after midnight. They created several brief, seemingly casual encounters between the faux Dr. Buchanan and other passengers aboard the ferry to ensure that there would be witnesses able to attest to Buchanan's presence on the boat that night. The pair exchanged a brief, almost passing, greeting with Holton as they boarded the ship. Shepard kept his face down and his words to a minimum during the exchange. Vanduser and Shepard then approached one of the passengers and proffered their fare—a minor incident intended to create another witness who might testify to having seen Buchanan alive and on board the ship before the suicide leap. While no meeting occurred between the fake Buchanan and Middleton, the other crew member who knew the doctor by sight, the conspirators prepared the ground for testimony from Middleton as well: at one point on the brief trip, when Middleton was within sight and hearing of Vanduser and Shepard, Vanduser made sure to clearly address Buchanan by name.

For his part, Vanduser had only to act naturally while steering the bogus Buchanan into the line of sight of potential witnesses and engaging in conversation that included speaking the doctor's name aloud. Vanduser played his role well, though too dramatically for the skeptical reporters who later descended on the scene of the suicide. Once Shepard (in his guise as Buchanan) had leapt from the ferry, Vanduser raised the alarm, shouting, "My God, Dr. Buchanan has jumped overboard!" His subsequent tears at the shocking demise of his friend—witnesses said he "cried like a child"—struck some as more theatrical than genuine.[17]

Meanwhile, Shepard timed his jump for the point in the river where the ferry approached the channel running between Smith and Windmill Islands. Once in the water, he swam for a small skiff waiting conveniently nearby in the shadow of some trees overhanging the bank of one of the islands. He grabbed the edge, and the man or men on board moved the craft silently downriver, aiming steadily toward the Jersey shore.[18]

The conspirators planned the fake suicide reasonably well. They had procured the necessary swimmer/impersonator, arranged for a skiff, checked the tides, and ensured that a sufficient number of witnesses would see the jump or at least be able to identify the jumper as Buchanan. More-over, in the days before the jump, the real Buchanan had set the stage with actions, both real and feigned, designed to create the portrait of a despon-dent man. Police special agent Thomas Barrett later recalled Buchanan receiving a letter while in police custody that left the doctor visibly upset. He recalled Buchanan looking up after reading the letter and telling him, "I have nothing to live for . . . Time was when they were glad to assist me. Now all have deserted me." When Buchanan broke down, seemingly on the verge of an apoplectic fit, Barrett found him sufficiently convincing that he sent for a doctor. Reporters flocked to interview Buchanan's wife Lucy after the suicide. She described her husband's increasingly distraught condition as he awaited his approaching court date. She said he had been behaving erratically, several times attempting to go out in public less than fully clothed, for example. She claimed to have found and taken from him a bottle of laudanum. And she said she had made it a practice to keep a firm hold on his arm when they were out walking, for fear that he might wander away, intending to harm himself.[19] Some of Buchanan's anguish must have been real, though his actions were probably a mix of genuine and sham behavior.

Despite these preparations, it soon became apparent that neither the local press nor the police believed the suicide. The *Philadelphia Inquirer* expressed early skepticism. "Death or Fraud?" blared the headline from its first story on the incident, and in the article that followed, the pur-ported facts of the suicide shared equal time with disclaimers and cau-tionary notes. Phrases like "the drowning ruse" expressed the press's suspicions about the story. The *Inquirer* commented skeptically on the timing of the jump, noting that it occurred near a "favorable point" in the river that made a safe landfall on Smith or Windfall Island as likely an outcome as drowning. The *Philadelphia Record* quoted a night watch-man for a chemical company located on the Jersey side of Windmill Is-land who claimed that he had seen a small boat containing three people at around 1:15 A.M. on the night in question. In the eyes of the press, Buchanan remained what he had been for years, a "slippery customer" whose entire career had been so "crooked" that one could easily believe that he might orchestrate such a fraud. Philadelphia's police chief, Samuel Givin, shared this skepticism, characterizing the entire affair as "fishy."[20] Givin then claimed to "know" that Buchanan had been in Philadelphia, as creditors or bailsmen were "looking for him."[21] While the *Inquirer* attributed skepticism of the story to others, the local press sounded the harshest notes. "Until the dead body of the world renowned 'doctor' is found," the *Philadelphia Inquirer* asserted, "there will not be many to believe that the reported suicide has any foundation in fact."[22]

While it was not commented upon publicly at the time, the same story related another small but telling detail in its account of the suicide. Buchanan allegedly "pulled off his coat" before throwing himself overboard. This behavior seemed odd for someone supposedly intent on self-instruction. Why take off the coat? Such an action was consistent, not with suicide but with an effort to avoid the weight of waterlogged clothing while feigning suicide and making a hurried swim to safety. The weight of a wet coat might turn an intended short swim into a genuine drowning. Ironically, Thomas Coyle later published a short work entitled *Everybody a Swimmer* (1884), in which he cautioned readers on the inherent danger of swimming fully clothed in deep water. "Very few persons, even good swimmers, ever try the experiment of swimming with their clothes on . . . [i]f they should try it once they would be convinced of the great necessity of getting out of their clothes the first thing on being dumped overboard."[23]

From the conspirators' perspective, the coat had been necessary to give added bulk to the impersonator attempting to pass for Buchanan. It had also provided a vehicle for planting evidence attesting to Buchanan's troubled state of mind. Vanduser made sure that others, including the press, saw the crumpled newspaper inside the coat with its margin notes scribbled on the pages. The marginalia contained directives to his children: "Isabella: You must do what is for the best. Save all you can out of the wreck . . . George and you should work together—blood is thicker than water. It is all over and I am mad. We will sell the museum first and then the college."[24]

While the coat and its contents served a practical purpose in the suicide ruse, in the context of the publicity Buchanan's case had received in recent months, no experienced police detective or astute journalist would have missed the curious detail of its removal before the jump. They immediately recognized it for what it was—a telling piece of evidence pointing to an elaborate ruse. John Norris and the *Philadelphia Record* not only shared the *Inquirer*'s skepticism, they soon commenced a surveillance operation that ultimately led them to Buchanan.

In the meantime, speculation abounded among those convinced that Buchanan had fled the state and perhaps even the country. One of the first public signals hinting that authorities had picked up Buchanan's trail came from Pittsburgh. Less than forty-eight hours after the alleged suicide, with no body having yet surfaced, a telegram arrived from John H. Skelton in Pittsburgh. He posed a blunt question to Philadelphia police: "Is there any reward for Dr. Buchanan? If so, how much? Answer." Within that same forty-eight hours, other telling details appeared in print indicating that the police and the press were making progress in their investigations. The overtures made to Thomas Coyle appeared in the newspapers, along with an account of the sighting of several men in a boat near the *Philadelphia* soon after the alleged suicide.

Further troubling evidence appeared when an investigation began on August 19 in federal court to determine the liability of the bondsmen who had provided Buchanan's bail. The *Philadelphia*'s engineer, John Holton, called the first day, testified that a man he believed to be Buchanan had approached him on the *Philadelphia* that night, shaking his hand and offering a quick pleasantry as he passed by. The judge pressed him for a definitive identification.

Judge: "Was it Dr. Buchanan?"
Holton: "That was my impression."
Judge: "What makes you doubt it?"
Holton: "I don't doubt it."
Judge: "Have you any reason to doubt it?"
Holton: "I have no particular reason to doubt it with the exception that when he spoke to me his voice was hoarse and his hand was rough and hard, but in every other way it was Dr. Buchanan."[25]

Holton's testimony appeared cautious at best. He seemed to be trying to identify the man who jumped from the ferry as Buchanan while leaving himself a small window through which to extricate himself should the unfolding circumstances warrant such an action.

Holton also told the press of a much earlier conversation he had had with Buchanan. Several years earlier, Holton recalled, the doctor had been aboard the same ferry when someone fell overboard and drowned close to the spot where the recent leap had occurred. A shaken Buchanan had commented, "If I dropped there I would sink like a stone."[26]

Given Holton's prior connection with Buchanan, many saw this anecdote as too convenient. Holton had probably conspired to some degree in a plot that was quickly and unexpectedly falling apart because so many people simply refused to accept the suicide as genuine. Now he was stuck. It was one thing to offer corroborating testimony of a death everyone quickly accepts without question; it was quite another to corroborate a death that few accepted and that both the police and the press were actively investigating as a fake. Holton's testimony showed the discomfort of someone struggling to follow the script of a cover story unraveling under public scrutiny.

In his court testimony the following week, Thomas Vanduser, the other key witness, stuck more closely than Holton to the script, but by then it was too late. The police and press had uncovered too much evidence inconsistent with a suicide. With Buchanan's home already under surveillance, watchful authorities noted a visit there by Vanduser, together with the delivery of "provisions" in quantities sufficient to arouse suspicion. Moreover, Martin Chapman had apparently left the city. Inquiries at his residence showed that he had been absent for a week already.[27] By August 20, Philadelphians were no longer asking, "Did you hear about Dr. Buchanan?" The question had become, "Do you think they'll catch Dr. Buchanan?"

Over the next few days, those who speculated that Buchanan had pulled off his escape began to think they might be right. The *New York Herald* published claims by a Pittsburgh veterinarian named Jennings asserting not only that Buchanan was alive but that he knew where he was hiding. However, rumors that Buchanan's arrest was imminent came to nothing.[28] With newspapers unable to confirm the various alleged sightings of Buchanan in New Jersey and Delaware, a brief public silence fell over the story. Yet one such sighting may well have been true: a barber in Wilmington, Delaware, claimed to have shaved Buchanan's muttonchop whiskers and dyed his hair.[29]

One of the few voices contradicting the skepticism regarding John Buchanan's purported death belonged to Lucy Buchanan. In an interview published August 23, the grieving widow asserted her belief in the doctor's death, citing the eyewitness testimony to the leap from the boat and her husband's "decrepit" physical and mental condition just before the incident, when he had displayed "fits of insanity." Several days earlier, she had posted an advertisement offering $150 for the recovery of her husband's body. It remains possible she was a coconspirator, but several of her statements to the press expressed concern that she would be held responsible for the $12,000 posted by the bail bondsmen, for which her home and property had been used as security. Her belief in the suicide was also supported by her bizarre story of being approached for money. She said she had been contacted by a stranger—a "man in a navy suit"—who met with her away from her home and claimed that her husband was safe with friends in Pittsburgh. The man then told her that he had been sent by Buchanan, who required money immediately, to collect $200 from her. When Mrs. Buchanan refused to pay the stranger and said he should go to the police, he hurriedly withdrew. Whether this episode was a botched extortion scam or a real attempt by Buchanan to contact Lucy is unclear. Her comments to the press and later divorce proceedings seem to imply that she was victimized by her spouse.[30]

Finally, on August 24, the *Detroit Free Press* carried the breaking news— John Buchanan had been located in the area, moving between hideouts in Michigan and across the border in Canada. At some time before the faked suicide, Buchanan had left Philadelphia for Camden, where he had boarded a train for New York and from there made his way west into Canada. Having traveled so far and so quickly, the doctor probably felt he had passed beyond immediate danger. That feeling did not last very long.

STRANGE WANDERINGS

On the evening of August 23, 1880, John Buchanan left his room at the International Hotel in Windsor, Canada, and sauntered up and down Sandwich Street, a cane in one hand, occasionally clasping both hands behind his back in a nonchalant manner. As he walked, he may have been reflecting on the chain of events that had turned his life upside down and brought him to this small Canadian town, just across the Detroit River. He may have been thinking about his family in Philadelphia. He may even have felt a little smug about having "slipped the shackles off" right under the noses of his pursuers. As he had once admitted to an acquaintance, years before, Yankee types had always irked him with their boastful veneration of American "wisdom" and their disparaging remarks about the "gillies" from Scotland. More than once, his opponents had believed they had caught him "dead to rights" and all but "bound and chained," yet now he seemed to have outwitted them all.[31]

John Buchanan had fled west hoping to reestablish himself. Traveling under the name Fairchild as a precautionary measure, he was attracted by the prospect of starting his life anew, without all the baggage of the diploma mill accusations associated with his real name of Buchanan. Talks with fellow eclectic physicians had made him hopeful about establishing a medical school in Michigan or Canada, but discussions nearly two weeks earlier with several Detroit-area physicians and businessmen had not borne immediate fruit.[32] He may have hoped that the arrival of his brother-in-law Martin Chapman would revive these prospects.[33]

As Buchanan approached Mackenzie Hall, he turned to retrace his steps. Then a young man addressed him with "Good evening, Dr. Fairchild." Buchanan stopped short.

"I beg your pardon, sir, but you have me at an advantage." The young man identified himself as a reporter for the *Detroit Free Press*, whose assignment was to obtain an interview with the infamous Dr. Buchanan of Philadelphia. "Well, young man," the doctor replied, "I am glad to meet you but I don't know how I can help you to find Buchanan."

The reporter pressed on. "Now, Doctor, you are all right over here; won't you tell me squarely, aren't you Buchanan?"

As the two men walked along, Buchanan showed no signs of breaking off the conversation—but also no intention of letting down his guard. "My name is Fairchild, . . . not Buchanan. Is that square enough for you?"[34]

The young reporter was already impressed. One of the men present at Buchanan's meeting with Detroit physicians had accompanied him to Windsor and then pointed out Buchanan (aka Fairchild) as he came walking down the street. The reporter had to think quickly. His journalistic ambush had failed to surprise or shake the man. So now the reporter tried a line of questioning designed to show Buchanan just how much the *Detroit Free Press* already knew about his whereabouts and activities. "Why did you leave Detroit so suddenly and secretly if you are Fairchild and not Buchanan?" the reporter asked.

"How do you know I have been in Detroit?" the doctor asked in return.

"Because I saw you there," the reporter replied, " . . . on two different occasions."

Thinking fast and speaking confidingly, Buchanan produced a quick and plausible lie based on mistaken identity. "Well, I'll tell you why I left. There is a reward of $600 offered for the arrest of Buchanan and I felt that as everybody who had been introduced to me believed me to be Buchanan, that out of them all there might be one who would cause my arrest on suspicion just for the sake of the reward. . . . I have business to do. I can't afford to be detained."

Having gained Buchanan's admission that he had been in Detroit, the reporter pressed further, asking for details, such as when had he left Detroit. Apparently content to continue the conversation, Buchanan confessed that he had been in Detroit the previous day. Recognizing that the doctor was not going to budge on his identity, the reporter now took a different tack, asking, "Do you know Buchanan?"

"I used to know a physician of that name in Philadelphia, and he was a talented man," the doctor replied.

The reporter picked up on the use of the past tense. "Do you think he committed suicide and is dead?"

By this time, the pair was approaching the depot yard. In the fading daylight, the older man paused, leaning against a fence, and offered a surprising reply. "Well, to be frank with you, young man, I do not think the suicide story is true."

The reporter now returned more forcefully to the question of identity. There was no reason to maintain the charade; each man understood that the other knew the truth. The reporter repeatedly pressed "Dr. Fairchild" to drop the pretense and admit his true identity as the fugitive doctor from Philadelphia. But while John Buchanan may have admired the young man's pluck in pursuing him and the story into Windsor, he was no innocent, rattled by a few questions. He had accumulated a decade of experience in parrying accusations and questions from the Philadelphia press, legislators, and local officials. He finally asked a question of his own that put an end to the interview. "Now, as a newspaper reporter and a man accustomed to the study of character and circumstances, would you expect me, even if I were Buchanan, to admit the fact to you or any other reporter, under the present circumstances?" The reporter acknowledged that such a confession to the press was too much to expect. He then offered a cigar to the doctor as they resumed their walk. The conversation grew more casual. The doctor commented on the beauty of the Detroit

River and the many virtues of the city until it was time for the reporter to board the ferry back to Detroit.

The reporter returned with his notes to the offices of the *Detroit Free Press* to write his story. Any disappointment he felt at failing to extract a confession was tempered by his certainty that "Dr. Fairchild" was in fact Buchanan. Not only had his companion positively identified Fairchild as Buchanan but the doctor's conversation seemed to obliquely confirm his identity while denying it. The doctor's responses to the reporter's questions had seemed like a ritual exchange: two men going through the motions of a charade in which each knows that the other knows the truth. Having taken the measure of the man, the reporter evinced an unexpected respect for the scoundrel, telling his readers that John Buchanan "is a shrewd, educated and self-possessed person and well-calculated to take care of himself."

Although the Detroit reporter came away impressed with his subject's apparently unflappable demeanor, it was merely a façade. Upon returning to his room, Buchanan packed his belongings, paid his bill, and departed the hotel. When the reporter returned on August 24 to continue the dialogue, he could not find Buchanan. Moreover the reporter soon learned that Buchanan or an accomplice had planted several false trails for pursuers to follow, involving the purchases of train tickets to multiple destinations, including New York; Toronto; and London, Ontario.[35] Buchanan had also dropped a letter in the mail to the *Detroit Free Press*. Writing as Dr. Fairchild, he claimed to be experiencing unfair harassment in a case of mistaken identity with Buchanan. To add verisimilitude, the doctor had had someone else write out the letter he had composed, so that its handwriting would confirm his separate identity from Buchanan. Later, Buchanan further disguised his trail by having a friend who was heading back to Philadelphia mail another letter by "Fairchild" from New York.[36]

Windsor, Canada, was the first of many stops in Buchanan's peripatetic journey through towns and villages in Ontario. Over a period of less than four weeks, Buchanan spent time in Windsor, Chatham, London, Bothwell, Courtright, and St. Clair. In part, these moves served to keep the doctor one step ahead of detectives anxious to collect the reward for his capture and reporters eager for a story, now that the *Detroit Free Press* had announced his presence. However, the primary reason behind these moves was the failure of Buchanan's original plans in Detroit.

Buchanan had intended to join forces with friends in the Detroit eclectic community as the first step toward opening a medical school, either there or across the river in Canada. It appears that Buchanan had for some time been considering abandoning Philadelphia entirely for a fresh start in Michigan. At the time of his arrest, Buchanan held a number of shares in a medical school incorporated that same year as the Detroit Eclectic College. Although the school never became operational, several individuals with connections to the EMC took part in a later effort to open it as the Detroit University for Rational Medicine and Surgery. This group included former EMC faculty members John J. Siggins and Phillip Bissell, as well as several EMC diploma holders—E. Payne, W. C. Roney, and F. C. Waters—now listed as faculty for the Detroit endeavor.[37]

After one or two meetings on the scene in Detroit, however, Buchanan was convinced the planned college would not materialize, and he decided to relocate to San Francisco instead. To do so, though, the doctor's dwindling finances would require an infusion of cash, and to raise that cash, Buchanan sold a pair of American University diplomas in the Detroit area for $30, holding several more blank diplomas in reserve.[38] Perhaps deeming further diploma sales too risky, he instead staged a series of lectures and exhibitions under assumed names as a way of raising money without staying too long in any one town.

After leaving Windsor, the doctor traveled approximately thirty miles east to Chatham, arriving on August 25. He checked into the Rankin House under the name of H. E. Darling and announced that he was acting as an advance man for W. W. Mumey,[39] a professor and lecturer on phrenology and the "science of new life." There "Mr. Darling" (aka Buchanan) set about distributing handbills and advertisements for a lecture by Mumey, scheduled for several days later. That lecture, entitled "Love, Courtship, Marriage and Divorce," came off as planned on Saturday, August 28, though it is unclear how much revenue the event raised. Buchanan served as the ticket taker but took no active part in the lecture otherwise.

Monday afternoon's *Chatham Planet* carried a tepid review of the lecture, or at least Mumey perceived it as such and sent word to the newspaper that he wished to discuss the notice at his hotel room. Surprised by the lecturer's immediate reaction to the piece, a journalist from the newspaper met Mumey and Buchanan at the hotel, only to be surprised by his unexpectedly "gracious" reception. Mumey did all the talking, while Buchanan stood to the side, quietly listening to the conversation.

While expressing his displeasure at the unfavorable review, Mumey acknowledged that he was "not much of a lecturer." Then he divulged the real source of his disappointment. Mumey and his colleagues planned to open an "electro-therapeutical institute" in Windsor, and his lecture in Chatham was the first in a series of talks designed to "introduce" him to the citizens of Ontario. He complained that the *Planet*'s notice had "killed him" in the eyes of the public and threatened an enterprise into which he had already invested several thousand dollars. Then, after remarking wistfully that he would gladly have paid money to have the notice buried, Mumey asked if the newspaper might be willing to omit the review from the material they would be forwarding to the Windsor and Detroit newspapers.[40]

Mumey and Buchanan were right to have been concerned about the effect of the tepid review. Between word of mouth and the *Chatham Planet*'s notice, the turnout for that night's lecture proved disappointing, and the following night saw another dismal result. On September 1, Buchanan made a day trip by train into Windsor for unknown reasons, and on September 2, Buchanan and Mumey traveled ten miles northeast of Chatham to the town of Bothwell. There the two distributed handbills for an evening lecture featuring Mumey as "Professor Robinson." Bothwell was a small town characterized by one reporter as "a sequestered nook," off the beaten path even by the standards of rural Ontario.[41] Apparently, the two men hoped the combination of a new name for the featured lecturer (Robinson) and the relatively isolated location would provide a venue untainted by their lackluster reception at Chatham. That same day, they were joined by Buchanan's brother-in-law, Martin Chapman.[42]

The Bothwell lecture, entitled "The Human Body and Its Illnesses," met with little more success than the earlier efforts at Chatham, however. Only a "small audience" paid to attend, and the sparse turnout so disappointed Buchanan that he refused to participate in the lecture as they had planned for that night. Instead, Martin Chapman entertained the audience for an hour, speaking and showing pictures using a "magic lantern" device.[43] Buchanan's refusal to participate signaled a growing sense of frustration. Lecturing as a fund-raising tactic was not going well.

Buchanan's prior trip into Windsor on September 1 may have included further talks with Detroit-area physicians about a medical school, but a more likely reason for the quick trip was to arrange for the arrival of Chapman and a young Philadelphia woman, Norah Leonard. Chapman's whereabouts had been a matter of interest to the police and the press for several weeks. He had vacated his residence at 323 South Eighth Street at some point before Buchanan's faked suicide, and although he did testify before a Philadelphia magistrate on August 25, on matters related to the Buchanan case, his whereabouts were otherwise unknown.[44]

Chapman may have been keeping Buchanan informed about events in Philadelphia, but the two men were together in Canada when Buchanan received a financially devastating piece of news. On September 4, 1880, the U.S. district court, in consideration of the mounting evidence contradicting Buchanan's alleged suicide, declared Buchanan's bail forfeited. With his bondsmen now responsible for the $12,000 bail, the doctor's home and property in Pennsylvania and New Jersey were at risk.[45] Subsequent press reports soon placed Buchanan, Chapman, Mumey, and Leonard forty miles away in London, Ontario, for the strangest event in the fugitive's lecture series—a séance before a crowd of several hundred people.

Nineteenth-century America offered fertile ground for spiritualism, a quasi-religious movement without the formal trappings of church credo or canon. The immediate origins of the spiritualist movement can be traced to upstate New York. The intense religious fervor and revivalism flaring up in the region during the early nineteenth century have led some historians to nickname the region the burned over district—an appellation signaling the smoldering aftereffects of the area's emotional religious revival activities. What spiritualism produced in bountiful supply were self-styled mediums, seers, and clairvoyants, who succeeded in sweeping up large numbers of credulous believers and depositing them in exhibitions of communications with the dead or spirit world. Skeptics saw nothing at work in spiritualism but the intersection of human foibles—specifically, naïveté and greed—with cranks, hoaxers, and hucksters separating a gullible public from their money. The national momentum behind spiritualism accelerated in the late 1840s, with widespread public notice of the writings of the Poughkeepsie seer Andrew Jackson Davis and the spirit rappings of the Fox sisters from Hydesville, New York.

Presuming that a fugitive on the run would prefer to keep a low profile and avoid publicity, Buchanan's decision to arrange for a spiritualist evening might seem irrational. Yet, the idea did possess some elements of logic. John Buchanan knew and understood many human motives and foibles. It was his comprehension of the human desire to gain an advantage through shortcut or subterfuge, for example, that allowed him to profit for so long from the sale of diplomas. Now Buchanan was displaying his knowledge of other elements of human nature: people's curiosity and excitement about the unknown and, for some, a willingness to suspend disbelief if doing so could assuage pain over loss. Both of these human traits were at work in making spirit evenings or séances so popular among nineteen-century Americans. People enjoyed participating in these events whether they genuinely believed in communication with the afterworld or simply found it entertaining to be "in on the hoax" amidst a group of true believers. Regardless of the audience members' motives for attending, self-styled mediums exploited these spirit evenings for profit.

John Buchanan had probably witnessed such performances firsthand, as an estimated three hundred self-styled mediums and clairvoyants were operating out of Philadelphia by 1870. In 1874, that city's newspapers devoted considerable column space to the massive popularity of the mediums Nelson and Jennie Holmes. The couple claimed to be channeling the spirit of Katie King, daughter of the pirate Henry Morgan, through a materializing cabin in their small apartment at Ninth and Arch Street—a leisurely walk from Buchanan's office and the EMC.[46] Now Buchanan—in desperate financial straits after his bond forfeiture several days earlier—agreed to the proposed séance. While he may not have relished the idea, he probably thought the event presented a guaranteed payday.

The program scheduled for Tuesday evening, September 7, called for a "spiritualistic entertainment" by renowned medium J. Foster (Buchanan) and his assistants, T. J. Peeples (Chapman) and Emma Stuart (Lucy Mumey).[47] They promoted the affair as "spiritualism on trial," with the audience serving as jurors. Their handbills threw out an entertaining challenge: "If there is any truth in spiritualism, it is your duty to know it." Unlike the magic lantern lectures the group had delivered elsewhere in Ontario, the spiritualist evening drew a large crowd of between four hundred and five hundred people. Unfortunately for Buchanan, though, the windfall from this crowd never materialized. Quite simply, he and his

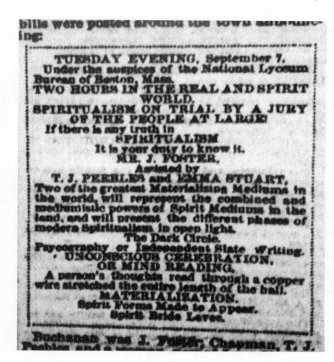

Fig. 14. A spiritualist evening. On the run and low on money, Buchanan tried to raise funds through public lectures conducted under pseudonyms, including the séance in London, Ontario, being publicized in this handbill. Image courtesy of Newspaper Department, Free Library of Philadelphia.

colleagues were out of their element. They failed to understand that their sizable audience had come looking for entertainment. The crowd wanted a theatrical performance, not a scientific lecture. Given that Chapman and Mumey had previously taken the lead in the lectures at Chatham and Bothwell, Buchanan's more prominent role in the London event seems surprising, but perhaps he was under pressure from his companions to take the lead. He may have embraced the opportunity, sanguine about his ability to talk his way through the part and confident that he could dazzle a backwater audience just as he had medical students, colleagues, and local officials in Philadelphia. He probably reasoned that the same voluble lecturing style that served him so well at the EMC would suffice for this Canadian audience.

The later press accounts of the evening portrayed John Buchanan in a highly unflattering fashion, however. Reporters claimed that he "mumble[ed] a few words" and beat a hasty retreat from the stage. Even if Buchanan was out of his element in such a theatrical setting, it remains striking that he faltered so badly in this venue and at a time when he needed money so urgently. One might expect that his experience and performance in other potentially nerve-racking scenarios (lecturing students, giving testimony before a senate committee, responding to ambush interviews by the press) would have adequately prepared him to at least get through his performance. Yet press accounts of the event leave some things unclear. Since they do not provide the chronology for that evening, Buchanan's turn on stage may have followed Chapman's. If so, Buchanan's poor performance might be explained as a reaction to the crowd's rowdy and suspicious reception of Chapman.

Chapman's turn in front of the audience started well. He recruited volunteers from the audience to tie his hands in multiple knots and then place him in a cabinet from which he would either "ring a bell" inside the cabinet or entice the spirits to "pull some fellow's ear." Chapman seemed pleased with what he and his colleagues had developed for their audience, believing he was giving the crowd "an elegant entertainment." Apparently, elegance was no substitute for more spectacular conjuring. The crowd soon started demanding that Chapman provide the kind of theatrical flourishes that audiences had come to expect from spiritualist performances. Hecklers began to interrupt Chapman with cries of "Give us a ghost!" and "Float an angel!" An exasperated Chapman later confided, "They wanted us to do some materializing . . . if we had known they wanted an angel, we would rigged one up." It seems Chapman had neglected to read the handbills they had printed for the affair. Buchanan and his colleagues had promised to deliver the standard fare of a spiritualist exhibition: "the dark circle . . . independent slate writing . . . mind reading" and "spirit forms made to appear . . . [and] levitate."[48] Chapman may have been ignorant of, or have forgotten, the extent of the theatrics hinted at in these handbills; clearly the audience had not.

Perhaps fearing the potential for physical mischief from the frustrated crowd, Buchanan cut short his turn on stage. He and Chapman slipped quietly out of the building at the first opportune moment. As the evening dissolved into an affair of "money be damned and every man for himself," the hasty departure of the two performers left Mumey, acting that night as ticket taker and cashier, to face a disgruntled audience seeking a refund. Authorities arrested Mumey, but soon released him. Newspaper reports of the evening were vague on the financial resolution to the matter but implied that Buchanan and Chapman had left town with at least some of the night's proceeds.

CAPTURED

John Buchanan's travels continued for several days after the debacle in London. He and Chapman remained in Ontario, first traveling to Komoka and then another forty miles to Sarnia, near where the St. Clair River drains into Lake Huron. By now, after nearly three weeks on the road and constant relocations from one town and hotel to another, Buchanan was tired. As his anxiety increased, so too did the precautions the group was taking. Buchanan traveled in disguise. Gone were his muttonchop whiskers and stylish collar-length hair. Now he was clean shaven except for a bristly black mustache, and his closely cropped hair was dyed to a dark hue. Buchanan continued to register at hotels under an assumed name, but now he spent even more time in his hotel room, venturing out in public less frequently. He also took another precaution: he made sure that his hotel room came equipped with a rope fire ladder. It would allow his escape should he be caught unawares on the second or third floor of a hotel.[49] If all these precautions were to fail and Buchanan was arrested, he had lined up several Detroit-area physicians willing to testify that he was not the fugitive, John Buchanan, but a physician colleague they had know for many years and the victim of mistaken identity.[50] Buchanan's fears were neither paranoid nor spiritualistic. They were realistic. As Buchanan moved around Ontario after the London séance, he was being hunted by John Norris and a small party of journalists and representatives of the law—and they were closing in.[51]

During his travels, Buchanan continued to communicate with friends back in Philadelphia. One press account claimed that he did so through letters in a disguised hand to a Job Green on Pine Street, and through unsigned telegrams to a George Lathrop. He may have routed other communications through an attorney he secured in Windsor or via Martin Chapman. Whatever Buchanan's methods, at least one line of communication was soon compromised. Norris, his colleagues, and the *Detroit Free Press* began tracking Buchanan through Norah Leonard. She had been in Windsor with Buchanan on August 23. When Buchanan slipped away after the encounter with the *Free Press* reporter, so, too, did Leonard. Norris's contacts picked up Leonard's trail, tracking her until she rejoined Buchanan, Chapman, and Mumey.[52]

Norris succeeded in tracking and capturing Buchanan for several reasons, including a large measure of good fortune. First, Norah Leonard apparently never suspected that she was being shadowed or her communications monitored. She inadvertently helped to close the net on Buchanan when she doubled back to the group before their London séance. Second, Norris had help from the *Detroit Free Press*. The Philadelphia journalist and the Detroit newspaper joined forces to maximize their chance of success. Norris had essential background information. He not only could identify Buchanan by sight but knew the doctor's contacts and connections in Philadelphia. For their part, the reporters of the *Free Press* had the physical proximity to Buchanan in late August to monitor his location and actions at various points, especially once they had found Norah Leonard's trail. Norris brokered a deal between his paper, the *Philadelphia Record*, and the *Detroit Free Press* that gave both papers first rights in printing all aspects of the story. Finally, despite Buchanan's many changes of location in Canada, the various Ontario towns he visited were all near the U.S.-Canadian border, making him easier to track. If Buchanan had moved farther inland or gone farther west, he might well have escaped. But by remaining so close to the border—within sixty miles and often much closer—Buchanan made it easier for Norris to coordinate the multi-jurisdictional efforts required to apprehend him.

John Norris's commitment to pursuing Buchanan is not hard to understand. From the moment the first reports of Buchanan's suicide hit the newsroom at the *Philadelphia Record*, Norris had doubted the story, and the details that emerged only heightened his suspicions. Having worked so hard earlier that spring to secure the original evidence against Buchanan, Norris had no intention of letting the doctor slip away from a likely conviction and sentence by the U.S. district court in Philadelphia. Norris approached his newspaper's publisher, William Singerly, and laid out his case for pursuing this new twist in the Buchanan saga. Singerly had already advanced Norris the funds required for his sting of Reverend Miller and Philadelphia University earlier that year, as well as providing the funds to purchase diplomas from Buchanan in Norris's scheme to catch Buchanan by charging him with mail fraud. Once again, Singerly did not disappoint. He assured Norris of sufficient funds to track Buchanan, secure his arrest, and return him to the U.S. district court in Philadelphia. Singerly's financial support allowed Norris and his reporters to thoroughly investigate the alleged suicide, monitor Buchanan's home, follow leads, and ferret out inconsistencies in the witness testimony. During the last week of August, as everyone awaited the decision of the judge in the bond hearing, Norris must have focused heavily on coordinating efforts with the *Detroit Free Press* to track the movements of Buchanan and his party.

The bond hearing was critical to Norris's efforts. While the techni-cal issue at hand was the bondsmen's responsibility for the $12,000 bail set to guarantee Buchanan's appearance in court, in a larger sense, the judge's decision was a *de facto* ruling as to whether Buchanan was alive or dead. If he was alive, he was in default of his bond for having failed to appear. If the judge believed he had committed suicide, his affairs would be more appropriately the business of the probate court. On September 4, the judge ruled Buchanan in default of his bond and ordered his bail forfeited. Norris now had the legal leverage to push authorities to arrest Buchanan—if Norris could find and apprehend him.

Once the bond issue was settled, Norris traveled to Harrisburg, pre-sumably to meet with the Pennsylvania state attorney general, Henry Palmer. The Philadelphia attorney J. Howard Gendell probably joined Norris for the meeting. Norris brought Palmer two critical pieces of in-formation and a key commitment: Buchanan's whereabouts in Ontario, the Pennsylvania district court's ruling that Buchanan was alive, and Sing-erly's financial commitment to fund the pursuit and arrest of the fugitive. Palmer lent a sympathetic ear. Though it was still early in his single term as attorney general, Palmer was establishing a track record that alienated him from the state's corporate and political powers: challenging the re-bates demanded by the railroads, pressing tax suits against large corpora-tions, and declaring unconstitutional a law passed by the state legislature to increase their own pay.[53] Bringing the infamous Dr. John Buchanan to justice would improve his standing in the public eye. Palmer agreed to support Norris and his allies. In his later account of the affair, he gave most of the credit for the state's success in bringing Buchanan to justice to Norris's sleuthing and "perseverance," Gendell's legal work, and the "public spirit" evinced by Singerly in advancing the necessary funds.[54]

Norris and Gendell then set to work to obtain the requisite legal au-thority to detain Buchanan. With Buchanan moving frequently both within Ontario and across the U.S.-Canadian border, this was not an easy task. Although the doctor stayed mostly on Canadian soil, Norris and Gendell hoped to avoid an arrest requiring extradition from Canada—a prospect liable to be time-consuming and potentially frustrating should

Buchanan flee the area before they could obtain the necessary authority for an arrest. They resolved instead to apprehend Buchanan in Michigan. This meant they must either bide their time until he voluntarily recrossed the border or somehow lure him back onto American soil. Deciding on this latter course, they opened communications with Michigan's governor, Charles Croswell.

Norris journeyed to Michigan to meet Croswell, with documents and evidence in hand. Shortly before midnight on the same evening as Buchanan's failed London séance, Norris gained Croswell's agreement to help them apprehend Buchanan as soon as he set foot on Michigan soil. Having gained the governor's pledge to help, Norris took an overnight train to make the seventy-five-mile journey from the governor's home in Adrian, Michigan, to the offices of the *Detroit Free Press*, arriving in Detroit on Wednesday morning, September 8. Norris and colleagues from the *Free Press* then crossed the Detroit River to Windsor, Ontario, where "final arrangements" were being made to lure Buchanan back across the border. That afternoon, Norris retraced his steps to Adrian to collect the "requisition" papers with Governor Croswell's signature and once again took the overnight train to Detroit. Accompanying Norris on this marathon of train trips and meetings was Charles F. Miller, a Philadelphia detective assigned to the case by that city's district attorney.

On Thursday morning, September 9, preparations to capture Buchanan and his colleagues were nearly complete. The doctor and his party were gathering that day at Courtright on the Canadian side of the St. Clair River. *Free Press* reporters journeyed fifty miles northwest to tiny St. Clair, on the U.S. shore immediately opposite Courtright. Meanwhile, Norris and Miller hurried farther north to Port Huron, where they obtained the services of a St. Clair County deputy sheriff who could legally execute the governor's order for Buchanan's arrest. The plan was for Norris, detective Miller, and Deputy Lansing to return to St. Clair by 8:00 P.M., where they would join forces with the *Free Press* reporters. There they all would await Buchanan and his party, who were scheduled to cross the St. Clair River and return to U.S. territory that evening.

At this point, an obvious question arises. How did Norris know that Buchanan would be reentering the United States at that particular time and place? When later pressed on the subject, Norris refused to divulge the details behind how Buchanan was enticed across the river. Instead he asserted reportorial privilege in protecting the identity of his source. The source almost certainly had to be someone within Buchanan's inner circle, and, given the fluid movements of Buchanan's troupe in Ontario, most probably one of Buchanan's traveling companions: Norah Leonard, W. W. Mumey, or Martin Chapman. Speculation at the time and thereafter fell heavily on Chapman. Since Chapman was listed in EMC and American University publications as a faculty member, he too faced potential legal charges once the schools' practices became public knowledge in the spring and summer of 1880. Moreover, a warrant for his arrest on felony perjury and conspiracy charges, stemming from his testimony in the U.S. district court on Buchanan's faked suicide, had already been issued, meaning that he, like Buchanan, was a fugitive. With the likelihood of capture increasing, Chapman may have decided the time had come to separate his fate from Buchanan's and salvage what he could of his own life. It would have been surprising if certain thoughts had not occurred to him. *What if I were to cooperate in returning Buchanan to U.S. soil for an arrest? Could I trade such cooperation for a reduced sentence or even get the perjury and conspiracy charges dropped?*

Chapman's involvement in Buchanan's capture and any possible motives are pure speculation. Moreover, his later actions seem inconsistent with his having reached any kind of bargain with authorities. Nevertheless, among Buchanan's three traveling companions, Martin Chapman was (1) the only one who was in Philadelphia in late August and thus in a position to appreciate how badly the suicide ploy had unraveled amidst press and police inquiries; (2) well-positioned in early September 1880 to know Buchanan's precise location and where he was headed next; (3) the only one besides Buchanan facing serious criminal charges, giving him the most to gain by cooperating with authorities; and (4) the only one of the three who had previously interacted directly with John Norris, an earlier contact that could have led Chapman to view Norris as a possible conduit for a bargain with authorities. However the trap was set up, and whichever member of Buchanan's inner circle helped set it, Norris hurried back to St. Clair that evening expecting to catch the fugitive doctor.

Given Norris's silence on how the trap was planned, the details of what transpired that night are difficult to piece together. Nevertheless, one point is clear. The fundamental lure enticing John Buchanan back to American soil was money: he and Chapman were almost broke. When the two were apprehended, they carried only $1.70 between them. According to one press report, an apparently bogus telegram reached Buchanan sometime earlier, telling him that Mumey and his wife Lucy would be awaiting the group in St. Clair with money to fund the party's travels farther west. Buchanan had been anticipating a money packet of $300 for several days, though its source is unclear. One of the key missives in the communication chain was a telegram, ostensibly from Lucy Mumey in St. Clair, saying, "Husband will be here."[55]

The night started badly for Norris, as he, Miller, and Lansing reached St. Clair well past the 8:00 P.M. rendezvous time. Their late arrival probably had Norris fuming. Arriving in St. Clair, the three men hurried to a hotel near the waterfront, where they joined forces with a pair of *Free Press* reporters who had secured a small skiff and an oarsman to bring Buchanan and his colleagues across the river.

By the time Norris and the others were making the short walk toward an old wharf in the shadows of an abandoned mill, darkness had fallen. On the opposite shore a few lights and the dim outlines of Courtright were just visible. Norris briefed the oarsman on the message he was to deliver to Buchanan's party, waiting at a wharf on the opposite bank. Then he and his fellows retreated into the shadows to watch as the skiff, its lantern twinkling on the water, slowly traversed the half-mile of water. Once the skiff reached the other shore, its light disappeared. Several minutes later, the lantern light reappeared. Unfortunately, as the skiff moved steadily closer to the St. Clair shore, it became apparent that the oarsman had returned alone.

Stepping ashore in the shadows of the abandoned mill, the oarsman delivered his "message" to Norris and the others. The *Free Press* reporters described the ensuing discussion as "earnest" but gave no hint as to its content or what had momentarily gone wrong on the opposite shore. The meeting ended with the group passing a written note to the oarsman to deliver to Buchanan and his party. Once again the skiff set out across the St. Clair River. Again the light from the skiff disappeared as it reached the wharf at Courtright. But unlike the few minutes of anxious waiting last time, this time the darkness lingered much longer and the boat did not reappear. The skiff's long delay on the Courtright side of the river had Norris's group worried. The tension finally eased as the faint light of the skiff reappeared on the water. But as the skiff slowly approached the near shore, those waiting saw that this time, it had two occupants—the oarsman and a single passenger. And when the boat reached shore, the passenger slowly clambering from the boat was not the portly figure of a middle-aged man but a young man looking for Norris's party.

The *Detroit Free Press* described how Norris and his colleagues retreated to the hotel with the young man, where a back and forth dialogue commenced. Norris's refusal to reveal the particulars of his plan means that we have no way of knowing who the young intermediary was, or even who he believed he was conversing with that evening. A *Free Press* reporter subsequently offered a terse description of the exchange as culminating in a final "proposition" that would be carried back to Buchanan on the far side of the river. But the proposition would not be carried by the young intermediary. The press account described Norris's group as holding the young man a "hostage" to ensure "faithful observance of certain conditions of the contract."

The skiff crossed the river to Courtright for a third time. Norris and Miller returned to the wharf, where they crouched behind a pile of bricks to wait for the response to their latest missive. The wait probably seemed interminable. The thought may have occurred to Norris that if they failed to lure Buchanan across that night he was liable to escape entirely. Once his suspicions were aroused, the doctor was unlikely to be enticed across the river again anytime soon and perhaps unlikely to remain longer in the area.

Finally those waiting saw the skiff returning from the opposite shore for the third time, and this time it contained three people. The skiff bumping into the wharf was followed by a gentle scraping as someone secured the boat to the dock. The oarsman came ashore first and led the way, lantern in hand. Behind him came Buchanan and Chapman. The group passed the brick pile, unaware of Norris and Miller a few feet away. Norris recognized the frame of the heavyset doctor walking past. He quickly stood up, stepped quietly behind Buchanan, and threw his arms over the man's shoulders, saying, "Doctor, I have a prescription for you." John Buchanan, after more than a decade of staying one step ahead of the authorities, was caught entirely unawares. He gave an involuntary, startled cry and offered a gesture of surrender. Detective Miller took him by the arm.

Chapman stammered out, "Who are you?"

Drawing closer, Norris responded, "You know me, Chapman, Norris." The brief exchange may have been genuine or a façade intended to protect Chapman and hide his role in the capture. Detective Miller pointed the two captives toward the hotel. As John Buchanan stepped inside, it was just past midnight on September 10, 1880. The former EMC dean had covered an exhausting six hundred miles during his recent travels; he had been on the run for more than three weeks. It would take Norris and Miller less than thirty-six hours to bring him back to Philadelphia.

"If I had followed the dictates of my
own mind I never should have done it."

—John Buchanan, *Philadelphia Inquirer*,

March 25, 1881

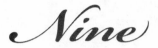

Trial and Imprisonment

RETURN TO PHILADELPHIA

John Buchanan sat slumped in a chair in the lobby of a St. Clair, Michigan,
waterfront hotel. The hour was well past midnight. Despite the excitement
stemming from the unexpected turn of events that evening, Buchanan had
surrendered to his fatigue—closing his eyes and soon nodding off into a
fitful sleep. John Norris felt exhausted too, but he did not have the luxury
of giving in to sleep. The two men awaited the *Milton Ward*, a side-paddle
steamer scheduled to reach St. Clair at 4:00 A.M. Norris planned for the
steamer to take them to Port Huron, Michigan; from there they would
make their way east to Philadelphia. Norris and reporters from the *Detroit
Free Press* had been jointly writing the account of Buchanan's capture that
would appear in both that paper and Norris's *Philadelphia Record*, in line
with the agreement the two newspapers had reached earlier in their hunt
for Buchanan.[1] Norris also carried with him several documents brought
from Philadelphia in preparation for Buchanan's examination before a
magistrate—a necessary step in the extradition process.

Fig. 15. John Buchanan after his arrest. While on the run, wanted by the law, and hoping to avoid detection, Buchanan cut and dyed his hair and shaved his beard. Image courtesy of Print Collection, Miriam and Ira D. Wallach Division of Art, Prints and Photographs, New York Public Library, Astor, Lenox and Tilden Foundations.

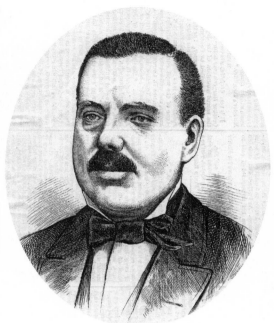

Norris noted the physical transformation in John Buchanan's appearance. The notorious doctor had long been recognizable not only by his muttonchop side whiskers and middle-aged paunch but by his air of self-confidence. The haggard man in the rumpled suit dozing across the room hardly resembled that well-known Philadelphia figure. His hair was cropped short, close to the scalp, and dyed black. The muttonchops were gone, replaced by a similarly dyed mustache that seemed anything but inconspicuous, especially surrounded by the white stubble of several days' growth of beard. Still, there was no confusion as to identity. In overseeing the search of Buchanan's person and possessions, Deputy Lansing and Detective Charles Miller had found plenty of corroborative evidence. This had included sixty shares of stock in the Detroit Eclectic Medical College, though Norris had no idea exactly how far the doctor's negotiations had progressed. It had also included a program from the failed séance in London, Ontario, and a letter of warning that might well have prevented Buchanan's capture that evening had he heeded it.

The *Milton Ward* arrived at almost precisely 4:00 A.M. Norris and his colleagues roused Buchanan and Chapman and promptly escorted them aboard the steamer. John Buchanan had little to say. He located a chair near a steam radiator in the enclosed cabin area and was soon sleeping again. Approximately two hours later, with the sun just beginning to crest the horizon, the steamer reached Port Huron. Soon after Buchanan's capture, Norris had sent a telegraph to Governor Croswell, notifying him of their success. The governor's office had arranged for formal extradition paperwork to reach Port Huron by eleven o'clock that morning.

After the party had disembarked from the steamer, Deputy Lansing guided Norris, Miller, and their two prisoners to Huron House for a few hours of rest. The group procured a pair of rooms that included what Norris described vaguely as adequate safeguards for the prisoners. While registering at the hotel, John Buchanan evinced his first moment of stubborn pique. As the men stood before the clerk, he refused to sign the hotel register. The delay keeping him from catching a few hours sleep in a bed exasperated Chapman. Curtly offering, "I'll fix that," he stepped forward and signed the register for Buchanan. Appropriately enough, he did so by giving his brother-in-law another fictitious name—Charles Smith—a touch wholly in keeping with the practices both men used while on the run in Ontario.

Several hours later, after lunch, Buchanan and Chapman stood before a local judge to satisfy a Michigan state law that required any individual accused of being a fugitive from justice to undergo an examination. Although the formal extradition paperwork had not yet arrived from the governor's office, an impatient Norris saw no reason to delay the required examination. Judge McKay asked Norris to provide his testimony and submit any evidence in his possession. Norris unpacked his documents and delivered a detailed factual account of recent events, commencing with Buchanan's indictment in Philadelphia on July 2, 1880, and fully describing the charges made against him in the Court of Quarter Sessions in Philadelphia County, Pennsylvania. Norris's language was precise, formal, and legalistic. John Buchanan faced four indictments in Pennsylvania stemming from his "making a . . . false instrument . . . commonly called a diploma" and "publishing . . . a false and fraudulent instrument." He then explained that Buchanan, after posting bail, had failed to return to court on August 18, prompting the court to order his bail forfeited on September 4.

John Norris then explained his use of assumed names (John William Fanning, George Austin Dawson, and Henry Dawson) in communicating with Buchanan via the U.S. mail to secure various diplomas. Norris gave the amounts he had paid for the diplomas and the types of diplomas he had received from each institution affiliated with Buchanan. One of these diplomas was from the EMC, but most bore the imprints of either the American University of Philadelphia or Livingston University, a lesser-known West Virginia school. Norris testified that all the diplomas he had bought from Buchanan had been "antedated" to a date of issue preceding the start of their correspondence and the purchase. Thus all the diplomas Norris had received under his various aliases in early 1880 bore dates between 1873 and 1879. All the correspondence about these transactions, Norris told the court, was being held by the U.S. postal inspector for Philadelphia.

Norris then testified that the John Buchanan before them was the same man who had sold him the diplomas and whose signature appeared on all of them, along with the signatures of other faculty members. Norris further asserted that Buchanan's signatures on the diplomas were authentic, being fully consistent with his handwriting and signatures on earlier letters to Norris. The judge now interrupted momentarily with a question of his own: Were the rest of the signatures on the diplomas authentic? Norris acknowledged that he could not give a definite opinion, and went on to discuss two specific signatures he knew something about. He said first that he believed a signature purportedly by Charles G. Polk to be a forgery, based on the writing sample for Polk he had in his possession. He then took an opposite view of the signature of Charles Kehnroth, saying he believed it to be authentic, also based on comparison with writing samples in his possession. Norris said he believed that the remaining signatures were probably forged, although he admitted that he could not offer evidence to back up this view.

After Norris's lengthy and legalistic account, Judge McKay turned to John Buchanan, who had remained silent during Norris's testimony, and asked him if he would like to pose any questions of this witness.

"I don't want to ask any questions," the doctor responded defiantly. "I think it is unnecessary to make a statement to show that whole thing is perfectly legal."

But then, as if he could not resist the temptation to contest the account of the man who had almost single-handedly ruined him, Buchanan found the energy to launch a counterattack, contesting Norris's testimony with assertions of his own. Addressing the judge directly, he stated that the Eclectic Medical College of Pennsylvania is a "perfectly regular institution," legally chartered by the Commonwealth of Pennsylvania in 1850. He avowed that the same was true for the American University, chartered by the same Commonwealth in 1867, and Livingston University, chartered by the state of West Virginia in 1874. Norris might cast aspersions on these colleges, but in fact all three were "perfectly regular" and legally empowered to issue their respective degrees.

Buchanan next turned to the diplomas that Norris had offered in evidence. Looking toward his accuser, he said, "Mr. Norris's name is not J. W. Fanning nor [is it] George Austin Dawson. Those names are on our books! The names attached to those diplomas are of parties who have attended our institution and I can prove this by persons who were in attendance." The judge nudged Buchanan's testimony along with a question of his own. How did Buchanan answer Norris's claim that the diplomas carried forged faculty signatures? Buchanan explained the discrepancies in the signatures as resulting from a common practice among many schools seeking to get their diplomas out to graduates in a timely manner. "It is usual in all cases for the names of the faculty to be appended by someone if they are not individually present." Then, apparently remembering Norris's allegation that he personally had forged the signatures of faculty members, Buchanan firmly denied doing any such thing. "There is nothing in the statement of Mr. Norris to show the commitment of forgery by me. I did not sign Polk's name or any other name to those diplomas."

The judge turned back to Norris. Responding to Buchanan's claim that EMC records would verify the attendance of a graduate named Fanning, Norris explained his use of the name John William Fanning. "I had some correspondence with Buchanan through the mails. [I] told him that I had studied medicine some and was practicing, but wanted a certificate and referred to an article I saw relative to the sale of diplomas in Europe. I received an answer from him saying he did not sell diplomas but he would send [a] *certificate of scholarship* [italics added]." Norris wanted the judge to appreciate Buchanan's clever use of nuanced language in his reply letter, and his caution in avoiding any written statement confirming the sale of a diploma. Norris then explained his choice of aliases. "John William Fanning was my grandfather's name," Norris said. "He is now dead and I assumed this name for the purpose of entrapping John Buchanan. I have visited Tippecanoe City where John William Fanning is stated to have lived and no such person lives there."

Judge McKay next turned to Detective Miller, asking for his statement. Miller briefly confirmed his identity as a detective, affirmed Norris's account of events, and testified that the alleged offense was a violation under Pennsylvania law. Satisfied regarding the validity of the request for extradition, McKay ended his examination. The defendant could either post $2,000 bail immediately or be committed to jail to await the arrival of the extradition paperwork and the judge's ruling. The prospect of contesting the extradition proceeding in this remote area of Michigan, far from any of his allies in Philadelphia, probably struck Buchanan as daunting and a waste of time and resources. Buchanan declined bail and asked to waive the extradition formalities. He wished to proceed immediately to Philadelphia in the custody of Norris and Miller. He must have calculated that the sooner he could reconnect with his many contacts back in the familiar confines of Philadelphia, the more effectively he could prepare his legal defense. By 3:30 that afternoon, Norris and Miller had left for Philadelphia with Buchanan and Chapman in tow.

The remainder of the return trip to Philadelphia proved uneventful, although one seriocomic moment did occur at the city's train station. At some point in the journey, Chapman learned that Thomas Vanduser had been arrested and charged with perjury for his statements to the police and his depositions in the matter of Buchanan's supposed suicide. Although the press had been characterizing the returning Chapman as a witness, it seems that Chapman knew better, fearing that he would soon face charges of his own in Philadelphia. During the return trip, Buchanan and Detective Charles Miller shared a berth with Chapman, but Miller's precautions to secure Chapman proved inadequate. As the train slowed in the outskirts of the rail yard in Philadelphia, Chapman managed to slip from the train. Despite the early hour, the tremendous publicity surrounding Buchanan's flight and capture had brought the local press out in force, waiting anxiously at the station in the hope of getting a statement or an interview with the fugitive physician.[2]

U.S. Postal Service Special Officer Thomas Barrett boarded the train as soon as it came to a stop and moved to secure John Buchanan for the trip to Moyamensing Prison and to arrest Martin Chapman for perjury.

But when Detective Charles Miller helpfully pointed Thomas Barrett to the berth where Chapman had spent the night, drawing back the curtain with a flourish, the men found only an empty berth. This in turn aroused suspicion from the reporters thronged around the train, convincing many of them that Chapman's arrest would turn out to be mere theater, with all charges against him soon to be dropped. Chapman's escape was successful but short-lived. After remaining at large for more than a month, an attentive Philadelphia police officer finally spotted and arrested him.[3]

One enterprising reporter for the *New York Herald* had jumped the gun by boarding the incoming train at a stop farther up the line. This won him a brief interview with Buchanan before the train reached Philadelphia, scooping the waiting throng of reporters. A reluctant Detective Miller had accompanied Buchanan and the reporter to the smoking compartment of their Pullman car for the interview. The reporter noticed the doctor's haggard look, the change in his physical appearance, and the "seedy" condition of his clothes. Though visibly distraught at times, Buchanan rallied sufficiently to admit to only the most obvious facts. While acknowledging that "Of course, it is impossible for me to deny that I ran away from Philadelphia," he avoided other admissions, instead talking willingly on topics that had no material bearing on the case, such as his initial escape route through Camden to New York City and from there to Canada. He balked at what he deemed wildly outrageous accusations. In particular, he denied a story that he was taking the women in his party to San Francisco to set up a brothel, calling the notion "untrue and absurd." Buchanan defended the women as "patients of mine," but offered nothing more to explain their presence.[4]

As the interview progressed, Miller periodically interrupted—sometimes to encourage Buchanan's halting efforts but at other times to offer biting comments. At one point, Buchanan offered a wistful expression for what might have been. "The fact is I have been hounded to death," the doctor said. "I hoped to escape to the Far West where, unknown and forgotten, I could have made an honest living." The hat Buchanan held in his hands moved with the erratic tremors of his body. Miller broke the silence by extracting a flask from his coat pocket.

"Doctor, you need bracing up."

Buchanan downed half a tumbler of whiskey as the reporter posed another question, "About the suicide . . ."

Buchanan cut him off. "About the suicide and the scene on the boat, I solemnly declare myself utterly ignorant. I was not there. Other people planned it, but I never paid a cent to anyone, or promised to pay anything." Then, perhaps sensing that he had been more vehement than he intended, Buchanan offered another possibility. "It is possible that, knowing I had fled, other persons, for motives of their own, may have arranged the pretended suicide."

The interview closed as the train slowed for its approach to the station. Buchanan was no stoic, but he had managed to remain sufficiently composed to admit only to known facts—specifically, those that were either benign or incontestable at this point. Nothing he said could incriminate him further. In fact, he had adroitly recognized that specifying precisely when he left Philadelphia could harm the prospects of his friendly witness, Vanduser. Buchanan may have been contemplating admitting that he had fled only *after* he himself had jumped from the ferry.

Chapman's escape from the incoming train should not have been the only drama surrounding Buchanan's return to Philadelphia. One story in circulation claimed that a friend of Buchanan's had hired a group of toughs to stage a diversion when the train arrived, so that the doctor and his brother-in-law could slip away.[5] The tale was probably nothing more than a rumor, though Chapman's actual slip from the train may have signaled an awareness on his part that no help would be waiting at the station.

John Buchanan's decision to waive extradition and his cooperative demeanor during the return trip to Philadelphia drew one small consideration from the local authorities: he was allowed a quick stop at his city residence at 1636 North Eighth Street to wash and change into clean clothes before being transported to Moyamensing jail. During this stop, he encountered one of his household servants who, according to the *Record*, expressed shock at her employer's sudden appearance. A brief homecoming exchange with his wife proved strained. When the meeting began with a warm embrace and the heartfelt cry, "Is that you? Can I believe my eyes?" it seemed that a quick reconciliation was imminent. But instead, Lucy Buchanan's demeanor turned markedly "cool" as she began venting her anger over the events of the prior month. She even went so far as to claim there were no clean clothes for her husband in the house.[6]

Detective Miller transported Buchanan to Philadelphia's Court of Quarter Sessions for a noon appearance before a judge. The judge read quickly through the bench warrant and remanded him to Moyamensing. So quietly were these legal formalities carried out that few inside the courtroom were aware of Buchanan's presence. The prisoner refused to speak with any of the assembled reporters from Philadelphia or New York. Once Buchanan had been loaded into the police wagon for transport back to Moyamensing, U.S. Postal Service Special Officer Thomas Barrett answered a few questions from the gathered reporters, mostly downplaying the idea that Buchanan would claim that he had jumped from the ferry.

Almost simultaneously with Buchanan's court appearance, Thomas Vanduser was giving testimony in a hearing before U.S. Commissioner Gibbons. Vanduser stuck doggedly to his story, perhaps hoping that his friend would ultimately claim that he was present on the ferry. When pressed by the commissioner, Vanduser repeated his conviction that it had been Buchanan on the ferry that night. After all, he said, he had known Buchanan for years. "If it was not him," he claimed, "it was his ghost!"[7]

In the days that followed, a flurry of activities surrounded Buchanan, keeping his name and story steadily in the newspapers. With Buchanan back in Philadelphia, the legal wrangling over his bail intensified. Judge Butler in the U.S. district court had to listen to long discussions concerning the bail money and its forfeiture, and to the protests of the bond insurers, who pointed to Buchanan's delayed presence in the city. Buchanan's wife met periodically with her husband's attorneys, but spent as much time as possible at their home in New Jersey to escape the steady stream of reporters knocking at the door of their Philadelphia house. A grand jury arraigned Thomas Vanduser on perjury and conspiracy charges. Meanwhile, John Buchanan sat in his Moyamensing cell awaiting trial on charges of conspiracy to defraud.[8]

One month later, Buchanan learned that his brother-in-law had been arrested. As the weeks had passed since Chapman's escape from the train, some thought the former dentist had departed for good. Then on October 23, an officer recognized and arrested Chapman only blocks away from his home. Seemingly sanguine at this turn of affairs, Chapman said only that during his absence he had spent an enjoyable time "fishing and gunning" in New Jersey. Now he joined Buchanan and Vanduser in jail to await formal arraignment on conspiracy to defraud charges.[9]

Jury selection took place in mid-November, with a trial date set for November 23. The trial lasted only a day and lacked any of the courtroom drama that newspaper readers or the large throng of reporters had anticipated. The scene certainly seemed set for high drama, with three defendants (Buchanan, Chapman, and Vanduser), their attorneys, the crusading newspaper editor Norris, an array of witnesses, and a "capacity" crowd. But despite the dramatic connotations of the charge—conspiracy to defraud—the facts of the case provided for a rather straightforward disposition of the matter.[10]

The fundamental question was simply whether Buchanan and his companions had conspired to fake the doctor's death as a means of getting him out of legal trouble without forfeiting any of the bail money or sureties they had provided to gain his initial release. The evidence offered to the court consisted largely of affidavits and restatements of testimony provided by many of the same witnesses who had already testified previously as part of the bail forfeiture hearings. The court concluded at 3:00 P.M.; the jury withdrew to deliberate and returned its verdict the following day. Buchanan and his brother-in-law Chapman were found guilty of conspiracy; Vanduser was acquitted. The district attorney, after consulting with defense counsel, dropped the perjury charges against Chapman and Vanduser, feeling that the outcome on the conspiracy charges had "substantially settled" the question of perjury. Buchanan and Chapman left the Court of Quarter Sessions and were returned to their cells to await sentencing later in December. In the interim, Buchanan began a new phase of his ordeal, as he entered a different courtroom the following week to answer the mail fraud charges that Norris had labored so hard to secure.[11]

The events of the late summer and fall of 1880 had provided the public with riveting reading. The ruin of John Buchanan and the demise of the EMC teemed with the plotlines that sold newspapers. Beginning with suicide, a staged death, and a criminal manhunt, the drama turned to comic farce with descriptions of a séance and a last-minute jump from a train. Not only newspapers cashed in on this story line. A local Philadelphia printer, A. W. Auner, saw the story as too good an opportunity to pass up. Working from the tune of a popular lullaby called "Baby Mine,"[12] Auner rewrote the lyrics to summarize the story Philadelphians were talking about.

Facing page: Fig. 16. Lyric sheet for "Bogus Dr. John." The dramatic elements of Buchanan's fake suicide and flight found a humorous outlet with one Philadelphia publisher. The lyrics accompanied a popular tune, "Baby Mine." Image courtesy of the American Antiquarian Society.

A. W. AUNER, SONG PUBLISHER & PRINTER,
Tenth and Race Sts., Philadelphia, Pa.

BOGUS DR. JOHN.

AIR:—BABY MINE.

I read an article in the paper,
　Dr. John, Dr. John;
Of your little steamboat caper,
　Dr. John, Dr. John;
But the story's sugar-coated,
'Cause your body would have floated,
Yes, to the top it would have floated,
　Dr. John, Dr. John;
For in the water you'd get bloated,
　Dr. John, Dr. John.

Still, it was a daring plan,
　Dr. John, Dr. John;
To put whiskers on a man,
　Dr. John, Dr. John;
With instructions to yell and bawl,
And for help to loudly call,
Now, that was an awful gall,
　Dr. John, Dr. John;
He jumped overboard for a stall,
　Dr. John, Dr. John.

Now, if a steamboat was in motion,
　Dr. John, Dr. John;
Aud if you took a little notion,
　Dr. John, Dr. John;
And $50 I would slide,
If you'd jump into the tide,
With intention of suicide,
　Dr. John, Dr. John;
Then you must skin out and hide,
　Dr. John, Dr. John.

Now the papers spread the news,
　Dr. John, Dr. John;
So you must mind your P's and Q's,
　Dr. John, Dr. John;
Or you'll get tripped up at last,
With all your glories of the past,
Then you'd get an awful blast,
　Dr. John, Dr. John;
So don't you go so fast,
　Dr. John,—Buchanan.

I read an article in the paper,
Dr. John, Dr. John;
Of your little steamboat caper,
Dr. John, Dr. John;
But the story's sugar-coated,
'Cause your body would have floated,
Yes, to the top it would have floated,
Dr. John, Dr. John,
For in the water you'd get bloated,
Dr. John, Dr. John.[13]

"Bogus Dr. John" gained nothing more than a temporary place around the saloons and pianos of Philadelphia. But it did signal a change: Philadelphians were now laughing at John Buchanan rather than with him in his colorful, long-running battle with local authorities.

ON TRIAL

Sitting in his jail cell on the evening of December 1, 1880, John Buchanan must have felt stunned by that day's turn of events. The mail fraud charges that he had feared most had proven innocuous. The judge had acquitted him.[14] His attorneys, William Mann and F. Carroll Brewster, felt that prosecutors had overreached in the case: that they could not prove their charge under the statute as written and that conviction would not be possible based upon the facts of the case. John Buchanan had sat through John Norris's testimony earlier that day as he detailed his correspondence with Buchanan using the Fanning and Dawson aliases, explained the nature of the inquiries, and described the culminating financial transaction, exchanging cash for diplomas. Postal agent Thomas Barrett had followed Norris on the stand and offered a mundane recitation of facts: Norris's letters as Fanning and two Dawsons, his sending these through the mail, the discovery of the same letters in Buchanan's desk drawer, and the local letter carrier identifying Buchanan's signature on a piece of registered mail that formed part of the Norris-Buchanan exchange. None of the testimony surprised Buchanan. He had heard variations on it during the abbreviated extradition hearing before a

Michigan magistrate and later in his attorneys' discussions of his case. The surprise was the discussion that ensued once the prosecution concluded its presentation of the evidence.

Brewster, one of Buchanan's attorneys who was himself a former judge, then addressed the court. Brewster asserted that under federal law, a conviction required a "scheme to defraud the persons directly addressed through the mail," not some unspecified third party. Brewster then read from the statute in question: "If any person having devised or intending to devise any scheme or artifice to defraud or to be effected, by either opening or intending to open correspondence or communication with any other person by means of the post office establishment of the United States, he shall be guilty of a felony."

Brewster followed this critical point by posing and answering a series of rhetorical questions. What is the actual fraud in this case? Was Norris defrauded? No, acting in his capacity as a reporter, he clearly understood the nature of the transactions being arranged in his correspondence with the defendant. The fact that he wrote to Buchanan using several aliases demonstrated the same understanding. How can it be fraud when both parties are aware of the value and nature of the item being transacted?

Brewster took the proceedings in just the direction he claimed they must invariably go, away from Norris's and Barrett's recitations of the details of the correspondence and back to a set of fundamental questions implicit in the law itself.

U.S. district court Judge Butler turned to the prosecution for a response. The prosecutors asserted there was no question that Buchanan's scheme sought to defraud through the mail. When Judge Butler expressed doubt as to whether Buchanan's interactions with Norris fell within the statute, the resulting protests and assertions from the prosecution seemed strong on emotion but weak on the point of law in question. Butler then asked a series of questions, homing in on the assertion that Buchanan sought to defraud. He pushed the prosecution to explain precisely who was being defrauded through the correspondence. Were these letters intended to defraud the ostensible recipients of Buchanan's letters?

The prosecution answered in the broadest possible terms: "Not to defraud them but the community through them." At this point, Judge Butler appeared satisfied that he had forced the prosecution to define precisely how they were interpreting fraud in this case—not as an act to deceive Norris or any other person seeking a Buchanan diploma but as a larger act of deception targeting the broader community of potential patients seeking to consult the holder of an EMC or American University diploma. From a legal perspective, these possible patients stood apart from the immediate transaction being carried out through the mail, but were the ultimate victims of the fraud. At best, they would be paying for expertise their so-called physicians lacked; at worst, they would be treated ineffectively or even injured, by untrained individuals naming themselves physicians solely on the basis of diplomas they had bought rather than earned. Butler understood how the prosecution wished to see fraud defined in this case. But his sympathy for their goal—ending diploma sales—did not deter him from adhering to the letter of the law—even if that law was poorly drawn. "The statute in question," Butler concluded,

> was awkwardly drawn but its meaning is easily reached. The scheme contemplated by it must be to defraud through the use of the United States mail. It must be a part of the scheme to use the mail . . . it must be an integral part as in the case where bogus warehouses are established and the mail is used to create the impression of a business that does not exist. Or in the case of a promise being made to mail articles of value when no articles of values are intended to be sent. It means a scheme that would be exploded at once if the victim were present. This case is alleged to have been a scheme to impose bogus physicians upon the public. But was there anything actually concealed in this scheme? What was the fraud? You are not alleging that the defendant is guilty of a fraud upon his correspondents. The correspondents knew as much of the fraud as the defendant did. The defendant did not contemplate any fraud of which the mail was a necessary part. The man who purchased the diploma was simply buying the means to impose upon others. There is no evidence that the defendant intended to deceive his correspondents by the use of the mail as is required in this statute. Therefore, I direct the jury to render a verdict of not guilty.

As the hearing progressed and the judge's line of questioning became clear, it was evident to Norris and the *Record* that the judge would not follow the prosecution's line of reasoning for a broad interpretation of the statute. Following the decision, the *Record* expressed in an editorial its disappointment that Buchanan had escaped punishment for the "great wrong" and "flagrant" fraud he had perpetrated. The *Record* lamented the crudely drawn statute that undermined the case and called on Congress to remedy what they perceived as a distinct defect in the law.

If John Buchanan felt relief at this favorable verdict, it must have been mixed with regret. The great irony of his legal situation was that if he had not panicked at the prospect of facing federal mail fraud charges, he would never have feigned suicide and bolted from Philadelphia, the actions that resulted in the conspiracy charge and conviction.

On December 7, 1880, Buchanan returned to Judge Butler's court for sentencing on the conspiracy conviction.[15] His brother-in-law joined him before the judge. Buchanan's attorneys made an "earnest" appeal to the court for leniency in the matter and pointed to several mitigating factors. They pointed out their client's age (fifty-three) and health as factors worthy of consideration. But the main thrust of their appeal was that Buchanan had been unfairly entrapped. Alluding to the strenuous efforts of Norris and the *Philadelphia Record* to target their client, they argued that he had been "harassed" and "entrap[ped]" through the machinations of the press. Then, once caught, he had been enmeshed in a legal labyrinth that threatened him with financial ruin. Imploring the court for leniency, Attorney Mann concluded with an emotional plea. "They piled upon him such excessive bail that it is no wonder human nature broke down and that [he] fled from justice."

Judge Butler proved sympathetic to the arguments of the defense and to Buchanan himself. In particular, he appeared convinced by defense evidence showing Buchanan's strenuous efforts to secure funds to cover his bail and repay the bondholders during the period of his flight. It is unclear what this evidence was but it resonated with the judge.

It is clear from the jury's prior decision to convict in this matter, that the defendant did wrong in attempting to fly from justice. The court is, however, aware of the peculiar circumstances surrounding this case and Dr. Buchanan specifically. I believe that he showed weakness and a want of courage in his decision to flee. I see this rather than wickedness and malignity of heart. In running away in the manner that he did and then attempting to secure his bail is commendable rather than otherwise. He might have fled without attempting to secure them. Never the less, the law is clear. This court hereby sentences the defendant to pay a fine of $500 and to undergo an imprisonment for ten months.

Turning to Chapman, Butler's sympathetic tone disappeared. He offered a recitation of Chapman's sins: actively conspiring with Buchanan to defraud, actively assisting the fugitive while he was on the run in Michigan and Ontario, and fleeing from justice himself by jumping from the incoming train bringing him back to Philadelphia. Butler concluded that Chapman's case "differed entirely" from that of his brother-in-law. He characterized Chapman as a dangerous man and sentenced him to twenty-two months in jail and a $500 fine.

An editorial in the *Record* sounded an entirely different note on Chapman's sentence. While the paper had lamented Buchanan's acquittal on the mail fraud charges, they now rued the penalty against Chapman. The newspaper characterized Chapman's sentence as "unduly harsh" and castigated the judge's "wholly inexcusable discrimination" against the man. In rationalizing its view, the *Record* cited Chapman's loyalty in "standing by his friend" and his willingness to forego any "personal interest" in the matter. It seems unlikely that John Norris shared the sentiments expressed in this editorial. Knowing as he did the extent of Chapman's involvement in the diploma trade, Norris more likely saw self-interest as Chapman's prime motivation.

EASTERN STATE PENITENTIARY

John Buchanan remained at Moyamensing for another two months following his sentencing. On February 5, 1881, he entered Pennsylvania's infamous Eastern State Penitentiary to begin serving a ten-month sentence for conspiracy to defraud the government.[16] He entered the massive prison complex located on what is now Fairmount Avenue in Philadelphia in the same unnerving manner suffered by all incoming prisoners. From the moment that authorities placed him in handcuffs for the roughly one-and-a-half-mile journey from Moyamensing jail to Eastern State, a black hood covered John Buchanan's head.

This practice of draping the head of an incoming prisoner in a black hood and removing it only upon entry into the facility was already an ancient practice by 1881. Nearly forty years earlier, Charles Dickens had visited the prison and commented on the tradition in his *American*

Notes for General Circulation. With a novelistic flourish, he described the practice as the prisoner's point of departure from the world of the living to that of the living dead—a reference to the prison's use of solitary confinement. John Buchanan experienced this firsthand from February through October 1881, although by then in a greatly altered form.

Eastern State Penitentiary originated in the minds of Philadelphia reformers in the late eighteenth century. The Society for Alleviating the Miseries of Public Prisons met in 1787 at the home of Benjamin Franklin. Their featured speaker that evening, Dr. Benjamin Rush, addressed the group on their common aspiration: to establish a *penitentiary*, a prison whose inmates would be expected to follow an everyday routine of quiet contemplation and penance of their misdeeds. The concept proposed contemplative penance as a route to genuine rehabilitation and reflected a conscious rejection of the corporal punishment and abuses typical of most prisons of the day. In seeing contemplative penance as the route to reform, the reformers naturally extended that concept to include solitary confinement for all prisoners, but Eastern State became infamous for the extent to which the practice was used.[17]

The group's first opportunity to apply their ideas came when Philadelphia authorities agreed in 1790 to reconstitute the city's Walnut Street prison along penitentiary lines. Previously, violent and nonviolent prisoners had been crowded together in large rooms and filthy conditions. Now the Walnut Street facility placed all prisoners in individual cells. Their only contact came via the guard delivering food and water daily. Even opportunities for reading were limited, since the idea was for prisoners to spend their time reflecting on the crimes that had brought them to Walnut Street.[18]

The initial results from the new regime at the Walnut Street Prison pleased both local authorities and reformers. The system eradicated the violence that had characterized Walnut Street Prison, along with the chaotic environment that had probably criminalized as many inmates as it reformed. While it was still unclear whether the reforms were bringing about true rehabilitation among the prisoners, the theory behind the new system struck the reformers as just, humane, and more likely to salvage productive citizens than the earlier system, which had been predicated solely upon physical punishment and mass, undifferentiated incarceration. Flush with their perceived success, ambitious reformers and state officials bided their time for an opportune moment to recreate this penitentiary on a larger scale.

This moment came in 1821, when the state legislature passed an act to create Eastern State Penitentiary at Cherry Hill, Pennsylvania. Over time, local citizens and inmates referred to the facility as "Cherry Hill," a name that became synonymous with its more formal title. John Haviland, a respected and highly successful Philadelphia architect, submitted the winning bid for the design of the facility and then oversaw its construction. Haviland's design proved genuinely revolutionary, later drawing formal visits from foreign governments and inspiring countless imitations throughout the world.[19]

Haviland built Eastern State on a radial design, featuring seven long cell blocks (the spokes) radiating from a central surveillance rotunda (the hub). The cell blocks contained two stories of numerous individual cells, where each prisoner would reside in private with a cot, a flush toilet, and a skylight—the only source of illumination. Each ground-level cell also featured a companion courtyard, a small area for exercise or gardening surrounded by a ten-foot wall. With a rudimentary system of hot water

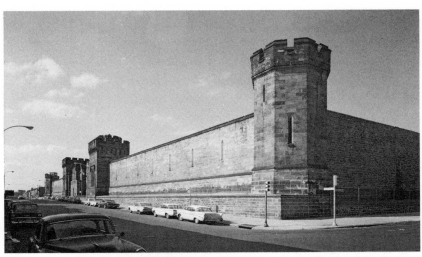

Fig. 17. Eastern State Penitentiary. This modern view shows the massive prison where Buchanan was held. After closing in the 1970s, the prison today serves as a popular tourist attraction. Image HABS, PA,51-PHILA,354-1 courtesy of the Library of Congress, Prints and Photographs Division, Washington, D.C.

piping, the cell blocks even provided a measure of warmth during the Philadelphia winters. The seven cell blocks converged at the central surveillance rotunda, where guards enjoyed a largely unobstructed view down each of the seven main corridors.[20]

Surrounding this interior structure were massive stone walls, giving the prison the ominous Gothic look of a medieval castle. Alexis de Tocqueville visited Eastern State in October 1831, only two years after its first prisoners had been installed. Like virtually all contemporary commentators on Eastern State, de Tocqueville responded to the building as something transported across time and space from the European Middle Ages, an impression reinforced by the scale of the structure and its placement atop a hill. Standing outside the "gigantic walls, gothic towers [and] ... wide iron gate," observers might shudder involuntarily at the horrors they imagined to be taking place inside.[21]

On the day John Buchanan entered Eastern State Penitentiary, the prison's meticulous record keeping began documenting all the pertinent facts of his incarceration. Through a series of records tracking prisoner admissions and discharges, population breakdowns, and sentence commutations, the prison recorded the facts about their newest inmate: John Buchanan—inmate A711—white male—physician—age 54—born in Scotland—convicted of conspiracy to defraud—sentenced to a ten-month term by the U.S. district court.[22] These facts were elicited by the warden, Edward Townsend, as part of the routine intake he performed with all inmates.

The data gathered at Cherry Hill went beyond demographic and statistical basics to include personal information that offered a more humanizing portrait of the individual. Thus, we learn that John Buchanan had gray hair and gray eyes, had a florid complexion, stood 5 feet 3½ inches tall, and weighed 178 pounds. Over the course of his time at Cherry Hill, Buchanan would lose five pounds. While he was overweight, he does not appear to be quite the "heavyweight" that the newspapers had so often described. Physical well-being was another matter. Both the admission and discharge books for the prison identified Buchanan as physically "impaired" but mentally in good health. This assessment of his physical condition may have been one factor in the choice of labor selected for Buchanan during his incarceration. There were many types of work to which prisoners were assigned, among them cordwaining, chair caning; sewing, knitting stockings, and various types of woodworking. Prison

Received.	Number.	Name.	Age.	Color.	Nativity	No. of convs.	Court.	Crime.
1881								
31	A.698	John M. Smith	29	B	Penna.	3	Dauphin	Larceny
"	699	Samuel Benson	25	"	"	3		"
1	700	Jacob L. Roren	27	W.	"	1	Phila.	Bigamy, Adul.
"	701	George Messick (7751)	27	"	Wilmington	2	"	Larceny
"	702	William McTague	30	"	Phila.	2	"	Ar+Btokill
2	703	Frank Ford	25	"	N. York	2	"	"
"	704	John Grey	38	"	Ireland	2	"	"
3	705	Henry Smith (9689)	26	B.	Penna.	3	"	Larceny
"	706	Andrew Miller	28	W.	Ireland	1	"	"
"	707	Abraham Mummert	21	"	Penna.	1	Adams	Larcy. Felo.
4	708	Chas. Lawrence	19	"	Phila.	2	Phila.	Burglary
"	709	James Dixon	29	"	"	1	"	"
"	710	James McAnnally	18	"	"	2	"	Larceny
5	711	John Buchanan (8390)	54	"	Scotland	1	U.S.D.C.	Conspiracy &dec
8	712	Fred. Eisenhower	39	"	Penna.	2	Chester	Burglary
"	713	Chas. Miller als Taylor (2884)	51	"	"	3	"	"
"	714	Tillie Biesecker	20	"	"	1	Lacka?	Larcy +Rec

Fig. 18. John Buchanan's prison record. Buchanan (fourth from the bottom) entered Eastern State Penitentiary in February 1881. He completed his sentence eight months later, only to begin serving twelve additional months in Moyamensing on state charges for selling diplomas. Prison population records; Eastern State Penitentiary; Record group 15; Records of the Dept. of Justice; Pennsylvania State Archives, Harrisburg.

officials assigned yarn winding to Buchanan, labor that was neither overly taxing nor physically demanding.

Prison records corroborated that Buchanan was married with two adult children and captured a little of his family background—specifically, that at age sixteen he was living at home with his parents in Scotland. We can assume that authorities elicited such biographical details to learn which inmates came from broken homes or were orphaned at a young age. Buchanan told prison officials that he abstained from alcohol, although at least one contemporary newspaper account hinted differently.[23] Not surprisingly, John Buchanan was far better educated than most of his fellow inmates. A random sample derived from the page containing Buchanan's reception record showed that one-quarter of incoming prisoners had never attended school and that nearly one-third were either illiterate or able to read and write "imperfectly." Buchanan claimed to have attended college and stated that he had completed his schooling at the age of twenty, an age greater than that of any other incoming prisoner in this sample.

Buchanan's fellow prisoners included the mixed lot one might have expected. The same random sampling showed that most other prisoners at Cherry Hill were laborers, mixed with some semi-skilled workers (e.g., clerks, cigar makers, boatmen, or waiters), and a few tradesmen (e.g., plumbers, barbers, jewelers, or printers). For some prisoners, the return to the Eastern State was a homecoming of sorts. Fully one-quarter of the incoming prisoners had served time previously. In addition, one-quarter of the incoming prisoners reported a family member in jail. Buchanan's fellow prisoners were also largely a nonviolent group. The same small random sampling shows that only 17 percent of the inmates had been incarcerated for a violent offense (e.g., assault and battery, manslaughter, or second-degree murder). The majority (62 percent) had been convicted of larceny, while the remainder were serving sentences for a range of nonviolent offenses (e.g., perjury, forgery, counterfeiting, and burglary). The records were less precise in a few instances, identifying such crimes as "keeping [a] bawdy house" and "adultery." Overall, this limited sampling creates a general picture consistent with that derived from a more extensive review of prison records published earlier by prison officials.[24]

While nonviolent offenders predominated within the prison, this did not rule out all violence. Suicides and attacks on fellow inmates did occur during Buchanan's time at Eastern State. The potential for violence was increased by the presence of mentally disturbed inmates, a state of affairs that had drawn public attention for many years. Only ten days after John Buchanan entered Eastern State, the *Philadelphia Inquirer* published an article on the dozen clearly "insane" inmates residing at the prison.[25]

For Buchanan and his fellow inmates, prison life relied heavily on a set daily routine. Buchanan would rise by 5:00 A.M., with breakfast to follow by 7:00 A.M. Dinner came at noon, supper at 6:00 P.M., and the lights were turned off by 10:00 P.M. at the latest, although within the cells, lit by skylight alone, the light disappeared with the setting sun. The prisoners spent their days working, reading, and in contemplation, although one hour of "exercise" was also provided daily. As Buchanan quickly learned, the prison's rules for inmates were simple: keep your cell and personal items clean, obey all directions and show respect for staff, apply yourself to your work, and stay silent. Regardless of the prison's religious overtones, any failure by inmates to comply with the rules brought swift consequences. For minor infractions, a meager diet of bread and water and a darkened cell were typical punishments. More intransigent prisoners were punished with physical restraint: a straightjacket, the iron gag, or the tranquilizing chair.[26]

The time for quiet contemplation undoubtedly proved a mixed blessing for Buchanan. While it did offer him the chance to reflect on his mistakes and plan a course of action to change his life direction upon his release, it also gave him ample time to indulge in self-pity, seated in a small stone cell that froze a prisoner in Philadelphia's harsh winters and suffocated him in summer's sweltering heat. John Norris and the other reporters following the case knew the extent to which John Buchanan had cooperated with local and state authorities after his capture. After his arrest and return to Philadelphia in September 1880, he had instructed his attorneys to raise no objections and pose no obstacles to the state's legal proceedings annulling the charters for the EMC and the American University.[27] This cooperative attitude had not extended to granting expansive interviews with the press, however. Norris and his *Record* colleagues still believed there was much to be learned from the former dean, if only he could be induced to speak freely. Now that Buchanan's court cases were settled, with the mail fraud charges against him dismissed, and given the solitude of his days in prison, perhaps Buchanan saw no reason to decline the interview Norris asked for. In March 1881, Norris arranged to visit Buchanan at Eastern State.[28]

A PUBLIC CONFESSION

Presumably the two men met in the narrow confines of John Buchanan's prison cell. Buchanan appeared to be in reasonably good health and spirits considering his imprisonment. His hair seemed a little grayer and he looked a few pounds lighter. Norris started with an obvious question, asking Buchanan how he had become involved with the EMC.

"Well . . . before I became connected with the Eclectic College I was respected. I was a member of the Nazareth Methodist Episcopal Church.

I had a good practice and was making a little money. After I joined the accursed thing I never made a dollar."

By word or expression, Norris must have signaled skepticism at this picture of Buchanan, property holder in both Philadelphia and New Jersey, in the role of pauper. Buchanan repeated his claim to penury. "During the last ten years my practice gradually left me—really I was making nothing. I had a heavy load to carry. Bread and butter had to be provided for three houses." Buchanan described his family obligations, including his wife, children, and parents. Norris brought the former dean back to the subject at hand by asking Buchanan to talk about the EMC.

"The college was mere farce—a sort of Free School. I struggled for ten years as no other struggled . . ." Norris prodded him to continue, asking how he came to be on the faculty.

"I became acquainted with the faculty in 1856 . . . and when Paine left in 1860 I commenced to lecture. Sites and Hollembaek got me in . . . and long have I struggled to get out!"

Buchanan warmed to the conversation, happy to share the thoughts he had nurtured in the solitude of his prison cell. He confided his own amazement in looking back at his career.

"I can assign no reason for my conduct. Insanity? Certainly every act, when I look at it, has been that of a crazy fool. When told to run, I ran. When two hundred diplomas were wanted, I ordered them to be printed. I lost all self-reliance. If I had followed the dictates of my own mind I never should have done it."

Once Buchanan brought up the diplomas, Norris encouraged him to talk of the sales, asking when they commenced.

Buchanan stressed his relative ignorance in the early years. "I knew very little of the workings of the concern then. The first sale of diplomas of which I was cognizant was that effected by Dr. Hollembaek in Canada." Norris pressed for specifics, but Buchanan was unable to recall the exact year this occurred. Then he offered a stronger assertion.

"The sale of diplomas dates back to 1853 . . . it was continually practiced from that date until the charter was annulled by the courts six months ago . . . the faculty were cognizant of these doings." This assertion was breathtaking in its scope, since it placed the start of the diploma trade much earlier than expected in the EMC's history. Buchanan may have been telling the truth but it seems equally likely that he was rationalizing his conduct by claiming it to be merely the continuation of a long-standing practice begun before his arrival at the EMC.

The two men's conversation continued along these lines, covering the formation of the American University and the political forces behind its establishment, ostensibly on behalf of Philadelphia's black population. An element of cynicism entered Buchanan's tone as he discussed the political maneuvering behind the school. Norris brought up the EMC's survival of the 1872 senate inquiry, asking how the school had kept its political influence.

Buchanan claimed that he or the school had paid $50 to each of the thirteen members of the Educational Committee of the State Legislature in 1871 and several thousand more to the Senate Committee in 1872. This astounding accusation apparently drew skepticism from Norris, who questioned the ability of Buchanan and the school to disperse such large sums.

Buchanan insisted that Norris did not fully appreciate the scale of the diploma trade in years past and even, to a lesser extent, to that very day in 1881. Buchanan claimed that more than two dozen concerns were selling diplomas in America and Europe. Then he offered his own personal estimate of its scale, speculating that twenty thousand bogus diplomas were circulating in America and twice that number in Europe. To back up this assertion, Buchanan offered an example from Missouri. "The Anthropological University of St. Louis. Fields, Sexton, Alford and Thrasher have an organization as perfect as the Catholic Church. They have penetrated every city of America and Great Britain with their agencies. The Eclectic [degree] is not popular and does not sell well but the University of Anthropology goes off like hot cakes. I have understood I could buy five hundred of its diplomas in bulk at any time. They deal largely. Alford approached me but I never answered the communication."

As for the European market, Buchanan claimed that "Scotch ministers take to these university degrees like a set of hungry wolves. They will not investigate. They have the degree mania badly." He claimed that Edinburgh degrees were easily obtainable during his time in Glasgow in the late 1840s. "They were around thick," he told Norris. "I could have bought [one] while attending Glasgow." Buchanan reminisced about sitting around a table with several EMC professors and signing diplomas in bulk, including a cache of five hundred diplomas intended for Europe through the Spanish consul. He seemed almost wistful. "Before the passage of the Medical Degree act in 1858 [*sic;* actually 1857] Great Britain carried off the plum for selling diplomas; since that time very little has been done. The Medical act . . . did this; it registered with one sweep all who had diplomas from a chartered college prior to that date."

As Buchanan continued, he stressed that the diploma business flowed in both directions. "I have been offered the degrees from all the institutions in Great Britain, but I never accepted one. I would not pay the expressage on them." He explained to Norris that the British diplomas were priced too dear, although the German degrees were tempting. "German degrees were cheap," he added. Buchanan thought this inexplicable considering that "German universities are more celebrated than the English." Buchanan's observations drifted back and forth on various aspects of the European diploma trade—from the various major universities and royal societies to the major brokers in the trade (Sturnam, Sayre, and Van der Vyver) and the inflow of these diplomas into America through Chicago. Buchanan's assessment of the trade expressed a deep-seated cynicism. "The same spirit haunts them all—they will sell degrees."

His observations on the diploma trade turned next to his eclectic colleagues. Buchanan claimed diploma sales were happening at the American Eclectic College of Cincinnati and intimated the same at the Eclectic College in Keokuk, Iowa. "They frankly told me how they did business. They make no secret of it. They sell like a grocer's shop. There are several thousand of their diplomas out in the West." The interview veered among the various players in the American diploma market before one of Norris's comments triggered another assertion from Buchanan. The former dean claimed that two-thirds of the doctors in Detroit held bought diplomas.

The shift in the conversation to the events in Michigan led Norris to inquire about Buchanan's contacts there—men like Henry Thomas and Henry Stickney. Both were close contacts over many years. Stickney even posed as Buchanan in 1876 to assist the latter in his flight from arrest that year.[29] Buchanan confirmed that he and Thomas had reached an understanding. Once Buchanan's presence was exposed in Detroit, if he were arrested, Thomas was prepared to swear an affidavit that Buchanan was actually his father. He had others prepared to swear to the same.

Norris then inquired about the medical school Buchanan had hoped to establish in Michigan. Buchanan acknowledged his efforts there, admitting that he had lined up several former Philadelphia eclectics for the venture, including John Siggins, Phillip Bissell, and Henry Stickney. Buchanan's mention of Stickney started him once again into the European diploma market. "It may have been possible that . . . Stickney sold some foreign degrees in this country. His opportunities were good—going back and forth frequently—and his associations were of that class. He knew the great diploma brokers—Sturman, Sayre and Van de Vyver."

At one point, Norris nudged Buchanan back to an earlier place in his narrative and the ferry on the Delaware River. He asked about the inspiration for the suicide ruse. Buchanan told the story of Foster, the former EMC student who had successfully pulled off the trick years earlier. He spoke of the laughs he and his friends had enjoyed in reminiscing about Foster's ruse, and how they had dusted off the ploy for his colleague, William Harbison, about five years ago. Buchanan admitted that his friend Vanduser had been behind that one too.

Norris asked Buchanan to confirm what everyone suspected about that night on the ferry: that an imposter made the jump. Buchanan admitted as much and then proceeded to reveal all about that night's events: the preparations ahead of time, the roles of Vanduser and Holton, and the swimmer they had procured known only as Shep. He also told Norris that by the time of Shep's leap, he was already en route to New York City by rail. Buchanan waved away the notion of any real danger. "Shep did not take ten strokes in the water before he caught hold of his partner's skiff!"

As they talked of the events of that infamous night, Buchanan revealed how he and his coconspirators had added touches of authenticity to the ruse: the scribbled marginalia on the newspaper left in the coat and Vanduser's continuing to New Jersey to deliver the fateful news to Buchanan's daughter. All that had been missing was a body. Buchanan confirmed that the lack of a body did not reflect an oversight. Once they had decided to try the fake suicide, they had simply been unable to secure one on such short notice.

This confessional tidbit led Buchanan to recall the EMC's many difficulties in securing cadavers for medical students. The Blockley Almshouse had proved a dependable supply over the years, but there had been times when circumstances and personal considerations hampered the school from obtaining bodies. On one occasion, he admitted, the school had been forced to secure (i.e., steal) five bodies surreptitiously from the institution.

Buchanan roamed aloud through his memories of life and medical practice in Philadelphia, speaking of the human foibles daily on display. Expressing his appreciation of human credulity, he recited a litany of scams he had witnessed firsthand: chicken gizzards pulverized into a compound to aid digestion, benign materials compounded at the shrine of Cupid in Minerva's Temple and advertised as aphrodisiacs, readings of the future performed by a Philadelphia fortune-teller in the light of flickering candles made ostensibly from human fat. He touched on the professional abortionists absolving their patients of shame along with a fetus, the wholesale druggists abandoning legitimate medicine to peddle "quack nostrums,"— and the EMC's sale of diplomas.

Perhaps these tales shocked even John Norris. When the newspaperman finished writing out his story, he added a brief postscript: "Owing to the present position of Buchanan, and the infamy of his career, anything that he may say will be likely to be taken cautiously by the public, especially where his statement involves the character of persons having the least claim to decency." Alternatively, this caution may reflect prudence by the *Philadelphia Record*, considering the numerous parties implicated by Buchanan and his claims of purchased influence with legislators.

Less than a week after the interview appeared in the *Record* and newspapers across the country, Buchanan issued a statement. He repudiated his alleged confession, calling it "bogus."[30] He may have done so upon advice of his legal counsel or in a fit of pique at the content and form of the published confession.

On October 10, 1881, John Buchanan left Eastern State Penitentiary in the company of the warden and an armed escort.[31] The group traveled to the Philadelphia Court of Quarter Sessions for a scheduled sentencing hearing before Judge Allison. Earlier in November 1880, while still awaiting trial on the conspiracy charges, Buchanan had pled guilty to state charges of selling diplomas. The state deferred sentencing on this conviction until the expiration of Buchanan's sentence for conspiracy. Once again, F. Carroll Brewster, one of Buchanan's attorneys, implored the court for leniency, citing the year his client had already spent in jail and his cooperation with authorities in the period since his conviction, including the relinquishment of the EMC and American University charters. Judge Allison acknowledged Brewster's plea but what followed contrasted markedly with the sympathetic tone adopted by Judge Butler the year before. Judge Allison began benignly with a dispassionate recital of the circumstances bringing Buchanan before the court: his prior guilty plea, the deferral of sentencing in this matter, and the specific language of the state law prohibiting the sale of diplomas that he had violated. To this point, the judge's comments and language had been precise and legalistic. If leniency were to be forthcoming, the judge would then have addressed the mitigating circumstances raised by Buchanan's lawyers. Instead, Allison proceeded down a different path.

> The power of the court to sentence an offender under this act of Assembly is restricted to what many persons would regard as an inadequate punishment for an offense which involves consequences most serious and far reaching, sacrificing health and life to the ignorance and incompetence of persons whose claim to practice medicine rests upon a false, and therefore fraudulent diploma or certificate. Of your connection with the commission of crimes of this character I need not here speak further than to say that it has been long continued and defiant of the law and right, and no punishment that I can impose under the power which the law places in the hands of the court can approach that measure of punishment which, in my judgment, you deserve. All that the law will permit me to do I feel myself required to impose on you, and therefore sentence you to pay a fine of $500 and undergo in imprisonment of six months in the County Prison on each of the two bills of indictment to which you had pleaded guilty.

We can only speculate on what Buchanan expected at this sentencing hearing. In consultation with his attorneys after his December 1880 conspiracy conviction, he had made a conscious decision to cooperate fully with state and local officials. He had answered all their questions regarding the EMC and the American University, clarified and resolved outstanding issues, and stood aside as the judicial process unfolded to revoke the schools' charters. He may have hoped that his cooperation would be recognized, producing a measure of consideration during his sentencing hearing. He may have hoped for nothing more than that the two sentences would run concurrently. Even this was denied. John Buchanan returned to jail, this time back to Moyamensing, where he remained until his release in fall 1882.

" . . . as long as fools and knaves shall seek to
buy diplomas we may expect that sharpers . . .
will continue to fabricate and sell them."
—"The Diploma Traffic," *Pacific Medical
and Surgical Journal*, June 1880

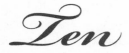

Old Tricks and a New Career

John Buchanan walked out of Moyamensing Prison in the fall of 1882
after two years of incarceration. He was fifty-six years old, his reputation
ruined and his career in shambles. To the general public, his name was
synonymous with the diploma trade, his infamy such that even the hint
of a prior association with him would subject any individual or group so
linked to unwelcome scrutiny. Eclectic physicians, in particular, eagerly
sought to put as much distance between themselves and the disgraced
doctor as possible.[1]

After his release, Buchanan proceeded to the office of the Philadelphia
prothonotary to have his name added to the local physician registry. In
June 1881, while John Buchanan sat in his cell at Eastern State Penitentiary, Pennsylvania had finally passed its first significant piece of medical
legislation—a modest medical registration law. Pennsylvania's law was
typical of those enacted in many other states. It required the county to
maintain a registry of physicians, laid out the criteria a physician must
meet to be added to the registry (e.g., presentation of a diploma), and
provided an exception for individuals lacking diplomas but able to show

that they had practiced continuously within the state for ten years or more. The law required a modest registration fee of one dollar and specified the penalty for violation of the law as a $100 fine and one year in jail.[2]

In the aftermath of the scandals involving Buchanan and the EMC, the local press followed the implementation of the law with interest. One *Philadelphia Inquirer* reporter interviewed Dr. Samuel Hoppin, the Jefferson Medical College graduate in charge of assembling the registry. When asked whether he had experienced any "trouble" with "bogus" diploma holders presenting themselves at his office, Hoppin quipped, "No; not I. They've had all the trouble." He then explained that a physician unable to produce a copy of a diploma, together with such corroborating evidence as course lecture tickets or a certification document from his medical school, would still be able to register by providing an affidavit or by invoking the clause making an exception based upon ten years' of continuous practice. The skeptical reporter then pressed Hoppin to explain how these multiple paths onto the register protected the public. Hoppin acknowledged the law's defects but sounded an optimistic note. "That is a many-sided question. The best part of the protection the public will get from the law is probably through its moral effect. The very fact that it is illegal to practice without registering will drive out of the city scores of quacks and charlatans who would otherwise prey upon the community. Then an occasional prosecution under the law will be likely to keep the general class in wholesome fear of its punishment."

Apparently unconvinced, the reporter pressed the point further, pointing out the inherent weakness of all medical registration laws. "But do not the old graduates of . . . Pennsylvania and Jefferson College and the ignorant experimenters from the schools of Paine and Buchanan and Miller all enjoy, equally, the benefits of registration?"

Hoppin answered truthfully. "Nominally, yes; but that is something the law cannot provide against." He then explained his plan to alleviate the deficiencies of the law. He intended to publish and make available an inexpensive copy of the register, listing the physicians alphabetically and naming the schools from which they had graduated. Furthermore, he promised, "the Buchanan and Paine doctors I shall classify by themselves." Several months later, the first edition of the registry appeared, with the newspapers republishing much of its contents, including the separate listing of the EMC and Philadelphia University graduates.[3]

Hoppin's disdain for the EMC proved so strong that in the final published version of the *Physicians' Protective Register*, he decided not to print the name of the EMC next to its graduates. In explaining this decision, he cited "reasons apparent to the profession." He did, however, acknowledge the *bona fides* of the school's early graduates: "These physicians . . . are in good standing and graduated from sixteen to twenty-four years ago, having completed the prescribed course of study and received their diplomas which bear the signatures of reputable and prominent physicians still practicing in this city and who then constituted the faculty."[4]

Despite Hoppin's zeal in publishing the registry and his clear desire to call out the EMC graduates for special attention, he followed the law scrupulously in registering Philadelphia's physicians, including John Buchanan. Hoppin had rebuffed Buchanan's initial attempt to join the registry based upon his diploma. Buchanan persisted, pointing to the clause of the law allowing him to present a certified copy of his diploma or an affidavit attesting to "a statement of this fact (i.e., diploma), together with the names of the professors whose lectures he attended and the branches of study upon which each professor lectured." When Buchanan presented an affidavit attesting to his attendance at Glasgow College in Scotland, Hoppin finally relented,[5] and Buchanan became one of nearly 1,500 physicians on the register. Nevertheless, as Hoppin acknowledged, the registry made no attempt to "discriminate between competent and incompetent practitioners."[6] In 1882, as in the past, *caveat emptor* remained the cautionary rule for patients in Philadelphia, as well as in most of America.

After his release from prison, John Buchanan retreated to the property he owned in Magnolia, New Jersey. Trouble followed, plaguing both him and his family. If his property dispute with his daughter Isabella and her husband is any indication, family harmony had been considerably undermined by John Buchanan's incarceration. Wrangling over property valued at $2,000, Isabella filed a complaint against her father in June 1883, claiming that he had "[illegally] seized" certain materials. Although he faulted his daughter for her action and remained extremely displeased, Buchanan believed that other parties had instigated the complaint. "I suspect there is more behind this," he told one reporter, hinting that unnamed individuals were determined to persecute him even after he had completed his jail term.[7]

This episode proved to be the first of several instances of the local press monitoring the affairs of John Buchanan and his family. Reporters attentive to anything involving the Buchanans published numerous pieces in the *Record* and the *Inquirer* detailing the tribulations of various family members during this period. While John pushed to be added to the physician registry in November 1882, his son George was facing charges stemming from the death of one of his patients. Sufficient evidence existed that the younger Buchanan stood trial in March 1883. Martin Chapman likewise drew public attention, featuring in a series of news articles reporting thefts and court proceedings for spousal support. As for John Buchanan himself, journalists gleefully reported on the apparent downturn in his fortunes, headlining their stories with titles like "Broken-Down Buchanan" and seasoning them with asides and innuendo. One Baltimore paper claimed that Buchanan was "barefoot and in rags" when arrested on his daughter's complaint. Another quoted "a friend" of Buchanan's, who claimed the doctor was being "persecuted and prosecuted" by members of his own family. The article then explained the family members' actions by alleging that these "former dependents" were no longer enjoying the largesse that had once flowed from the doctor's business enterprises. It concluded that Buchanan's relatives were anxious to see him back in jail "to get rid of him and to get possession of his money."[8]

During this period, Buchanan continued work on another book, *The Family Physician and Domestic Practice of Medicine*, which was published in 1884. The medical content of this work remained fairly consistent with that of previous books. However, the new book featured a long introductory passage. Over the course of twenty-five pages, Buchanan delivered a wide-ranging jeremiad on racial and national differences, gender distinctions, and the dangers of sexual depletion and germ theory, views wholly consistent with the deterministic Social Darwinism of his day. Before all of this, however, Buchanan unleashed a screed on the state of medicine, medical education, and the emerging system of medical regulation. This long passage reveals far more about Buchanan and his mental state than it does about any of the medical topics he addressed.

Buchanan's assessment of the state of medical science in America seems particularly revealing of his mind-set after his release from prison. He claimed that the medical profession was steadily deteriorating, resulting in a deplorable state of affairs for American doctors. "A physician does

not command the honor and respect . . . awarded him in other countries;
neither is he the recipient of brilliant rewards, nor does his talent . . .
engender . . . warm recognition and appreciation."[9] Though ostensibly
speaking in generalized terms, Buchanan, in the span of a few sentences,
shared what was perhaps his own personal sense of grievance. He probably
viewed his past in this manner: former colleagues had invited him to join
the faculty of what turned out to be a lesser school where questionable
practices were taking hold; once targeted by the local and medical press
he had been subjected to unceasing scrutiny of his personal and professional life; under this steady barrage of negative publicity, his once-sizable
private practice had disintegrated; and his critics were content with nothing less than his conviction and imprisonment.

Buchanan's description of the profession included an element of self-
pity as he listed what he believed to be the major contributors to this state
of affairs. The medical profession suffered from a continuing onslaught of
self-inflicted wounds, starting with the rampant sectarianism of the era.
Buchanan had abandoned his championing of eclectic medicine. Instead
he declared that "systems, cures, pathies, and isms . . . have been permit-
ted to grow, like poisonous weeds. . . . The art of healing is not a sect or
system, and never can be made one." Because the profession had toler-
ated and even fostered this splintering, the inevitable by-product was a
pool of poorly educated graduates lacking a true dedication to a "rational," unbiased study of medicine. Consequently, Buchanan argued, half
of all the graduates of American medical schools were sham doctors, little
more than a "burlesque" of true physicians. In Buchanan's mind, medical
education had fallen to its "lowest ebb," with only a handful of schools
providing quality education and the rest offering nothing but "incompetent" instruction.

Buchanan's lament on the state of American medicine and medical education, while hypocritical considering his part in producing unqualified
physicians, was an assessment shared by many. Mid-nineteenth-century
luminaries like Drs. Nathan Davis and Daniel Drake shared similar concerns about the "deficiency of talent" characterizing the medical profession,
with its subsequent impact on the "social position" of physicians. These
men recognized the cruel irony of a "learned" profession woefully short
on learning. A small number of schools were making significant strides
in educating and training future physicians; Harvard, for example, intro-

duced a three-year graduated curriculum in 1871. Given the proprietary model for medical education still prevailing at most schools, however, such practices were adopted only fitfully by other schools. Faculty and students alike understood that the proprietary system, under which small independent schools operated for profits based on student fees for lecture tickets, placed greater emphasis on a student's purchase of the ticket than on his attendance at the lecture. The typical absence of "practical" or clinical application of medical science further contributed to the woeful educational offerings at many schools. While change was under way in 1884, when Buchanan delivered his assessment of medical education, it is fair to state that much of American medicine was lacking in substance and generally provincial in outlook.[10]

Buchanan leveled some of his harshest criticism at homeopathy. "What educated man," he asked scathingly, "can talk with a fool who argues that a grain is, for potency, nothing, but the decillionth part of a grain is dangerously powerful?" As he saw it, "designations" like homeopathy, with their accompanying philosophies of treatment, were nothing more than "trade-marks for gain." In modern parlance, Buchanan might have called this *branding*, designed to secure patients and their fees. While his animus may in part have reflected jealousy that homeopathy had flourished in Philadelphia while eclectic medicine had withered, he nevertheless turned the same critical eye toward his own eclectic colleagues. One doctor he targeted specifically was John Scudder of the EMI in Cincinnati. Scudder had long been critical of the EMC, and of Buchanan in particular. Tired of having to clarify that the "Buchanan" in Philadelphia was not the EMI's Joseph Buchanan and anxious to disavow any recognition of the EMC, Scudder either ignored the Philadelphia doctor entirely or castigated him as "notorious."[11] Stung by such contempt, Buchanan in turn called Scudder's espousal of "specific medication" a "monstrosity" borne of homeopathy, deriding it as just another of the "trade-marks by which infamous scoundrels catch trade."

What Buchanan lamented most was the presence of "rogues, knaves, and illiterate[s]" populating the ranks of American physicians. In the span of three printed pages, Buchanan repeatedly brandished the word *charlatan* or a variation of it as a weapon against the incompetence characterizing so many practitioners. He labeled one-half of American physicians as "frauds or imposters . . . botch barbers . . . swindlers; uneducated asses [and] vipers living on the credulity of the people." According to Buchanan, their accomplices were the medical press of the day, whose "trashy" journals lent credence to the charlatans by publishing their advertisements championing "nefarious remedies." This tirade was all the more remarkable in the absence of any acknowledgement or recognition on his part that the vast majority of physicians and the public would readily have applied to the same epithet of *charlatan* to him.

With the venom finally emptied from his pen, Buchanan concluded his diatribe with a surprising recommendation: "Medical matters, so degraded and mixed up, could easily be rectified by the enactment of a United States registration law." What he proposed was more than simply a national version of the medical registration laws enacted by many states. He called for a medical examining board, composed of navy surgeons, in each state. All physicians would undergo an examination whose content would be tailored to the level of experience attained by the practitioner. Physicians with fewer than ten years' practice experience would be examined in all branches of medicine. Those with eleven to twenty years' experience would be assessed more narrowly on medicine, surgery, and midwifery. Those with more than twenty years' experience in practice would be grandfathered in without having to take an examination. In all cases, however, the medical degree would not be considered in the decision making behind the legal practice. Buchanan proposed that "the diplomas of all schools . . . be ignored, no questions, even, asked, as to whether he is a graduate or not—the test to be ability, irrespective of any worthless document." Perhaps nothing written by John Buchanan in the years after his arrest and imprisonment better reflects his jaded view of the medical degree and what it purported to represent. His skewed first-hand experiences underscored the reality that too often there was nothing educationally substantive behind the diploma; with so many institutions issuing medical degrees, most of them private endeavors driven by the inevitable need for profit, one should never presume that the diploma signified mastery of even a minimum educational standard.

The publication of his *Family Physician and the Domestic Practice of Medicine* had another significance. It marked the final chapter in Buchanan's diploma trade career. Moreover, it introduced a new business colleague, the book's publisher. Most of Buchanan's prior works had been self-published, but the publisher of *Family Physician* was listed as "R. Russell," otherwise known as Rebecca Russell, Reba Russell, and Rebecca R. Hurff. Buchanan had dedicated his book to her under this last identity, a dedication that read, in part, "To "R. R. Hurff, M.D., in token of her many scientific achievements" and "the brilliant powers of her mind." In Russell, a thirty-two-year-old New Jersey native, Buchanan had found a companion who would remain his partner in business ventures for the rest of his life. For at least a brief period, they also worked together to revive Buchanan's diploma trade.

At this time, Buchanan was maintaining two business locations in Philadelphia. At 2210 North Twenty-Ninth Street, he operated an enterprise called the Ozone Chemical Works. Apparently recognizing the difficulties of supporting himself solely as practicing physician and author, Buchanan joined forces with Russell in the manufacture of medicines—an endeavor that would in time become his primary employment; yet, Buchanan was reluctant to foreswear medical practice entirely. From his other office at 149 Fourth Street, Buchanan ostensibly continued his medical practice, seeing patients and steadily scribbling away on text destined for his *Journal of Progressive Medicine*. He also carried on a smaller-scale version of the diploma trade from this office. Despite the alleged protests of his wife, the pull of easy money from the trade still proved irresistible to him. Conflict between them over his resumption of the trade ultimately led to a final arrest.[12]

The first hint that Buchanan had resumed his old activities appeared as a brief mention in the *Philadelphia Inquirer* of January 19, 1885. Under the small heading of "All Sorts," listing "Items of Local and General Interest," a single sentence stated, "Dr. John Buchanan, it is alleged, is still negotiating the sale of crooked diplomas." The following day, police arrested Buchanan and Russell and charged them with illegally selling diplomas and with forgery, for signing them with false names. In fact, they had brazenly signed the diplomas in the names of at least three prominent—and recently dead—Philadelphia physicians: Joseph Pancoast, Samuel Gross, and Charles Miegs.[13]

Buchanan submitted to his arrest "coolly." His colleague Russell was far less "composed"—the first hint of the combative personality of Buchanan's new partner. Swallowing his anger, Buchanan used the subsequent visit from a *Record* reporter to make his case. When asked to respond to the charges arising apparently from his wife's intercession with the police, Buchanan offered a strenuous denial. "It is all a lie—every word of it. My wife is not a respectable woman and I am trying to get a divorce from her." Then he made a sensational counter-accusation, asserting his wife's complicity in the 1880 suicide ruse by referring to it as that "drowning scheme of hers." For her part, she denied her husband's accusations, asserting that it was she who had left Buchanan upon his refusal to give up his "former practices." In contesting the divorce proceedings, she also accused her husband of adultery—presumably with Russell.[14]

In a series of hearings before magistrates on January 20 and February 6, the main outlines of the case emerged. Buchanan and an old acquaintance named Robert Moore had reestablished contact in late 1883. Their discussions turned to diplomas with the result that the two men, along with Russell and an engraver and calligrapher named William Hamilton, began producing and selling diplomas soon thereafter. Russell acted as courier, mailing the diplomas through an express office, an appropriate precaution given Buchanan's prominence and the possibility of his being recognized. A later disagreement between Moore and Buchanan led the former to approach Buchanan's wife, who was already engaged in divorce proceedings with the doctor. Buchanan acknowledged the argument but said it had arisen when he had fired Moore for drunkenness after hiring him to perform odd jobs around the office. Buchanan's attorney claimed that Moore's testimony was driven by financial interest, since he was collecting a "witness fee" from Mrs. Buchanan in the divorce proceeding. Both Buchanan and Russell entered "not guilty" pleas.

When their trial took place in mid-March, it was Russell who attracted the attention of jurors, the press, and the audience. This was partially because of her defiant tone. But public interest was primarily aroused by an unexpected genealogical twist to the case.[15] Under cross-examination at their trial, the prosecution pressed Russell on the multiple names by which she had been known at various times—Russell, Hurff, and King. Russell's responses displayed a be-damned attitude to Victorian notions of feminine sensibility.[16] When the prosecuting attorney asked why she did not use her married name, King, she replied, "I never did. We married and agreed to separate. That was ten or twelve years ago. I don't know whether my husband is dead or alive."

The prosecution shifted to Russell's business relationship with Buchanan. She then startled everyone present by claiming that she had known Buchanan since the age of six and that he was actually her biological father. When asked why she had not revealed this information previously or in signing the "article of co-partnership" for her business arrangement with Buchanan, she claimed she had hoped to avoid a "terrible scandal," since her mother was a "respectable woman."

Almost certainly surprised by this assertion and perhaps seeking less sensational ground to cover, the prosecutor queried Russell on her medical background. Russell proved to be an extremely combative witness.

"When did you study medicine?"

"I have studied medicine for ten years in Salem, New Jersey and in this city."

"Where did you graduate?"

"I have not graduated."

"Are you a doctor? You had a sign out with an 'M.D.' to it."

"I have no diploma. The M.D. stood for money down."

This seemingly flippant reply drew a strong reaction from the courtroom crowd. The prosecutor remonstrated with Russell, but she refused to back down.

"Do you understand the sanctity of an oath?"

"I do."

"Do you mean to say that when you put 'M.D.' on the sign that you meant money down?"

"I do. That is exactly what I meant. I say that under oath. It didn't make any difference to me what people believed—I am not responsible for what they believe." After a lengthy deliberation, the jury returned with a guilty verdict on Buchanan. Russell was acquitted.

Despite the conviction, it appears that John Buchanan served no jail time. A review of subsequent issues of the *Inquirer* and the *Record* uncovered no further mention of the case or of a sentencing hearing. Instead, a brief note six months later claimed that a gravely ill Buchanan was near death at a friend's home in New Jersey as he "await[ed] trial for issuing bogus diplomas."[17] This may be an indication that the legal objections raised by Buchanan's defense team during the hearings and trial earlier that year actually prevailed, overturning the jury's decision. Buchanan's defense team had objected specifically to the "uncorroborated statements" of the witness Moore, who was technically *particeps criminis* to the alleged crime. Buchanan's lawyers also filed a demurrer on the original indictment, apparently claiming that evidence—specifically the forged diplomas in question—were not presented.[18] Their efforts appear to have been successful. In any case, John Buchanan had already determined to make a major life change.

Exodus from Philadelphia

In late 1885 or early 1886, John Buchanan left Philadelphia after approximately thirty-five years in that city. Together with Russell, he moved to New York City, where the two passed themselves off over the next twenty years as father and daughter or as business partners. Buchanan finally understood that his infamy not only had ended his sale of diplomas but also made it impossible for him to practice as a doctor, especially in Philadelphia. It was time for a change of scene—and a change of occupation. Buchanan decided to dedicate his energies to manufacturing medicines, in addition to writing and publishing. By relocating to New York, he entered an environment in which almost no one knew him on sight and even those who might were unlikely to encounter him in a metropolitan area of several million people.

Before committing wholly to the manufacturing and sale of medicines, Buchanan made at least one more foray into the diploma trade. A brief item in the *New York Medical Journal* from April 3, 1886, carried a letter from a reader inquiring about an obscure publication he had recently stumbled upon—the *Journal of Progressive Medicine*. The publication was edited by John Buchanan, M.D., and published by R. R. Russell at 77 Greenwich Avenue in Brooklyn. Most of the publication's contents extolled the virtues of medicines produced by their "manufacturing chemist," John Buchanan. What most caught the reader's eye, however, was a small announcement concerning the "Medical Department of Ohio University" with its "graded course of study" and "tuition in private classes." Interested parties were directed to make all inquires through "Professor Buchanan" at the same Greenwich Avenue address.[19] As an indication of just how brazen Buchanan had become in his diploma trade, it is worth noting that while the school was a legitimate institution, an 1885 course catalog confirmed that it did not even possess a medical school![20]

Perhaps more than one reader made the connection between the announcement about Ohio University and Philadelphia's "bogus Dr. John." In any case, Buchanan apparently cast no more lures to doctors wanting quick and easy diplomas. Instead, he and Russell spent the next twenty-odd years quietly working together in Brooklyn to build a business in herbal remedies. The business, known as Buchanan and Company, remained in operation until Buchanan's death in January 1905.[21] There is something almost aesthetically pleasing about John Buchanan's shift from medical education to patent medicines. Both fields were either loosely regulated or wholly unregulated in the mid-1880s. Buchanan's motives in shifting from one to the other reflected pragmatism and opportunity.

America at that time was awash in potions, lotions, ointments, and elixirs of every type and variety. Whether euphemistically described as patent or proprietary medicines or denigrated by critics as snake oil or nostrums, such products flooded the American marketplace. Some—such as Lydia Pinkham's Herb Medicine—captured the imagination and favor of the purchasing public. Although such products are often casually referred to as patent medicines, this term is a misnomer; proprietary medicines were seldom patented, as that would have required disclosing their ingredients. Generally, the only protection sought for such products were copyrights or trade rights to their product names and label images. Surviving samples of marketing for these medicines date as far back as the colonial era, but the real explosion in their availability and popularity came after the Civil War, when a boom in print media produced on steam presses gave them a platform through journals, magazines, pamphlets, and flyers. A commercial advertising culture developed to "facilitate trust" through the medium of the printed word. Those selling these medicines recognized that only nonstop advertising kept their products viable in a congested market, while the owners of penny press publications recognized in turn the financial boon this advertising gave to them.[22]

The attraction of the patent medicine field to Buchanan and Russell was simple: Americans were spending vast amounts of money on these products. In the year 1900 alone, Americans spent an estimated $75 million on so-called patent medicines. For manufacturers of such products, the potential revenues were temptingly lucrative. One well-established Wisconsin manufacturer, the Reinhardt Brothers, achieved sales worth $35,000 in 1904, a year they described as a "lean" one for business.[23] Buchanan and Russell developed sales through their own publication, *The Germicide*, through advertising, and, like many others in the field, by placing their informational literature with druggists across the country.[24]

Since promotional literature like *The Germicide* is ephemeral by nature, few copies of that publication survive to provide a systematic assessment of

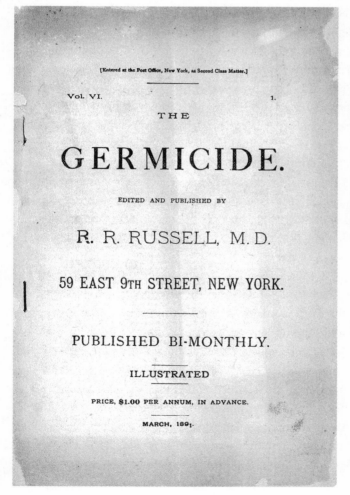

[Entered at the Post Office, New York, as Second Class Matter.]

Vol. VI.   1.

THE

GERMICIDE.

EDITED AND PUBLISHED BY

R. R. RUSSELL, M. D.

59 EAST 9TH STREET, NEW YORK.

PUBLISHED BI-MONTHLY.

ILLUSTRATED

PRICE, $1.00 PER ANNUM, IN ADVANCE.

MARCH, 1891.

Fig. 19. *The Germicide*. One of the few surviving copies of a publication by John Buchanan and Rebecca Russell, reflecting Buchanan's late career transition from selling diplomas to selling patent medicines. Image courtesy of the author.

Buchanan's and Russell's approach to sales. One edition from 1891 identified Buchanan and Company as a manufacturer, importer, and exporter
of "bactericides, rare drugs and chemicals," which Buchanan priced from
fifty cents to two dollars. The title of the publication, its drawings of mi-
crobes, and its various articles explaining the role of bacteria in disease
helped to sheath the work in a mantle of scientific respectability sufficient
to impress the public. Meanwhile, the product line of Buchanan and Company ranged from multiple "ozonized" offerings (e.g., clay and sulphur
water) to products that were clearly botanically based, like saw palmetto
and eucalyptus. The claims for treatment were extravagant—for example,
chloride of gold for venereal disease or a cocaine suppository for impo-
tence. Occasionally, a qualifying statement hints that purchasers should
exercise caution in self-treating their conditions. The company's ozone
paste is a case in point. While advertisements claimed that the paste possessed a "special affinity for [treating] the cancer germ," they noted that
it was "destructive to healthy tissue as well."

How did Buchanan fare in his new career in proprietary medicines? If
the later battle over his estate is any indication, his business was lucrative.
In large part, this success reflected Buchanan's good timing. He entered
the field in 1885, more than twenty years before the 1906 passage of the
Pure Food and Drug Act. Even then, this federal legislation did not put
an end to proprietary medicines as it only prohibited false labeling and
required that potentially dangerous ingredients (e.g., alcohol and cocaine)
be specifically listed. Despite the disparagement of these products, some
of America's best-known twentieth-century products originated as patent
medicine, including Coca-Cola, Dr. Pepper, Hire's Root Beer, Geritol,
Phillip's Milk of Magnesia, and Luden Brothers cough drops.[25]

In 1885, John Buchanan transitioned from being an outlier in one
aspect of medicine to winning success in another by shifting from irregular practitioner and diploma trader to a physician advertising proprietary medicines. As time went on, however, the same determination
to safeguard the public that had impelled the regulation of medical
education began to impinge on the field of patent medicines. With the
AMA's injunction against physician advertising and its steady campaign
against the patent medicine industry in the first decades of the twentieth century, Buchanan found that he had moved from being a pariah in
one field (medical education) to becoming an outcast in another through

Buchanan and Company. However, Buchanan did not survive to see the 1906 passage of the Pure Food and Drug Act, and his timing may have proved fortuitous. By dying in 1905 (at the age of seventy-six), he avoided having to reinvent himself or his career once again.

ALL THINGS CONSIDERED

The final denouement in the story of John Buchanan's career threatens to reduce the serious issues embedded in his story to a farce. Admittedly, some aspects of his life and career read like episodes from a novel, but these elements should not trivialize what was at stake. The actions of John Buchanan and the EMC directly impacted the careers of hundreds, if not thousands, of individual physicians and physician hopefuls in the United States and overseas, and indirectly affected the lives of many more patients. In the broadest sense, his career and the devolution of the EMC into a diploma mill impacted multiple causes and communities: eclectic medicine, medical legislation, and medical education. Furthermore, Buchanan's long career in the medical diploma trade underscored the failure of physicians to work collectively against one of the most fundamental threats to their emerging profession.

The eclectic movement within medicine represented a major dissenting branch in the American practice of nineteenth-century medicine. Eclectics were always a minority among physicians in the United States. One contemporary estimate placed their numbers at 5 percent of all U.S. physicians in 1873.[26] In Philadelphia, they comprised only 2 percent of doctors in 1886.[27] Yet on multiple levels they embraced their identity as a dissenting minority, even turning it into a virtue. More importantly, the eclectics' milder therapeutic stance proved timely and popular with patients. Despite this popularity, eclecticism remained locked in what the head of the National League for Medical Freedom described as a "battle for its life" against the "intolerance" and persecution of medical regulars.[28]

At the same time, the eclectics' small numbers and the persistent antagonism they faced from medical regulars left their movement highly vulnerable when Buchanan's activities drew increasing national scrutiny. Leaders within the eclectic movement fought a persistent battle against the guilt by association that invariably crept into the reporting of John

Buchanan's exploits. In fact, Buchanan contributed to this by deliberately sowing confusion in the press, as when he promoted a National Medical Eclectic Association, a title using the same words (in a different order) as the name of the legitimate, original national organization based in New York. He also benefited from a serendipitous confusion with Joseph R. Buchanan, an early and well-known leader in the eclectic movement.[29]

Alexander Wilder's 1887 history of the eclectic movement underscored the difficulty of "outliving the Philadelphia scandal." As Wilder described it, Buchanan's activities brought a "great onslaught upon Eclectics" and offered critics an easy opportunity to tarnish them with "ridicule and condemn[ation]."[30] Eclectic leaders lamented the "misfortune" to their movement's "reputation" but could not escape acknowledging some culpability of their own through the "loose . . . management" practices at some of their colleges.[31]

Similarly, despite the periodic hue and cry over Buchanan's activities in the 1870s, medical regulars often behaved as if there were little to gain from joining with legal authorities to vigorously move against the EMC. In the prevailing atmosphere of rancorous medical factionalism, Buchanan and the EMC delivered more serious wounds to the eclectic cause from the inside than any that medical regulars could administer from outside. While action against the EMC might prompt public praise, medical regulars saw a judicious application of silence and inaction as their optimal course; they understood that direct assaults on the EMC might just as easily trigger a backlash by eclectics accusing them of persecution arising from professional jealousy. In essence, the profession seemed partially paralyzed by its divisions in dealing with Buchanan. As one Cincinnati physician summed up the situation, "It is vain to hope that these things [diploma sales] can be corrected by the profession itself."[32]

As for John Buchanan, his activities grew so infamous that his name became a byword for fraud. A contemporary medical journal on the American West Coast—thousands of miles from Philadelphia—could disparagingly describe a medical degree as little better than the "average Buchanan diploma," and be confident that its physician readership would understand the implication of fraud.[33] So deeply engrained was the association of Buchanan diplomas with fraud that even a decade after the height of the scandal, writers were still using terms like "Buchanan's disciples" or "Buchananistic" degrees with confidence that their readers would recognize and understand the connotation.[34]

The sheer numbers involved in Buchanan's diploma trade figured prominently in his infamy. At the time of his arrest alone, authorities uncovered evidence for the sale of three thousand diplomas, though one contemporary journal commented upon the *Philadelphia Record* publishing a list of nearly nine thousand graduates from the Eclectic Medical College.[35] Whatever the actual numbers, for years after his arrest and the shuttering of the school, Buchanan's diplomas resurfaced repeatedly and periodically in the United States and abroad.[36] This resulted in a regular stream of queries to Philadelphia officials from state medical boards across the country (e.g., Texas and New York) and from government authorities overseas.

This is not to say that the EMC was the only operation of its kind in post–Civil War America. Competitors in the diploma trade littered the field across all regions of the country. Edinburgh University, originally established in Missouri before shifting operations to Chicago, presented itself as a "branch" of the Scottish institution. The Illinois Board of Health ultimately pressed local authorities for the arrest of its proprietor, Nathan S. Dodge.[37] Yet Edinburgh faced stiff competition from other schools in other states. Illinois ultimately became a national hotbed for the diploma trade. A retrospective list compiled by the AMA in 1918 revealed at least a dozen medical diploma mills based in that state alone.[38]

Bellevue Medical College of Massachusetts received a state charter in 1880 only to see its "dean," Rufus King Noyes, arrested in December 1882 for mail fraud and diploma sales. Noyes subsequently prevailed in the courts by presenting his legally held charter, which empowered the school faculty as the "sole judges" of a student's fitness for a diploma. This legal turn of affairs spawned a brief interlude in which scam artists regarded Massachusetts as the perfect place to incorporate diploma mills; these included the American University of Boston, Excelsior Medical College, and the Druidic University, among others.[39] Neighboring states in New England fared no better, with diploma mills or fraudulent institutions later appearing in New Hampshire and Vermont.[40]

Two of John Buchanan's colleagues established paper institutions similar to his American University: Henry Stickney, who set up the New England

University, and Henry S. Thomas, who set up the Detroit Eclectic Medical College.[41] Within the fold of eclectic medicine, the American Eclectic Medical College in Cincinnati offered further embarrassment when the Illinois Board of Health classified the school as "fraudulent" and a diploma mill.[42] So, too, did the Wisconsin Eclectic Medical College, whose owner/proprietor, Fred Rutland, was arrested in 1897 after selling nearly one thousand diplomas.[43] The physiomedical leader William H. Cook identified two Cincinnati schools, Alva Curtis's Physio-Medical College and William Nicely's Physio-Eclectic Medical College, as having connections to Buchanan, strongly hinting that they were diploma mills, if not outright labeling them as such.[44]

Medical diploma mills popped up in numerous states and territories from the Atlantic coast to the Pacific, operating with varying degrees of success and longevity. The schools mentioned here were among the approximately forty institutions identified as fraudulent by the AMA Council on Medical Education in its 1918 review of U.S. medical colleges.[45] Yet even if this discussion demonstrates that the EMC did not stand alone as a diploma mill, it remains the single most significant example of one, both because of the sheer volume of diplomas it granted fraudulently and because of the broad national and international attention it garnered during the critical period when state laws to regulate the practice of medicine were being introduced. No other medical diploma mill approached the scale and impact of the EMC until the 1920s, when the exposé reporting of Harry Brundidge and the *St. Louis Star* implicated two Missouri medical schools and licensing boards in three states: Arkansas, Connecticut, and Missouri.[46]

The persistence of medical diploma sales underscored the frustrations facing legitimate medical educators. With state laws governing the issuance of educational charters wholly outside of their control, educators could only implore legislators to craft or revise these laws with appropriate attention to the potential for abuse. Meaningful efforts to reform education were making headway in much of the country in the late nineteenth century, but a dark corner of pseudo-medical education persisted despite the efforts of organized medical professionals (the AMA) and educational associations (the AAMC).

Buchanan and the EMC served also as a stalking horse for those seeking to justify medical regulatory legislation and as a cautionary tale highlighting the potential for abuse in the absence of regulatory constraints. Within the eclectic community, this steady drumbeat for medical legislation created a strategic quandary. Eclectics generally opposed any form of medical law as "class legislation" that would create a "close[d] corporation of medicine." They regarded regular or "old school physicians," working through the AMA, as the driving force behind such legislation, motivated by a determination to consolidate the advantages they already held through their larger numbers.[47] Prominent among the eclectics leading this cause was Joseph Buchanan, who spearheaded the National Constitutional Liberty League. Buchanan and the league fought against all medical licensing legislation, launching a successful campaign that long delayed such legislation in Massachusetts.[48]

Steady backing for medical legislation from the AMA only intensified after the U.S. Supreme Court decision in *Dent v. West Virginia* (1889), in which the court affirmed a strong set of powers for medical licensing boards. Even before this decision, however, some in the eclectic community recognized that continued opposition to such laws meant potentially forfeiting any role in crafting medical legislation at a time when the push for such laws was gaining momentum. Once reconciled to the inevitability of regulation, eclectics first pushed for registration laws, but when the Buchanan scandal underscored the inherent weakness of such laws, they grudgingly supported the creation of state medical boards provided that regular physicians were not a majority on the board and thus in a position to exploit their advantage along sectarian lines.[49] Unfortunately for the eclectic community, one of the major seeds for the regulatory system they had initially opposed sprung from an insufficiently tended patch of ground within their community in Philadelphia.

Once they were firmly established, state medical boards began making their influence felt among proprietary and substandard medical schools, especially those operating as little better than diploma mills.[50] As the only entities legally empowered to issue medical licenses, these boards were uniquely positioned to encourage educational reform by gradually raising standards for licensees and by creating and publicizing formal lists of approved medical schools. These lists served as precursors to the de facto recognition and accreditation efforts of later groups, such as the AMA Council on Medical Education and the Association of American Medical Colleges (AAMC).[51] In 1906, the council conducted the first of

Table 6: Number of U.S. Medical Schools by Classification
(Including percentage accounting for all medical students)

	1905	1915	1920	1927
Class A schools	82*	66 (76%)	70 (89%)	62 (95%)
Class B schools	46	17 (18%)	7 (5%)	3 (3%)
Class C schools	32	12 (6%)	8 (6%)	6 (2%)

* Percentage data unavailable for 1905
Adapted from "Medical Education in the United States," *JAMA*, August 17, 1929, 533; Morris Fishbein, *History of the AMA, 1847–1947*, 898.

several surveys of U.S. medical schools. The woeful collective state of American medical education was reflected in the three-tier classification system established by the council in the early twentieth century. The council categorized "acceptable" schools as Class A, those schools whose deficiencies were remediable fell into Class B, and those schools deemed wholly unacceptable or requiring "complete reorganization" were listed as Class C.[52]

The significance of this role for state medical boards should not be discounted, as the ability of medical schools to facilitate collective change in medical education within the confines of a voluntary association had already proven inadequate. The first iteration of the AAMC collapsed in 1882 over the issue of requiring a three-year program for a diploma. It is coincidental but symbolically apt that a reorganized AAMC did not reemerge until 1890, the same year that the first national association of state medical boards was founded.[53]

Taking all of this into account, the labors of medical educators and medical regulators presented mixed results. Even in a state like Illinois, whose medical licensing law and Board of Health were regarded as templates for best practices, it proved exceedingly difficult to fully extinguish the dubious practices of borderline or outright fraudulent schools. Educational chartering laws were outside the purview of the state medical board responsible for issuing licenses. Thus, while Illinois might refuse to recognize and license graduates from a school like the EMC or Edinburgh, they had no power to shut down these institutions. Accordingly, the holders of degrees granted by diploma mills sought licenses in states whose licensing body lacked statutory authority to recognize or approve medical schools and thus held no power to deny a license based upon the source of the diploma presented. Further complicating this landscape for medical licensing was the continued presence and practice of older physicians whose many years in practice predated licensing laws. These individuals were often statutorily exempted or granted special consideration.

The growth of medical regulation in the 1880s to include examining boards marked the next step in a steady progression away from reliance on the medical diploma as a credential sufficient by itself to legitimate the practice of medicine. John Eaton, the U.S. commissioner of education, pointed specifically to the Illinois board as an exemplar for medical regulation, citing the inclusive composition of its board; the inclusion of lay members; and its determination that a candidate's understanding of human health and disease should form the basis for granting licensure, irrespective of sectarian education.[54] In essence, a shift was under way, both in medical regulation and education, from reliance on an outcome measure, such as a diploma, to a focus on the underlying educational process that the outcome measure ostensibly represented. However, this transition took time—playing out over many years in some instances.

Reflecting on the state of American medical education and regulation, and with John Buchanan and the EMC clearly in mind, Commissioner Eaton summarized the story this way and offered his own call to action. "We have seen unscrupulous and infamous men . . . in control of the charters of American medical schools, advertising and selling their wares in three continents, disgracing the profession of medicine . . . we have seen even the officers of justice conniving with these scoundrels to shield them from punishment . . . we have seen tardy justice . . . a pretended suicide, fleeing from justice . . . we have seen him [Buchanan] captured and inadequately punished for his long career of knavery by a short imprisonment."[55]

With all this in mind, Eaton proposed an ambitious funding strategy in each state to put medical schools on a sound financial basis and thus remove the temptation to promote dubious education. This strategy would require every legally chartered medical school, as part of the basic requirements for medical licensure, to secure sufficient capital to operate ($300,000) through bonds or other securities and to mandate an entrance examination for matriculants, a three-year curriculum, professors capable of clinical as well as didactic instruction, and a specified minimum number of hours of instruction that included laboratory work and hospital attendance. Eaton's goal was ambitious but was one that ultimately aligned with the progressive movements in both medical education and regulation.

Finally, John Buchanan's story is that of a criminal enterprise launched within the confines of a legitimate medical school, where it flourished discreetly before growing so large that it corrupted the entire institution and spilled into the public spotlight. His activities and the devolution of the EMC into a diploma mill operating purely for profit provided educators, legislators, and members of medical licensing boards with direct evidence of the vulnerabilities of their existing educational and regulatory systems. Although John Buchanan and the EMC were not the sole causes for systemic changes in medical regulation and education, their activities, and the ensuing scandal, which reached international proportions, imparted a high-profile impetus to reform that coincided with corresponding efforts already unfolding in both arenas.

"Nothing so difficult as a beginning . . .

except perhaps the end."

—Lord Byron, *Don Juan*

Epilogue

Despite his infamy in the diploma trade two decades earlier, John Buchanan's death went unreported in any of the newspapers at the time—a reflection at first glance of just how far Buchanan had drifted from the social and medical mainstream. This surprising silence actually had a different explanation. The lack of public notice regarding Buchanan's death stemmed not from a disinterested press and a forgetful public but from an overt and prolonged effort by Reba Russell to conceal her business partner's death, and an estate estimated at $25,000, from his children. Buchanan's patent medicine enterprise had flourished, a fact that emerged from the well-publicized and heavily contested probate case concerning his estate.[1]

In August 1907, George Buchanan received a letter from a stranger informing him of his father's death.[2] The younger Buchanan could not have been entirely surprised at this news. When he had last visited his father, in 1904, the old man had been in poor health. The date of his father's death did surprise him, however: John Buchanan had died more than two years earlier. At the subsequent Chancery Court hearing on the Buchanan estate, held in Camden, New Jersey, in January 1908, George testified that it had become impossible to see or visit his father without the permission of Russell. He then described how she had impeded his efforts to see his father and claimed that she made any visits he did manage to achieve extremely "unpleasant," asserting that on one occasion Russell "practically had me ejected" from the premises.

Buchanan's two children suspected both Russell's motives for this behavior and her role in their father's personal and business affairs. They knew of his foray into patent medicines late in his career and believed that Russell's failure to inform them of their father's death signaled her intent to pilfer the estate's assets. At the first day of the court hearing on January 9, 1908, attorneys for George Buchanan and Isabella Buchanan McGarvey laid out their case, alleging that Russell had unlawfully collected and withheld funds from John Buchanan's estate.

This first day featured two surprises: the appearance of another claimant to the estate—Buchanan's second wife, Lucy—and Russell's elaborate testimony centered on her upbringing as Buchanan's illegitimate child. Lucy's appearance probably caught the two Buchanan siblings off guard. Their former stepmother testified that she had married John Buchanan in July 1873, several months after the death of his first wife.[3] In support of her claim, she submitted a certified copy of her marriage certificate. She acknowledged commencing divorce proceedings between herself and her husband in the mid-1880s but asserted that these were dropped in consideration of a financial settlement from Buchanan. The younger Buchanans offered a weak protest, but to no avail. With a marriage certificate entered in evidence, the judge ruled Lucy Buchanan as a claimant.

While this development captured attention in the courtroom, the main story line presented by the newspapers focused on Russell. Reporters played up her claim to be Buchanan's daughter as a stunning revelation. In fact, Russell had first made this assertion more than twenty years earlier, during court proceedings in 1885 against her and John Buchanan on charges of diploma sales. Now Russell added elaborate elements to her testimony. Stating that Buchanan was her biological father, she claimed that he had placed her with the Hurff family in New Jersey to avoid disgracing her biological mother. Russell told how she had finally learned as a teenager of Buchanan's identity as her father and how, after this revelation, she had been visited periodically by a heavily veiled woman who often gave her money but always concealed her identity by refusing to lift her veil or give her name. Russell claimed that she had used this money, together with funds she had earned from painting and writing, as the capital for the patent medicine business she operated with Buchanan. According to Russell, John Buchanan's role had been minimal, and it was only because of her daughterly devotion that she supported her increasingly incapacitated father.

Attorneys for Buchanan's adult children ridiculed Russell's story and worked steadily to discredit her. They pressed her concerning the multiple names by which she had publicly presented herself: Hurff, Russell, King, and Buchanan. They offered to subpoena her husband, Winfield King, whom she had claimed was dead. Ridiculing her assertion that she had sold individual paintings for thousands of dollars, they entered one such work into evidence to show that she lacked the requisite talent. They also provided evidence of her financial assets, which included holdings in various New York and New Jersey banks. They also worked steadily to rattle her under cross-examination. After first establishing her age, for example, they asked when Buchanan arrived in America, insinuating that her supposed father's arrival to America came well after her birth.

The attorneys saved their most dramatic attack on Russell for the second day of the hearing, when they called her brother, Daniel Hurff, to the stand. He testified growing up with his sister, Rebecca or Reba, and their parents, Reece and Ann Hurff, and recalled her addressing their parents as "pop" and "mother." In harsher terms, he called his sister's testimony an "outrage" explicable only through insanity.[4] Russell's attorney counterattacked by claiming that Daniel's testimony missed the point: Rebecca Russell may well have been raised by the Hurff family as one of their own children, but given that Daniel Hurff was only eighteen months older than Rebecca, he could not testify to witnessing her birth as his sister. Either from stress or as a dramatic ploy to undermine Daniel and gain sympathy, Russell fainted toward the end of Daniel Hurff's testimony, causing the judge to call a recess that delayed the court proceedings.

Although Russell's attorney did his best to put forward a plausible case for his client, several facts were damning—in particular, her failure to alert the Buchanan siblings of their father's death and John Buchanan's sale of one piece of property to Russell for $1. To divert attention from this evidence, her attorney instead focused much of his closing statement on the plausibility of Russell's explanation. He pointed out that Russell had heard the story of her true identify directly from Buchanan and argued that since John Buchanan was a "bad man," it was perfectly "credible" that he had been capable of such an affront against social mores as fathering an illegitimate child. The attorney went on to argue that Buchanan, to his credit, had protected the identity of Russell's mother, who had later made a respectable marriage and had a family.

The attorney making the closing argument for Buchanan's legitimate children, George and Isabella, mocked Russell's entire story. Calling it a "fabrication," he closed with several challenging rhetorical questions of his own. "Is it conceivable that this country girl could . . . without training have painted pictures . . . for large sums, one of them bringing $1000? Is it conceivable she could have established by her own resources a manufacturing business in New York of world-wide scope?"

On January 12, 1908, at the conclusion of testimony and closing statements, the judge dismissed all parties and retired to consider his decision. The *Philadelphia Record* aptly labeled the matter a "strangely tangled" case and offered its opinion that the judge would have some "deep thinking" to do in order untangle the bizarre story, with its multiple claims and counterclaims. Ultimately, and perhaps unsurprisingly, the judge ruled in favor of Buchanan's legitimate children.[5]

When John Buchanan—physician, educator, author, entrepreneur, convicted criminal—died in 1905, the days of his greatest national notoriety were more than two decades in the past. However he did not slip into the poetical good night unnoticed. Not only had he returned to the newspapers in 1908 with a final melodramatic flourish as the offstage presence in a bizarre probate case, but he continued to cast resounding echoes into the personal and professional affairs of family, friends, and colleagues.

For some friends and colleagues, the association with John Buchanan and/or the EMC gave them their sole moment in the public spotlight, welcome or unwelcome, and once it had passed, they melted back into the mass of humanity, busily getting on with daily life, largely unknown and anonymous. For others, the nexus with Buchanan and the EMC constituted merely one episode in long and successful careers. The experiences of Buchanan's family members were equally varied. Some suffered from the relationship, propelled by their link to Buchanan into personal and professional missteps that his notoriety aggravated through the glare of public attention. Other friends and family members managed to rise above their association with John Buchanan and the EMC, so that the scandal surrounding him became nothing more than a footnote to their careers, or in some cases, a chapter they omitted entirely from their personal histories. Following are brief notes on the later fortunes of a few of the people whose lives intersected John Buchanan's.

After the Civil War, the financial strains acting on the EMC and its increasingly unprofessional and erratic policies provoked corresponding upheaval among its faculty. Most of the school's early leaders did not live to see the ignominy of the EMC's public disgrace. One of the original founders, Joseph Sites, died in 1878, after a long and successful medical career in Philadelphia.[6] Another early EMC leader, Henry Hollembaek, later left the area, settling in Burlington, Vermont, where he died in 1896.[7] Marshall Calkins, whose addition to the faculty had been something of a feather in the EMC's cap, left during its heady early days, before any hint of the scandals to come. After settling for a time in Springfield, Massachusetts, he took up a faculty position at the University of Vermont. His 1922 obituary in the *Boston Medical and Surgical Journal* offered no hint of his prior connection to Buchanan's school.[8]

The fortunes of William Paine were considerably more checkered. Once a member of the EMC faculty, he later became Buchanan's rival in the diploma trade through his leadership of Philadelphia University and joined him in the ensuing scandal. Unlike Buchanan, however, Paine— described by one former student as possessing "more brains" than any of his eclectic colleagues—worked to disassociate himself from Philadelphia University and for a time enjoyed a good measure of professional and financial success. Acquiring an impressive building at Ninth and Chestnut in Philadelphia, he founded his own business, which operated initially under the grandiose title of the William Paine Medical and Surgical Institute. Whether Paine's practice waned or he sought to supplement his income through nonmedical activities is unclear, but he later converted the building into the Peabody Hotel. Then in 1892, Paine ran into trouble with local health officials when it became known that a man with leprosy was working in the hotel kitchen. Paine suffered the embarrassment of being charged with "maintaining a nuisance prejudicial to public health." Perhaps the timing was coincidental, but several months later he sold the building and relocated to Virginia.[9]

William Bowlsby, whose connection with Jacob Rosenzweig during the trunk murder trial of 1871 had threatened his career, drifted away from the orbit of the EMC soon thereafter. He remained in Brooklyn, continued to practice medicine, and became deeply active in the Knights of Pythias, a fraternal order founded in 1864. Bowlsby apparently lived down his association with the abortionist Rosenzweig and in his old age was sufficiently respected in his community that in 1901 the *Brooklyn Daily Eagle* carried an article on the surprise party given for his seventy-third birthday. When he died several months later, the same paper published a laudatory obituary, calling him a "shining light" among physicians. The intervening thirty years and many subsequent sensational murder cases seem to have crowded out the 1871 trunk murder and Bowlsby's brush with notoriety from New Yorkers' memories.[10]

If human memory worked in William Bowlsby's favor, simple human error did Jacob Rosenzweig an even greater service. After his 1871 conviction under New York's malpractice law for the manslaughter of Alice Bowlsby, he entered prison resigned to serving a seven-year sentence. In spring 1872, however, his astute attorney, William F. Howe, took note of a change in New York state law that had replaced the statute under which Rosenzweig was convicted. Howe's close reading of the law found that its drafters had failed to include the usual provision that convictions for past crimes applied under the primary or preceding statute should remain in force. Howe challenged Rosenzweig's conviction and sentence on this basis, and succeeded in getting it overturned by the New York State Supreme Court. On November 12, 1873, after serving only two years and six months, Jacob Rosenzweig left his cell at Sing Sing. At the final hearing in a protracted legal process, Rosenzweig listened impassively to the judge's decision, offered a deep "bow to the Court"—and walked out a free man.[11]

Those closest to John Buchanan did not fare so well. In March 1883, his son George endured a nerve-racking trial of his own for malpractice. Five months previously, one of his dental patients had died after a surgical procedure performed by the younger Buchanan. The young woman's aunt testified that on her deathbed, her niece removed a set of false teeth from her mouth and, pointing to them, said, "The man who made these is the cause of all my suffering." A jury agreed, finding George Buchanan guilty of causing Elizabeth Holstein's death by malpractice. It is unclear whether he served any jail time for this conviction, since his attorney immediately filed a motion for a new trial on grounds unspecified in the press. Whatever the outcome, George's troubles in dentistry were far from over.

The younger Buchanan next appeared in the news in 1891, nearly a decade later, on charges of practicing dentistry without a license. After the jury acquitted him, George apparently tried to transition out of dentistry, running a retail shoe business with a brother-in-law, W. L. Fitzpatrick. In that same year, however, this business ran afoul of creditors, one of whom was George's own father-in-law. Thus Buchanan's venture into a family-run business ended in another public embarrassment. The *Philadelphia Inquirer* highlighted the failed business endeavor, and disparaged George's title of doctor by enclosing it in quotation marks.[12]

Martin Van Buren Chapman, John Buchanan's brother-in-law and accomplice in his suicide ruse and escape to Michigan and Canada, experienced even greater troubles. He continued to practice dentistry at various locations in Philadelphia and New Jersey until the early part of the twentieth century. Like George Buchanan, however, Chapman ran afoul of authorities for unlicensed practice. In 1902, a court convicted him of practicing dentistry without a license in Bridgeton, New Jersey. This case was merely the most recent in a series of legal troubles that Chapman periodically brought upon himself. In 1883, the newspapers had reported his failure to appear in court to answer charges of financial nonsupport of his wife. In that same year, Chapman faced a more serious charge, alleging that he and a female companion had "robbed" one of her relatives of more than $1,000. Chapman never appeared for the court hearing and forfeited his bail. He was twice arrested on assault charges in 1885 and 1886, one of the victims being his own mother.[13]

A profound and uncharacteristic silence surrounds the life of Rebecca (Reba) Russell, who remains one of the most fascinating characters surrounding John Buchanan. Russell, a self-taught woman from New Jersey who became Buchanan's longtime business partner in the manufacture of patent medicines and occasional periodical literature, comes across in the surviving press accounts as anything but quiet or demure. In fact, she emerges instead as pragmatic but avaricious. She could strike a defiant tone and assume a pugnacious posture even within the otherwise quiet confines of a courtroom. After the flurry of news coverage over Buchanan's estate, Russell disappeared entirely from all records, taking with her whatever funds she managed to retain from her long association with Buchanan.

The *Philadelphia Record* editor John Norris proved to be John Buchanan's greatest nemesis and the instigator of his downfall. While the Buchanan affair might have been the crowning achievement of a career for many a reporter, it was for Norris merely one of many successes. Recognized for his tenacity, determination, and talent, Norris soon caught the eye of those giants of the publishing industry, Joseph Pulitzer and William Randolph Hearst. Norris served as Pulitzer's "personal representative" on newspaper matters, worked directly for Hearst at the *New York Journal,* and later served as business manager for the *New York Times.* In 1908, as chairman of the American Newspaper Publishers' Association, he launched himself with crusade-like fervor into busting up the "paper trust" that was inflating wood pulp prices throughout the newspaper industry. In September 1913, Norris sat in the gallery of the United States Senate listening to final debate on the issue before the vote that ultimately lifted duties on paper and wood pulp. Utah Senator Reed Smoot, who was on the losing side of this particular political struggle, turned at one point in his comments from the Senate floor and waved to Norris, seated in the gallery above. Smoot acknowledged that "my friend Norris is safe in leaving the Senate gallery" knowing that he had won this particular fight. Norris's devotion to work and total commitment to fighting for what he felt were just causes may have compromised his health and contributed to his early death. Family members reported that he simply would not rest when engaged in these political crusades. Norris's son recalled that his father, perhaps remembering the technicality that had once allowed John Buchanan's American University charter to slip past the Pennsylvania state legislature, obsessed over the legislative process and its language in his fight against the paper trust. "He seemed to be afraid that some comma would be left out of the bill, some slight mistake made, that would defeat all of his efforts." John Norris died in 1914, not yet fifty-eight years old.[14]

Henry Palmer, the Pennsylvania attorney general and Civil War veteran who benefited from Norris's and Singerly's commitment to prosecuting John Buchanan, experienced considerable political success. After leaving his position as the state's attorney general in 1883, he practiced law, and then in 1900 ran successfully for a seat in the U.S. House of Representatives in 1900. He was twice re-elected (in 1902 and 1904) and regained the office once more in 1908.[15]

J. Howard Gendell, the Philadelphia attorney who assisted Norris in his investigation and capture of Buchanan, went on to enjoy a prominent legal career in that city. He later served with distinction as special assistant to the city solicitor and then was elected to the position of city solicitor himself. He held this last position at the time of his death in 1910.[16]

The seemingly inexhaustible wealth of *Philadelphia Record* owner and publisher, William Singerly eventually dissipated under the strain of the financial panic and depression of the mid-1890s. The national economic downturn caused two of his Philadelphia banks to collapse. Singerly, once a nominee for Pennsylvania's governorship and for many years the state's leading Democrat, died in 1898 shortly after finalizing arrangements for the sale of the *Philadelphia Record*.[17]

Dr. John Rauch, who had carefully monitored the actions of the EMC and swiftly moved to add the school to the list of those disapproved by Illinois's board of health, remained in his position as secretary for that board until 1891. The Illinois board served as the primary exemplar for broadly empowered medical licensing boards in the nineteenth century with a set of expansive powers that went beyond merely licensing physicians to actively determining which medical schools' graduates would be eligible for licensure in that state. Rauch was a lifelong bachelor dedicated to his work, yet despite his many successes, he managed to alienate friends and foes alike with his forceful pronouncements and firm hand in guiding the board. According to his successor, critics "hounded" Rauch from his position with the Illinois board, leaving him "broken hearted" at the "ingratitude" of former political allies who stood by when attacks upon his leadership reached a crescendo between 1889 and 1891.[18]

Finally, what of the EMC itself? Today, the 500 block of Pine Street in Philadelphia is lined with attractive brownstone buildings. Like much of the city's center, the area has become gentrified, vibrant with upscale restaurants, small businesses, neighborhood bars, and the lively comings and goings of young professionals and families. No trace remains of the building at 514 Pine Street that once housed the Eclectic Medical College of Pennsylvania. There are no historical markers to give even momentary pause to local residents or to entertain interested tourists who have strayed from the nearby landmarks of Independence Hall and the Liberty Bell to explore the city on their own. There is just a story, fast receding in time and fading in the city's collective memory, a dim recollection from an era long past, of an oddly named school and the notorious criminal physician whose exploits once tarnished the image of Philadelphia.

Appendix

Lyrics to "Bogus Dr. John"

I read an article in the paper, Dr. John, Dr. John;
Of your little steamboat caper, Dr. John, Dr. John;
But the story's sugar-coated, 'cause your body would have floated,
Yes, to the top it would have floated, Dr. John, Dr. John;
For in the water you'd get bloated, Dr. John, Dr. John.

Still, it was a daring plan, Dr. John, Dr. John;
To put whiskers on a man, Dr. John, Dr. John;
With instructions to yell and bawl and for help to loudly call,
Now, that was an awful gall, Dr. John, Dr. John;
He jumped overboard for a stall, Dr. John, Dr. John.

Now if a steamboat was in motion, Dr. John, Dr. John;
And if you took a little notion, Dr. John, Dr. John;
And $50 I would slide if you'd jump into the tide,
With the intent of suicide, Dr. John, Dr. John;
Then you must skin out and hide, Dr. John, Dr. John.

Now the papers spread the news, Dr. John, Dr. John;
So you must mind your P's and Q's, Dr. John, Dr. John;
Or you'll get tripped up at last with all your glories of the past,
Then you'd get an awful blast, Dr. John, Dr. John;
So don't you go so fast, Dr. John—Buchanan!

Source: "Bogus Dr. John," Air: Baby Mine. [Philadelphia]: A. W. Auner,
ca. 1880–81. Imprint held by the American Antiquarian Society, Boston,
Massachusetts.

Notes

ABBREVIATIONS FOR PERIODICALS

Source material for *Diploma Mill* draws heavily on journals and newspapers, predominantly from the nineteenth century. Titles for those sources cited frequently in the endnotes are abbreviated as follows.

AJP	*American Journal of Pharmacy*
BHM	*Bulletin of the History of Medicine*
BMRHP	*Botanic Medical Reformer and Home Physician*
BMSJ	*Boston Medical and Surgical Journal*
ChRec	*Christian Recorder*
CMG	*Cincinnati Medical Gazette*
DetFrP	*Detroit Free Press*
EJM	*Eclectic Journal of Medicine*
EMJ	*Eclectic Medical Journal*
EMJP	*Eclectic Medical Journal of Pennsylvania*
EMJPh	*Eclectic Medical Journal of Philadelphia*
Fed Bull	*Bulletin of the Federation of State Medical Boards*
JAMA	*Journal of the American Medical Association*
JHMHS	*Journal of the History of Medicine and Allied Health Sciences*
JPM	*Journal of Progressive Medicine*
MSR	*Medical and Surgical Reporter*
NEJM	*New England Journal of Medicine*
NYH	*New York Herald*
NYT	*New York Times*
NYTrib	*New York Tribune*
PET	*Providence (R.I.) Evening Telegram*
PhInq	*Philadelphia Inquirer*
PhPL	*Philadelphia Public Ledger*
PhPr	*Philadelphia Press*
PhRec	*Philadelphia Record*
PhT	*Philadelphia Times*
SFBul	*San Francisco Bulletin*
SpRep	*Springfield (Mass.) Republican*
WR	*Wheeling (W.Va.) Register*

Introduction

1. Many of the arguments put forth here first appeared in David Alan Johnson, "John Buchanan's Philadelphia Diploma Mill and the Rise of State Medical Boards," *BHM* 89, no. 1 (Spring 2015): 25–58.

2. See James C. Mohr, *Licensed to Practice: The Supreme Court Defines the American Medical Profession* (Baltimore, Md.: Johns Hopkins Univ. Press, 2013), 16–17, 169; Paul Starr, *The Social Transformation of American Medicine: The Rise of a Sovereign Profession and the Making of a Vast Industry* (New York: Basic Books, 1982), 12–13, 17–19; John Harley Warner, *The Therapeutic Perspective: Medical Practice, Knowledge, and Identity in America, 1820–1885* (Cambridge, Mass.: Harvard Univ. Press, 1986), 13.

3. Kenneth M. Ludmerer, *Learning to Heal: The Development of American Medical Education* (New York: Basic Books, 1985), 15; John Duffy, *From Humors to Medical Science: A History of American Medicine* (Urbana: Univ. of Illinois Press, 1993), 133–34.

4. John S. Haller Jr., *American Medicine in Transition: 1840–1910* (Urbana: Univ. of Illinois Press, 1981), 222; David A. Johnson and Humayun J. Chaudhry, *Medical Licensing and Discipline in America: A History of the Federation of State Medical Boards* (Lanham, Md.: Lexington Books, 2012), 28.

5. Ludmerer, *Learning to Heal*, 15–16.

Prologue

1. "Philadelphia's Daily Temperature, Precipitation, and Snowfall by Year," Phillyweather.net (website) at http://phillyclimate.blogspot.com/2007/07/1880 -philadelphia-daily-weather-data.html, accessed on Mar. 6, 2017.

2. Unless otherwise cited, events for Aug. 16–17, 1880, are taken from "The Pine Streeter," *PhInq*, Sept. 14, 1880, 3; "Dr. Buchanan Drowns Himself," *NYT*, Aug. 18, 1880, 2; "The Alleged Suicide," *PhInq*, Aug. 21, 1880, 2; "Buchanan—The Rumpus the Little Fat Doctor Is Kicking Up," *PhInq*, Aug. 20, 1880, 2; "Death or Fraud?" *PhInq*, Aug. 18, 1880, 2.

3. Correspondence between St. John Watkins Mintzer and Thomas Vanduser, MSS 2/1009, Series 6, St. John W. Mintzer Papers, 1847–1912, Historical Medical Library, College of Physicians of Philadelphia, Philadelphia, Pa.

4. "The Pine Street College," *PhInq*, June 17, 1880, 2.

5. "United States District Court," *PhInq*, Aug. 17, 1880, 2.

6. *Dictionary of American Biography*, s.v. "White, Andrew Dickson."

7. "Bogus Diplomas—the American University Again," *PhInq*, Mar. 31, 1880, 2.

252 NOTES TO PAGES 5–8

1. The Rise of Eclectic Medicine

1. Mona Nasser, Aida Tibi, and Emilie Savage-Smith, "Ibn Sina's Canon of Medicine: 11th Century Rules for Assessing the Effects of Drugs," *Journal of the Royal Society of Medicine* 102, no. 2 (Feb. 1, 2009): 78–80.

2. Paul Strathern, *A Brief History of Medicine: From Hippocrates to Gene Therapy* (London: Robinson Publishing Co., 2005), 34. For the transition to and impact of Galenic theory on Western medicine, see Mark Harrison, *Disease and the Modern World: 1500 to the Present Day* (Cambridge, UK: Polity Press, 2004), 16–19; Roy Porter, *The Greatest Benefit to Mankind: A Medical History of Humanity* (New York: W. W. Norton, 1997), 73–77.

3. John S. Haller Jr., *Medical Protestants: The Eclectics in American Medicine, 1825–1939* (Carbondale: Southern Illinois Univ. Press, 1994), 24–30; Russell M. Jones, "American Doctors in Paris, 1820–1861: A Statistical Profile," *JHMHS* 25, no. 2 (Apr. 1970): 150. For more on the Parisian school of medicine, see Erwin Ackerknecht, *A Short History of Medicine* (Baltimore, Md.: Johns Hopkins Univ. Press, 1982), 145–53; W. F. Bynum et al., *The Western Medical Tradition, 1800–2000* (Cambridge, UK: Cambridge Univ. Press, 2006), 37–53. For the Parisian school's alteration of medical discourse, see Michel Foucault, *The Birth of the Clinic: An Archaeology of Medical Perception* (New York: Vintage Books, 1994), x.

4. Johnson and Chaudhry, *Medical Licensing and Discipline*, 16.

5. John S. Haller Jr., *Kindly Medicine: Physio-Medicalism in America, 1836–1911* (Kent, Ohio: Kent State Univ. Press, 1997), xiii, 16; Duffy, *From Humors to Medical Science*, 81–82.

6. John Wesley, *Primitive Physick: or, An Easy and Natural Method of Curing Most Diseases*, 2nd ed. (London: G. Woodfall et al., 1747), ix–x; Nicholas Culpeper, *The English Physician—Enlarged* (London: A. and J. Churchill, 1703), cited in Haller, *Medical Protestants*, 8.

7. Haller, *Medical Protestants*, 37–40; Haller, *Kindly Medicine*, 18; Samuel Thomson, *A Narrative of the Life and Medical Discoveries of Samuel Thomson*, 9th ed. (Columbus, Ohio: Jarvis Pike and Co., 1833), 116–17.

8. Naomi Rogers, *An Alternative Path: The Making and Remaking of Hahnemann Medical College and Hospital of Philadelphia* (New Brunswick, N.J.: Rutgers Univ. Press, 1998), 1–3.

9. For an engaging overview exploring this ferment of sociomedical experimentation, see Erika Janik, *Marketplace of the Marvelous: The Strange Origins of Modern Medicine* (Boston: Beacon Press, 2014). See also ch. 2 of Roy Porter's *Blood and Guts: A Short History of Medicine* (New York: W. W. Norton, 2002).

10. William Rothstein, *American Physicians in the Nineteenth Century: From Sects to Science* (Baltimore, Md.: Johns Hopkins Univ. Press, 1985), 158; Rogers, *Alternative Path*, 4; John S. Haller Jr., *The History of American Homeopathy: The Academic Years, 1820–1835* (New York: Pharmaceutical Products Press, 2005), 40, 53.

11. Duffy, *From Humors to Medical Science*, 81–84. Regarding the efficacy of homeopathic treatments, a recent meta-analysis of 225 studies and 1,800 papers published by the National Health and Medical Research Council of Australia concluded there was "no reliable evidence" for the effectiveness of homeopathy. See *NHMRC Information Paper: Evidence on the Effectiveness of Homeopathy for Treating Health Conditions* (Canberra: National Health and Medical Research Council, 2015).

12. Rothstein, *American Physicians*, 157.

13. Haller, *Kindly Medicine*, 10.

14. Rothstein, *American Physicians*, 159–60, 232–33.

15. Haller, *Medical Protestants*, 33, 47, 57.

16. For a nuanced look at the Thomsonian movement as the origin for eclectic medicine, see Haller, *Medical Protestants*, ch. 2.

17. John S. Haller Jr., *Alternative Medicine: The Eclectic College of Cincinnati, 1845–1942* (Kent, Ohio: Kent State Univ. Press, 1999), 16.

18. Alexander Wilder, "Outline History of Eclectic Medicine," *Transactions of the National Eclectic Medical Association for the Years 1875–76* (New York: Gaylord Watson, 1877), 44.

19. Popular fears of grave robbing, murder, and dissection were prevalent in the United States and elsewhere. A notorious trial implicating Edinburgh surgeon Robert Knox led to Britain's 1832 Anatomy Act.

20. The statistics on medical schools are drawn from N. S. Davis, *Contributions to the History of Medical Education and Medical Institutions in the Unites States of America, 1776–1876* (Washington D.C.: GPO, 1877), 41. For more on Wooster Beach and the origins of eclectic medicine, see Haller, *Medical Protestants*, 69–82; Haller, *Alternative Medicine*, 21–23; Rothstein, *American Physicians*, 217–21; and *Dictionary of American Biography*, s.v. "Wooster Beach." On American dissection riots and popular fears, see Linden Edwards, "Resurrection Riots during the Heroic Age of Anatomy in America," *BHM* 25 (1951): 178–84.

21. Alva Curtis, *A Fair Examination and Criticism of All the Medical Systems in Vogue* (Cincinnati: Printed for the Proprietor, 1865), 105, qtd. in Haller, *Kindly Medicine*, 20.

22. "National Eclectic Medical Convention, Second Annual Session," *EMJ* 1, no. 6 (June 1849): 243.

23. Haller, *Kindly Medicine*, 20–21.

24. Alexander Wilder, "The Eclectic Platform," *The Medical Eclectic* 1, no. 4 (July 15, 1874): 109–10.

25. W. H. Cook and Alva Curtis, "What is Eclecticism?" *Physio-Medical Record* 21, no. 6 (June 1856): 85–88; *Transactions of the National Eclectic Medical Association for . . . 1875–76*, 351.

26. Mark Jackson, *The History of Medicine* (London: Oneworld Publications, 2016), 68–69; Porter, *Blood and Guts*, 81. A more comprehensive review of bacteriology's impact can be found in Ackerknecht's *Short History of Medicine*, 175–85.

27. William Paine, Editorial, *EMJPh* 2, no. 3 (Mar. 1859): 99–103.

28. Thomas Miller, "Case of the Late William H. Harrison, President of the United States," *BMSJ* 24, no. 17 (June 2, 1841): 261–67.

29. Thomas Cooke, "The Death of President Harrison," *BMRHP* 1, no. 11 (Apr. 1841): 172.

30. "President Harrison's Last Illness," *BMSJ* 25, no. 2 (Aug. 18, 1841): 25–32.

31. See Jane McHugh and Philip Mackowiak, "Death in the White House: President William Henry Harrison's Atypical Pneumonia," *Clinical Infectious Disease* 59, no. 7 (Oct. 2014): 990–95; and, by the same authors, "What Really Killed the President?" *NYT,* Apr. 1, 2014, D3. On Willie Lincoln's death from "bilious fever" (typhoid), see David Herbert Donald, *Lincoln* (New York: Simon and Schuster, 1996), 336.

32. Other proposed diagnoses of Washington's condition include quinsy and diphtheria. See Michael Hébert, "What Killed George Washington?" posted Feb. 16, 2009, Doctor Hébert's Medical Gumbo: Internal Medicine, Pediatrics, and Philosophy (weblog), http://drhebert.squarespace.com/dr-hberts-medical-gumbo /2009/2/16/what-killed-george-washington.html (accessed Mar. 6, 2017); and Vibul V. Vadakan, "A Physician Looks at the Death of Washington," *The Early America Review* 9, no. 1 (Winter/Spring 2005), http://www.earlyamerica.com /early-america-review/volume-9/washingtons-death/ (accessed Feb. 6, 2017).

33. David M. Morens, "Death of a President," *NEJM* 341, no. 24 (Dec. 9, 1999): 1845–49.

34. Thomas Cooke, "Sickness and Death of Gen. Washington," *BMRHP* 1, no. 7 (Dec. 19, 1840): 97–98.

35. "Circular Address of the Faculty of the Eclectic Medical Institute," July 1849, in Joseph R. Buchanan and Thomas V. Morrow, *EMJ* 8 Old Series, 1 New Series (Cincinnati: Wm. Phillips and Co., 1849): 319, 323.

36. "President Harrison's Last Illness," 25.

37. Owen Whooley, *Knowledge in the Time of Cholera: The Struggle over American Medicine in the Nineteenth Century* (Chicago: Univ. of Chicago Press, 2013), 3.

38. Charles E. Rosenberg, *The Cholera Years: The United States in 1832, 1849, and 1866* (Chicago: Univ. of Chicago Press, 1962), 153.

39. A. P. Cawadias, "The Mid-Nineteenth-Century Clinical School of Paris," *Proceedings of the Royal Society of Medicine* 45 (May 1952): 308; Ludmerer, *Learning to Heal,* 22; W. F. Bynum, *Science and the Practice of Medicine in the Nineteenth Century* (Cambridge, UK: Cambridge Univ. Press, 1994), 42–44.

40. Rosenberg, *Cholera Years,* 151–52.

41. *Transactions of the National Eclectic Medical Association for . . . 1875–76,* 318.

42. Joseph R. Buchanan and Thomas V. Morrow, "Statistics of Cholera Practice" (editorial), 314–16, quotation on 314; and "Circular Address of the Faculty of the Eclectic Medical Institute to the Medical Profession of the United States," 319–29, esp. 326, both in *EMJ* 8 (Old Series) or 1 (New Series) (July 1848). See

NOTES TO PAGES 21–27   255

also J. H. Jordan, "Cholera Epidemic in Cincinnati: Its Successful Treatment by Eclectics in 1849," *Transactions of the National Eclectic Medical Association of the United States of America for the Years 1885–86* (Orange, N.J.: Chronicle Book and Job Printing Office, 1886): 310–17; and L. C. Dolley, "Eclectic Physicians and Colleges," *EMJ* 4 (March 1852): 95.

43. William Paine, *History of the Rise, Progress, and Principles of the American Eclectic Practice of Medicine* (Philadelphia, Pa.: N.p., 1862), 18–22; *Transactions of the National Eclectic Medical Association for . . . 1875–76*, 332.

44. National Convention of Eclectic Physicians, 1849, *Transactions of the National Eclectic Medical Association for . . . 1875–76*, 320.

45. "Circular Address of the Faculty of the Eclectic Medical Institute," 319–21.

46. Henry E. Firth, "The Origin of the American Eclectic Practice of Medicine, and Its Early History in the State of New York," *Transactions of the Eclectic Medical Society of the State of New York for . . . 1877* (Albany, N.Y.: Jerome B. Parmenter, State Printer, 1878): 168–221, quotations on 189.

47. Rothstein provides a tabular overview of pre–Civil War licensing laws in *American Physicians*, 332–39.

48. Rothstein, *American Physicians*, 74–76.

49. Ibid., 106; Richard Shryock, *Medical Licensing in America, 1650–1965* (Baltimore, Md.: Johns Hopkins Univ. Press, 1967), 28.

50. Shryock, *Medical Licensing in America*, 25–26; Rothstein, *American Physicians*, 106.

51. Duffy, *From Humors to Medical Science*, 180; Rothstein, *American Physicians*, 78.

52. Rothstein, *American Physicians*, 145.

53. "Appendix: History and Proceedings of the National Eclectic Medical Association . . . Prior to the Late Civil War . . . ," *Transactions of the National Eclectic Medical Association for . . . 1875–76*, 307, 328–29.

54. "The Hospital Bill," and "Medical Politics in Cincinnati," *EMJ*, Old Series 3 (Cincinnati: William Phillips and Co., 1849): 142–44, 263–64.

55. Ronald Hamowy, "The Early Development of Medical Licensing Laws in the United States, 1875–1900," *Journal of Libertarian Studies* 3, no. 1 (1979): 75–77; Duffy, *From Humors to Medical Science*, 220.

2. The Rise of the Eclectic Medical College of Pennsylvania

1. Haller, *Medical Protestants*, 159–60.

2. Ibid.; Alexander Wilder, "The Medical Colleges in Philadelphia," *EMJ* 59, no. 7 (July 1899): 361–67, and (Aug. 1899): 417–22.

3. Harold J. Abrahams, *Extinct Medical Schools of Nineteenth-Century Philadelphia* (Philadelphia: Univ. of Pennsylvania Press, 1966), 29, 112, 162; Rogers, *Alternative Path*, 13.

4. Steven J. Peitzman, *A New and Untried Course: Woman's Medical College and Medical College of Pennsylvania, 1850–1998* (New Brunswick, N.J.: Rutgers Univ. Press, 2000), 1.

5. "To the Profession," *EMJP* 1 (Mar.–Apr. 1863): 48–49.

6. Haller, *Alternative Medicine*, 20.

7. "Report of the Select Committee of the Senate, appointed to investigate into the facts, concerning the alleged corrupt issuing of medical diplomas by medical colleges . . . ," *Session of 1872: Miscellaneous Documents Read in the Legislature of the Commonwealth of Pennsylvania* 2 (Harrisburg, Pa.: B. Singerly, State Printer, 1872), 1153.

8. Daniel Garrison Brinton, "Who's to Blame for the Bogus Diploma Business?" *MSR* 43, no. 17 (Oct. 23, 1880): 368–69.

9. The historical record gives various spellings of this surname, e.g., Hollemback, Hollenback.

10. See advertisement, *PhInq*, Sept. 15, 1851, 2; *Transactions of the National Eclectic Medical Association for . . . 1875–76*, 329–30, 336–41, 346–48.

11. *Transactions of the National Eclectic Medical Association for . . . 1875–76*, 306; Abrahams, *Extinct Medical Schools*, 45, 84, 160; Alexander Wilder, *History of Medicine: A Brief Outline* (New Sharon, Maine: New England Eclectic Publishing Co., 1901), 533.

12. Wilder, *History of Medicine*, 579–84; Haller, *Medical Protestants*, 107, 141, 173.

13. "Necrology," *JAMA* 27, no. 22 (Nov. 28, 1896): 1169; Alexander Wilder, "Eclectic Medicine in New Jersey," *Transactions of National Eclectic Medical Association* 26 (Columbus, Ohio: Nitschke Brothers, 1898): 324; *Charter of the City of Burlington with Ordinances* (Burlington, N.J.: S. C. Atkinson, 1851), title page ff.; *Charter of the City of Burlington with Ordinances* (Burlington, N.J.: S. S. Murphey, 1879), title page ff.

14. *List of the Post Offices in the United States* (Washington, D.C.: J. Shillington, 1855), 21; *Journal of the Executive Proceedings of the Senate of the United States of America* 11 (Washington, D.C.: GPO, 1887), 178.

15. "Joseph Sites" (manuscript), Box 33, Folder 956, Eclectic Medical College Records, 1845–1942; Collection No. 3, Series 10, Lloyd Library and Museum, Cincinnati, Ohio; *Transactions of the National Eclectic Medical Association for . . . 1875–76*, 338–41, 346–48.

16. Abrahams, *Extinct Medical Schools*, 256; "Eclectic Medical College," *PhPr*, Aug. 29, 1857, 2.

17. Marshall Calkins, *Valedictory Lecture to the Students of the Eclectic Medical College of Pennsylvania, 1855* (Worcester, Mass.: Charles Hamilton, 1856), 1–26; quotes on 23.

18. Haller, *Kindly Medicine*, 6.

19. "An American Medical Museum," *PhInq*, Feb. 13, 1857, 2; Abrahams, *Extinct Medical Schools*, 335. See also manuscript holdings of the College of Physicians, Philadelphia, MSS 2/0019, Series 3 (2) for Mintzer's papers and correspondence regarding the museum endeavor.

20. Abrahams, *Extinct Medical Schools*, 233–34.

21. Ibid., 237.

22. Calkins, *Valedictory Lecture*, 13–14.

23. John Fondey, *A Brief and Intelligible View of the Nature, Origin and Cure of Tubercular or Scrofulous Disease* (Philadelphia, Pa.: W. C. and J. Neff, 1855), 214–15.

24. Abrahams, *Extinct Medical Schools*, 259, 267; "Thirteenth Annual Session, 1863–64," *EMJP* 1, no. 2 (Mar.–Apr. 1863): 64ff.; "Sixteenth Annual Session, 1866–67," *EMJP* 4, no. 2 (Mar.–Apr. 1866): 104ff., "Sessions 1869–70," *EMJP* 7, no. 7 (July 1869): 336ff.

25. Ackerknecht, *Short History of Medicine*, 225.

26. Abrahams, *Extinct Medical Schools*, 265–66; "Thirteenth Annual Session, 1863–64," *EMJP* 1, no. 2 (Mar.–Apr. 1863): 64ff.

27. Wilder, "Medical Colleges in Philadelphia," *EMJ* 59, no. 7 (July 1899): 362; Wilder, *History of Medicine*, 593–94; Abrahams, *Extinct Medical Schools*, 335.

28. "Eclectic Medical College," *PhPr*, 2; Wilder, "Medical Colleges in Philadelphia," *EMJ* 59, no. 7 (July 1899): 362.

29. Wilder, *History of Medicine*, 735; "Book Notices," *American Observer: A Monthly Journal of Homeopathic Materia Medica* 9 (1872): 583.

30. "Marshall Calkins, M.D.," *BMSJ* 187, no. 24 (Dec. 14, 1922): 906.

31. Wilder, "Medical Colleges in Philadelphia," *EMJ* 59, no. 7 (July 1899): 363.

32. William Paine Papers, box 32, folder 905, Eclectic Medical College Records, 1845–1942; Collection No. 3, Series X, Lloyd Library and Museum, Cincinnati, Ohio.

33. Wilder, *History of Medicine*, 583, 593–95.

34. Ibid., 595.

35. William Paine, *History of the Rise, Progress and Principles of the American Eclectic Practice of Medicine* (Philadelphia, Pa.: n.p., 1862), 11–12.

36. Abrahams, *Extinct Medical Schools*, 235, 267.

37. Ibid., 561.

38. "Eclectic Medical College of Pennsylvania," *EMJP* 7, no. 8 (Aug. 1869): 368.

39. "The Philadelphia Diploma Trade," *SpRep*, July 24, 1880, 4.

40. "Tickets to the Healing Arts: Medical Lecture Tickets of the 18th and 19th Centuries," Penn University Archives and Record Center, http://www.archives.upenn.edu/histy/features/medical_lecture_tickets/narrative.html (accessed Feb. 23, 2017).

41. James McClintock Papers, box 31, folder 873, Eclectic Medical College

Records, 1845–1942, Collection No. 3, Series X, Lloyd Library and Museum, Cincinnati, Ohio.

42. Abrahams, *Extinct Medical Schools*, 111–14, 335–36.

43. Ibid., 244–46, 350, 360; Wilder, "Medical Colleges in Philadelphia," *EMJ* 59, no. 7 (July 1899): 366–67; Wilder, *History of Medicine*, 643–45.

44. Paine, *Rise, Progress and Principles of the American Eclectic Practice of Medicine*, 11–12; John Buchanan, "To the Profession," *EMJP* 1 (Mar.–Apr. 1863): 46; Abrahams, *Extinct Medical Schools*, 247–49.

45. Rogers, *Alternative Path*, 43–44.

46. Luke Poethig, "The Evolution of Penn's Medical School in the Middle and Late Nineteenth Century," Penn University Archives and Records Center (website), http://www.archives.upenn.edu/histy/features/medschool_evolution/1_intro .html (accessed on Mar. 6, 2017); Russell F. Weigley, "The Border City in Civil War, 1854–1865," in *Philadelphia: A 300-Year History*, ed. Russell F. Weigley, Nicholas B. Wainwright, and Edwin Wolf (New York: W. W. Norton and Co., 1982), 399.

3. THE RISE OF DR. JOHN BUCHANAN

1. U.S. Census Bureau, 1860 Federal Census, Philadelphia, Pennsylvania, 15th Ward, 255; U.S. Census Bureau, 1880 Federal Census, Philadelphia, Pennsylvania, Enumeration District (ED) 102, 5; U.S. Census Bureau, 1900 Federal Census, Manhattan, New York, ED 861, Sheet 5.

2. "Old Bogus: Statement from the 'Dean,'" *PhInq*, Mar. 25, 1881, 8; "60,000 Bogus Diplomas," *PhRec*, Mar. 25, 1881, 1.

3. U.S. Census Bureau, 1860 Federal Census, Philadelphia, Pennsylvania, 15th Ward, 255–56; U.S. Census Bureau, 1880 Federal Census, Philadelphia, Pennsylvania, ED 102, 5; U.S. Census Bureau, 1900 Federal Census, Manhattan, New York, ED 861, Sheet 5.

4. "Letter from Philadelphia," *BMSJ* 103, no. 3 (July 15, 1880): 65.

5. "Ready for Business," *PhInq*, Nov. 23, 1882, 2. A prothonotary is a principal or chief clerk of a court. Once a common term for such an office, it has fallen out of favor in the United States

6. See "Ready for Business," *PhInq*, Nov. 23, 1882, 2; "60,000 Bogus Diplomas," *PhRec*, 1; John Buchanan Papers, box 27, folder 732, Eclectic Medical College Records, 1845–1942; Collection No. 3, Series X, Lloyd Library and Museum, Cincinnati, Ohio.

7. D. Hayes Agnew, *Valedictory Address to the Anatomical Class of the Philadelphia School of Anatomy* (Philadelphia, Pa.: William S. Young, 1859), 24; Abrahams, *Extinct Medical Schools*, 294.

8. John Buchanan, *The Treatment of Venereal Disease* (Philadelphia, Pa.: W. B. Selheimer, 1865), 15; A. McElroy, *McElroy's Philadelphia City Directory 1860*

(Philadelphia, Pa.: E. C. and J. Biddle and Co., 1860), 113; U.S. Census Bureau, 1860 Federal Census, Philadelphia, Pennsylvania, 15th Ward, 255.

9. A. McElroy, *McElroy's Philadelphia City Directory 1859* (Philadelphia, Pa.: E. C. and J. Biddle and Co., 1859), 873; Buchanan, *Venereal Disease*, 15; John Buchanan, *The Eclectic Practice of Medicine and Surgery*, 3rd ed. (Philadelphia, Pa.: John Buchanan, 1867), 5–820 passim, index vii.

10. "Eclectic Medical Society of the State of Pennsylvania," *EMJP* 4, no. 2 (Mar.–Apr. 1866): 77; "Eclectic Medical Society of Pennsylvania," *PhInq*, Jan. 29, 1870, 2.

11. John Buchanan, *The American Practice of Medicine* (Philadelphia, Pa.: John Buchanan, 1868), xxxi; John Buchanan, *A Practical Treatise on the Diseases of Children* (Philadelphia, Pa.: John Buchanan, 1866), 16.

12. Nicholas Culpeper, *The English Physician* (London: Peter Cole, 1652); and Nicholas Culpeper, *The Complete Herbal*, (London: 1653); Genesis 1:29 *KJV:* "And God said, Behold, I have given you every herb bearing seed, which [is] upon the face of all the earth, and every tree, in the which [is] the fruit of a tree yielding seed; to you it shall be for meat."

13. Haller, *Medical Protestants*, 8; John Buchanan, *The Centennial Practice of Medicine* (Philadelphia, Pa.: John Buchanan, 1867), 52.

14. Buchanan, *Centennial Practice*, 168.

15. Buchanan, *Diseases of Children*, 16; Buchanan, *Venereal Disease*, 13; Buchanan, *Centennial Practice*, 101.

16. Buchanan, *American Practice*, xxx.

17. Buchanan, *Venereal Disease*, 11.

18. See the following works by Buchanan: *Diseases of Children*, 29; *American Practice*, 324; and *Eclectic Practice of Medicine and Surgery*, 14, 23, 25, 28, 650.

19. Buchanan, *Diseases of Children*, 5–7, 12, 74; Buchanan, *American Practice*, 125.

20. Buchanan, *Centennial Practice*, 148, 386–88; Buchanan, *American Practice*, 214.

21. Fondey, *Brief and Intelligible View*, 33.

22. A bougie is a smooth, slender, flexible instrument inserted into a canal of the body, often to remove an obstruction.

23. Buchanan, *Centennial Practice*, 296; Buchanan, *Eclectic Practice*, 135; Buchanan, *American Practice*, 35, 73, 188.

24. Buchanan, *Centennial Practice*, 108, 218; Buchanan, *Eclectic Practice*, 113.

25. Buchanan, *Venereal Disease*, 138–39.

26. An examination of passages in Buchanan's *American Practice* finds verbatim duplication of work attributed to others in the Feb. 1868 issue of the *Eclectic Medical Journal of Pennsylvania*. Cf. passages on brain inflammation in *American Practice*, 81, and *EMJP* 6, no. 2 (Feb. 1868): 49; on cancer in *American Practice*, 91, and *EMJP* 6, no. 2 (Feb. 1868): 53; and on elephantiasis in *American Practice*, 73, and *EMJP* 6, no. 2 (Feb. 1868): 71.

27. Buchanan, *Eclectic Practice*, 28–31; Buchanan, *Centennial Practice*, 44–46; Buchanan, *American Practice*, 351–52.

28. "Editorial," *EMJP* 7, no. 3 (Mar. 1869): 131.

29. Haller, *Medical Protestants*, 153–54.

30. "Editorial," *EMJP* 7, no. 1 (Jan. 1869): 3.

31. "Editorial," *EMJP* 7, no. 4 (Apr. 1869): 191.

32. "60,000 Bogus Diplomas," *PhRec*, 1.

33. Ibid.

34. Ibid.; Abel Charles Thomas, *A Century of Universalism in Philadelphia and New York* (Philadelphia, Pa.: J. Fagan and Son, 1872), 159.

35. Abrahams, *Extinct Medical Schools*, 342.

36. See *EMJP* 13, nos. 11 and 12 (Nov. and Dec. 1875), advertisement, title page ff.

37. These often appeared in Southern newspapers; see, for example, the *Augusta Chronicle*, Feb. 9, 1872, 3; and the *Weekly Louisianan*, June 13, 1874, 3.

38. For faculty rosters reflecting the departure of most of the early EMC faculty, see the advertisement preceding the title page in Buchanan, *Venereal Disease; EMJP* 4, no. 2 (Mar.–Apr. 1866), advertisement, 104ff.; *EMJP* 7, no. 7 (July 1869), advertisements at end of the issue.

39. Analysis of faculty turnover is derived from Harold Abrahams's research on the EMC's faculty, 1850–80. See Abrahams, *Extinct Medical Schools*, 269–86.

40. This analysis is based on the author's review of historical matter on various U.S. medical colleges, including school closings and suspension of classes. See AMA Council on Medical Education, *Medical Colleges of the United States and Foreign Countries* (Chicago, Ill.: American Medical Association, 1918), 6–16.

41. On the war's disruption, see Luke Poethig, "The Evolution of Penn's Medical School in the Middle and Late Nineteenth Century," Penn University Archives and Records Center (website), http://www.archives.upenn.edu/histy/features/med school_evolution/1_intro.html (accessed on Mar. 6, 2017); J. Woodrow Savacool and Frederick B. Wagner, eds., *Thomas Jefferson University: A Chronological History and Alumni Directory, 1824–1990* (Philadelphia, Pa.: Thomas Jefferson Univ., 1992), Part I: Jefferson Medical College 1855 to 1865, 89–124, available digitally at Jefferson Digital Commons, Scott Memorial Library, Thomas Jefferson Univ. (website), http://jdc.jefferson.edu/wagner1/17/; Peitzman, *New and Untried Course*, 21.

42. Weigley, "Border City in Civil War," 399; Alexander Wilder, "Medical Colleges in Philadelphia," *EMJ* 59, no. 7 (July 1899): 361–67 and (Aug. 1899): 417–22.

43. Hamowy, "Early Development of Medical Licensing Laws," 113–14, 119.

44. Haller, *American Medicine in Transition*, 201.

45. Kenneth Allen De Ville, *Medical Malpractice in Nineteenth-Century America: Origins and Legacy* (New York: New York Univ. Press, 1990), 76.

46. Data are derived from "Medical Colleges of the United States: Sessions 1861–62," *The American Medical Times* 3 (Sept. 28, 1861): 194–212.

47. See John L. Wilson, *Stanford University School of Medicine and the Predecessor Schools: An Historical Perspective* (Stanford, Calif.: Stanford Univ. Lane Medical Library, 1999), Part IV: Cooper Medical College, 1883–1912, available digitally at Stanford Medical History Center, Stanford Univ. (website), http://lane.stanford .edu/med-history/explore.html, (accessed Feb. 23, 2017); *Report of the Commissioner of Education for the Year 1875* (Washington, D.C.: GPO, 1876), 793.

48. Robert S. Newton, Alexander Wilder, and E. S. McClellan, eds., *American Eclectic Medical Review* 7, no. 1 (July 1871): 60–61; Alexander Wilder and Robert S. Newton, "Names of the Graduates of This College from Its Commencement in 1866 to Date," *The [New York] Medical Eclectic* 1 (1874): 29–31.

49. See William Frederick Norwood, *Medical Education in the United States before the Civil War* (Philadelphia, Pa.: Univ. of Pennsylvania Press, 1944), 79–80, 269.

50. Thomas Lindsley Bradford, *History of the Homeopathic Medical College of Pennsylvania; the Hahnemann Medical College and Hospital of Philadelphia* (Philadelphia, Pa.: Boericke and Tafel, 1898), 96, 138.

51. For examples of honorary degrees issued, see *EMJP* 4, no. 2 (Mar.–Apr. 1866): 75; and Abrahams, *Extinct Medical Schools*, 289–331. John Buchanan testified to issuing *ad eundem* degrees before a Pennsylvania senate committee in 1872. "Report of the Select Committee of the Senate, appointed to investigate . . . the alleged corrupt issuing of medical diplomas . . . ," *Session of 1872*, 1223.

52. "Testing the Doctor," *EMJ* 38, no. 6 (June 1878): 279–81.

53. "Editorial," *EMJP* 4, no. 2 (Mar.–Apr. 1866): 74.

54. Rothstein, *American Physicians*, 87–88; Duffy, *From Humors to Medical Science*, 134. On commercial and business colleges, see ch. 1 of A. J. Angelo, *Diploma Mills: How For-Profit Colleges Stiffed Students, Taxpayers and the American Dream* (Baltimore: Johns Hopkins, 2016).

55. Ludmerer, *Learning to Heal*, 15, 19.

56. The eight were the University of Pennsylvania School of Medicine (1765–); Jefferson Medical College (1824–); Pennsylvania Eclectic Medical College of Pennsylvania (1850–81); Philadelphia University of Medicine and Surgery (1860–81); Pennsylvania Medical University (1850–81); Medical Department of Pennsylvania College (1840–61); Homeopathic Medical College of Pennsylvania (founded 1848); and Female Medical College of Pennsylvania (founded 1850). In the 1990s, the last two were absorbed into a new entity originally called the Allegheny University of the Health Sciences and renamed Drexel University College of Medicine in 2002.

57. Calvin Newton, "Address to the National Eclectic Medical Association," *Transactions of the National Eclectic Medical Association for . . . 1875–76*, 344–45.

4. YEAR OF REVELATIONS, 1871

1. "The Times of Bagg," *Yale Alumni Weekly* 21, no. 1 (1911): 263–64.

2. "A Philadelphia Humbug," *The College Courant* 8, no. 13 (Apr. 1, 1871): 146–48. Unless otherwise cited, descriptions of the EMC and its faculty, as well as of the reporters' meeting with Buchanan in the opening section of this chapter, are derived from this article.

3. John Scudder, "The Curiosities of College Announcements," *EMJ* 37, no. 8 (Aug. 1877): 384–85.

4. Michael Sappol, *A Traffic of Dead Bodies: Anatomy and Embodied Social Identity in Nineteenth-Century America* (Princeton, N.J.: Princeton Univ. Press, 2002), 59, 142–43.

5. Ibid., 277, 281, 312.

6. "M.D., $40.—C.O.D.," *NYH*, May 3, 1871, 4.

7. S. N. D. North, *History and Present Condition of the Newspaper and Periodical Press of the United States* (Washington, D.C.: GPO, 1884), 105–8.

8. "The Terrible Tragedies," *NYH*, Sept. 2, 1871, 1; Thomas Dunphy and Thomas J. Cummins, comps., *Remarkable Trials of All Countries* (New York: S. S. Peloubet and Co., 1882), 15.

9. Arthur Pember, *The Mysteries and Miseries of the Great Metropolis* (New York: D. Appleton and Co., 1875), 82–83; "Medical Murderers," *NYH*, Feb. 27, 1872; "The Trunk Murder," *NYH*, Aug. 30, 1871, 1; "Bogus Diplomas: How Philadelphia Medical College Prostitutes Itself," *New York Herald-Tribune*, Oct. 25, 1871, 1–2.

10. Numerous authors and historians of today have found the story of Mary Rogers as irresistible as did nineteenth-century American readers. See Amy Gilman Srebnick, *The Mysterious Death of Mary Rogers: Sex and Culture in Nineteenth-Century New York* (New York: Oxford Univ. Press, 1997).

11. "The Evil of the Age," *NYT*, Aug. 23, 1871; "Something More Concerning Ascher's Business," *NYT*, Aug. 30, 1871.

12. Pember, *Mysteries and Miseries*, 82–84.

13. The Bowlsbys, living in Brooklyn, were not related to the deceased Alice Bowlsby of Patterson, N.J. In his closing arguments, William Howe, Rosenzweig's attorney, made use of the "singular coincidence" of two Bowlsby families intersecting in the case. Speculating that Alice Bowlsby's lover may have actually murdered her, he asserted that this theory was no more "extraordinary" than the involvement of the two unrelated Bowlsby families.

14. Dunphy and Cummins, *Remarkable Trials of all Countries*, 19–20.

15. Ibid.

16. "60,000 Bogus Diplomas," *PhRec*, 1; Pember, *Mysteries and Miseries*, 86–93.

17. Pember, *Mysteries and Miseries*, 86–93.

18. "Eclectic Murderers," *NYH*, Nov. 30, 1871, 8.

19. Johnson, "Buchanan's Philadelphia Diploma Mill," *BHM*, 39–40.

20. Brinton, "Who's to Blame for the Bogus Diploma Business?" 368–69; *Proceedings of the Board of Commissioners for District of Kensington* (Philadelphia, Pa.: Lever and M'Kee, 1852), 166, 222, 255; Agnew, *Valedictory Address*, 23–24; "The Bogus Diploma Business," *The Hahnemannian Monthly: A Homeopathic Journal of Medicine and Surgery*, new series 2, no. 9 (Sept. 1880): 574–75.

21. *Transactions of the National Eclectic Medical Association for . . . 1875–76*, 11.

22. Dorothy Gondos Beers, "The Centennial City, 1865–1876," in *Philadelphia: A 300-Year History*, ed. Weigley, Wainwright, and Wolf, 436–37; Peter Mc-Caffery, *When Bosses Ruled Philadelphia: The Emergence of the Republican Machine, 1867–1933* (University Park, Pa.: Pennsylvania State Univ. Press, 1993), 3–4.

23. Jack M. Treadway, *Elections in Pennsylvania: A Century of Partisan Conflict in the Keystone State* (University Park, Pa.: Pennsylvania State Univ. Press, 2005), 21; Harry C. Silcox, "William McMullen, Nineteenth-Century Political Boss," *Pennsylvania Magazine of History and Biography* 110, no. 3 (July 1, 1986): 391, 398; Alexander Kelly McClure, *Old Time Notes of Pennsylvania*, 2 vols. (Philadelphia, Pa.: John C. Winston Co., 1905), 2: 238.

24. "Local Affairs," *PhPL*, Oct. 6, 1870, 1; Abrahams, *Extinct Medical Schools*, 436.

25. Daniel R. Biddle and Murray Dubin, *Tasting Freedom: Octavius Catto and the Battle for Equality in Civil War America* (Philadelphia, Pa.: Temple Univ. Press, 2010), 416.

26. Roger Lane, *Roots of Violence in Black Philadelphia, 1860–1900* (Cambridge, Mass.: Harvard Univ. Press, 1986), 23.

27. Elizabeth M. Geffen, "Industrial Development and Social Crisis, 1841–1854," in *Philadelphia: A 300-Year History*, ed. Weigley, Wainwright, and Wolf, 309; Weigley, "Border City in Civil War," 385.

28. "Table III: Population of Civil Divisions less than Counties," *United States Federal Census 1870* (Washington, D.C.: GPO, 1872), 254; "Kinnard Appointed Agent," *ChRec*, Sept. 11, 1869, 2; advertisement in *ChRec*, Mar. 4, 1856, 155.

29. "Report of the Select Committee of the Senate, appointed to investigate . . . the alleged corrupt issuing of medical diplomas . . . ," *Session of 1872*, 1197.

30. John Buchanan, *To My Colored Brothers of the Fourth Legislative District* (Philadelphia, Pa.: n.p., 1871), 1–3. A partial version of this pamphlet is in the holdings of the Library Company of Philadelphia.

31. Ibid; advertisement, *PhInq*, May 11, 1870, 5; advertisement, *PhPL*, June 29, 1868, 2.

32. Beers, "Centennial City," 438.

33. "Voting and Rioting," *PhInq*, Oct. 11, 1871, 2; Silcox, "William McMullen," 400–401.

34. "The Legislature," *PhInq*, Oct. 13, 1871, 2.

5. Senate Inquiry and a Supreme Court Case, 1872

1. "Report of the Select Committee of the Senate, appointed to investigate . . . the alleged corrupt issuing of medical diplomas . . . ," *Session of 1872*, 1171–72.

2. Ibid., 1158–59.

3. Ibid., 1166.

4. Ibid., 1165.

5. Ibid., 1173, 1189.

6. Ibid., 1190, 1193–94.

7. Ibid., 1208.

8. Ibid., 1207–13, 1237–38.

9. Ibid., 1221–23. All subsequent descriptions of Buchanan's testimony are taken from this source.

10. The transcriber used the term *addendum* rather than *ad eundem*.

11. "Report of the Select Committee of the Senate, appointed to investigate . . . the alleged corrupt issuing of medical diplomas . . . ," *Session of 1872*, 1209–13, 1221–23.

12. Ibid., 1219–20.

13. Ibid., 1268.

14. Ibid., 1212, 1244, 1251.

15. Buchanan, *To My Colored Brothers*, 1–3.

16. "Report of the Select Committee of the Senate, appointed to investigate . . . the alleged corrupt issuing of medical diplomas . . . ," *Session of 1872*, 1232–33.

17. Ibid., 1201, 1246, 1248, 1281.

18. Ibid., 1228–30.

19. Joseph M. McClure, *The Evans Embezzlement; or, the History of a Bold and Successful Conspiracy to Defraud the State of Pennsylvania* (Philadelphia, Pa.: n.p., 1872).

20. Hylton later left medicine, gaining local and regional renown as a poet of epic verse. Not everyone found merit in his work. Bret Harte found Hylton's work "pretentious." See "Recent Poetry," *Overland Monthly* 10, no. 58 (Oct. 1887): 441–42.

21. "Report of the Select Committee of the Senate, appointed to investigate . . . the alleged corrupt issuing of medical diplomas . . . ," *Session of 1872*, 1198–1202.

22. Ibid., 1171, 1199, 1204, 1270.

23. Ibid., 1158–60.

24. Ibid.

25. *Philadelphia Sunday Dispatch*, Mar. 24, 1872, qtd. in "Bogus Diploma Business," *AJP* 44, no. 4 (Apr. 1, 1872): 191; "60,000 Bogus Diplomas," *PhRec*, 1.

26. "Old Bogus," *PhInq*, Mar. 25, 1881, 8; *Allen v. Buchanan, Legal Intelligencer* 9 (1873): 283.

27. See "Are We Progressing?" *EMJP* 12 (1874): 280; and "Rotten Foundations," *EMJP* 12,(1874): 91.

28. John Buchanan, "Profession and Retrogression," *JPM* (Sept.–Oct. 1872): 238.

29. Joseph Sites, "To the Profession," *JPM* (May–June 1872): 115–16.

30. "The Cure of Cancer" (advertisement by John Buchanan), *JPM* (May–June 1872): 117.

31. Joseph P. Fitler, *A Regular Physician's Specialty Forty Years* (Philadelphia: n.p., 1873), title page; see Fondey, *A Brief and Intelligible View.*

32. "The Diploma Trade," *PhInq*, Sept. 5, 1873, 2; "Are They Bogus?" *PhInq*, Sept. 4, 1873, 2.

33. "Death from Malpractice," *PhRec*, Sept. 17, 1874, 1; "Alleged Malpractice," *PhInq*, Sept. 17, 1874, 3.

34. "Death from Malpractice," *PhRec*, Sept. 17, 1874, 1; "60,000 Bogus Diplomas," *PhRec*, 1.

35. De Ville, *Medical Malpractice*, 2–3, 25. See also chapter 8 in James Mohr's *Doctors and the Law: Medical Jurisprudence in Nineteenth-Century America* (New York: Oxford Univ. Press, 1993).

36. Abrahams, *Extinct Medical Schools*, 439.

37. Silcox, "William McMullen," 401.

38. "Philadelphia and Suburbs," *PhInq*, Apr. 19, 1876, 3; "Dr. Buchanan Sent to Prison," *PhRec*, Apr. 19, 1876, 1.

39. "Dr. Buchanan Sent to Prison," 1.

40. For the broader sociopolitical context surrounding passage of the Comstock Law (known in full as *An Act for the Suppression of Trade in, and Circulation of, Obscene Literature and Articles of Immoral Use*, Mar. 3, 1873, ch. 258, § 2, 17 Stat. 599), see Helen Lefkowitz Horowitz's "Victoria Woodhull, Anthony Comstock, and Conflict over Sex in the United States in the 1870s," *Journal of American History* 87, no. 2 (Sept. 2000), 403–34; Nicola Beisel's *Imperiled Innocents: Anthony Comstock and Family Reproduction in Victorian America* (Princeton, N.J.: Princeton Univ. Press, 1997); Leigh Ann Wheeler's *Against Obscenity: Reform and the Politics of Womanhood in America, 1873–1935* (Baltimore, Md.: Johns Hopkins Univ. Press, 2004); and Paul Boyer's *Purity in Print: Censorship from the Gilded Age to the Computer Age*, 2d ed. (Madison: Univ. of Wisconsin Press, 2002).

41. "Rumored Flight of Dr. Buchanan," *PhInq*, May 27, 1876, 2; "Buchanan's Diploma Mill," *PhInq*, June 20, 1876, 2.

42. "Rumored Flight," 2; "Buchanan's Diploma Mill," 2; "The Last of the University of Philadelphia," *PhRec*, June 20, 1876, 1.

43. Brinton, "Who's to Blame for the Bogus Medical Diploma Business?" 369.

44. "The Police," *PhInq*, Sept. 18, 1876, 3; "At the Central," *PhInq*, Sept. 21 and 22, 1876, 3.

45. "Matters in the Court," *PhInq*, Feb. 16, 1877, 3. Postponements in the case appeared in the *Philadelphia Record* over the following two days.

46. "60,000 Bogus Diplomas," *PhRec*, 1; "Old Bogus," *PhInq*, Mar. 25, 1881, 8.

47. See *EMJP* 16, no. 7 (July 1877): 165–66, 172–73.

48. Ibid., 168–69, 171–72.

49. Ibid., 170.

50. Ibid., 171.

6. THE RETURN OF MEDICAL LICENSING LAWS

1. Rogers, *Alternative Path*, 2.

2. Mohr, *Licensed to Practice*, 156–59.

3. Lawrence Meir Friedman, *A History of American Law*, 3rd. rev. ed. (New York: Touchstone, 2005), 342–43.

4. Morris M. Kleiner, *Reforming Occupational Licensing Policies*, Hamilton Project, Discussion Paper 2015–01 (Washington, D.C.: Brookings Institution: Jan. 2015), 7, online at https://www.brookings.edu/wp-content/uploads/2016/06/THP_KleinerDiscPaper_final.pdf.

5. Stanley J. Gross, *Of Foxes and Hen Houses: Licensing and the Health Professions* (Westport, Conn.: Quorum Books, 1984), 55–56.

6. Elizabeth Fee, "Public Health and the State: The United States," in *The History of Public Health and the Modern State*, ed. Dorothy Porter (Atlanta, Ga.: Editions Rodopi B. V., 1994), 224–75, especially 232.

7. See W. G. Smillie, "The National Board of Health, 1879–1883," *American Journal of Public Health* 33, no. 8 (Aug. 1943): 925–30; David Rosner, Ronald H. Lauterstein, and Jerrold M. Michael, "The National Board of Health, 1879–1883," *Public Health Reports* 126, no. 1 (Jan.–Feb. 2011): 123–29.

8. Chief Justice John Marshall used the term *police powers* in *Brown v. Maryland* (1827). The U.S. Supreme Court further refined the state's distinct role in public health matters through a series of decisions, for example, *Thurlow v. Massachusetts* (1847) and *Mugler v. Kansas* (1887). Text cited here is from *Jacobson v. Massachusetts*, 197 U.S. 11 (1905).

9. Starr, *Social Transformation*, 103; Friedman, *History of American Law*, 340.

10. Christina Apperson, *Protecting the Public, Strengthening the Profession: A One Hundred Fifty Year History of the North Carolina Medical Board, 1859–2009* (North Manchester, Ind.: HF Group, 2009), 4–5.

11. Hamowy, "Early Development of Medical Licensing Laws," 80–81.

12. U.S. Census Bureau, *1870 Federal Census*, vol. 1: *The Statistics of the Population of the United States* (Washington, D.C.: GPO, 1872), 676.

13. Haller, *American Medicine in Transition*, 201.

14. "Registration Laws and Their Operations," *Philadelphia Medical Times* 13 (July 14, 1883): 72, qtd. in Hamowy, "Early Development of Medical Licensing Laws," 81.

15. Cited in Rothstein, *American Physicians*, 306.

16. Everett Hughes, qtd. in Starr, *Social Transformation*, 23.

17. Linda A. McCready and Billie Harris, *From Quackery to Quality Assurance: The First Twelve Decades of the Medical Board of California* (Sacramento: Medical Board of California, 1995), 2–3.

18. Mohr, *Licensed to Practice*, 45.

19. Samuel Baker, "Physician Licensure Laws in the United States, 1865–1915," *JHMHS* 39 (Apr. 1984): 178.

20. By 1881, there were nineteen state boards of health and a national board of health created by the U.S. Congress. Mohr, *Licensed to Practice*, 65.

21. *Dictionary of American Biography*, s.v. "Rauch, John Henry."

22. Clinton Sandvick, "Enforcing Medical Licensing in Illinois: 1877–1890," *Yale Journal of Biology and Medicine* 82, no. 2 (June 2009): 67–68.

23. Illinois State Board of Health, *Second Annual Report of the State Board of Health of Illinois, 1879* (Springfield: H. W. Rokker, 1881), 12, 19.

24. John M. Scudder, "The Illinois Medical Board," *EMJ* 37, no. 12 (Dec. 1877): 581.

25. Illinois State Board of Health, *First Annual Report of the State Board of Health of Illinois, 1878* (Springfield: Weber, Magie and Co., 1879), 12.

26. In October 1879, Illinois's attorney general, J. K. Edsall, clarified the board's scope of authority relative to the "in good standing" clause of the 1877 law. Edsall claimed that determining whether a school was in good standing was "a question of fact to be determined by your Board" with a requisite "duty to refuse" licenses to graduates of schools "fall[ing] materially below the average standard," even if legally chartered. See Illinois State Board of Health, *Second Annual Report, 1879*, 16.

27. Illinois State Board of Health, *First Annual Report, 1878*, 5, 16.

28. Ibid., 17–18.

29. Ludmerer, *Learning to Heal*, 99, 234, 327n.

30. Johnson and Chaudhry, *Medical Licensing and Discipline*, 88.

31. Illinois State Board of Health, *Third Annual Report of the State Board of Health of Illinois, 1880* (Springfield: H. W. Rokker, State Printer, 1881), 42–44.

32. Ibid., 44–45, 95. A 2008 study applied survival analysis methodology to assess the impact of a school's inclusion on the Illinios disapproved list. Inclusion on the list proved highly correlated with school closures. See Lynn E. Miller and Richard Weiss, "Medical Education Efforts and Failures of U.S. Medical Schools, 1870–1930," *JHMHS* 63, no. 3 (2008): 348–87.

33. Awareness of the trepidation felt by eclectics nationally can be seen in editorials by John Scudder of the Eclectic Medical Institute of Cincinnati. See his editorials "Proposed Board of Medical Examiners" and "Legislative Frauds," *EMJ* 37, no. 3 (Mar. 1877): 126, 146.

34. Illinois State Board of Health, *First Annual Report, 1878*, 5, 16.

35. Illinois State Board of Health, *Third Annual Report, 1880*, 15–16, 44–95.

7. JOHN NORRIS AND THE *PHILADELPHIA RECORD*

1. "Report of the Attorney General," *Reports of the Heads of Departments of the Commonwealth of Pennsylvania, 1880–81* (Harrisburg: Lane S. Hart, state printer, 1881), 3.

2. Ibid.

3. Charles Doyle, *Mail and Wire Fraud: A Brief Overview of Federal Criminal Law* (Washington D.C.: Congressional Research Service, 2011), 1n.

4. This account of Norris's visit with Miller is taken from "The Diploma Mill," *PhRec*, Mar. 1, 1880, 1.

5. "John Norris Dies in His 58th Year," *NYT*, Mar. 22, 1914.

6. Sam Hudson, *Pennsylvania and Its Public Men* (Philadelphia: Hundson and Joseph, 1909), 13–14; J. Thomas Scharff and Thompson Westcott, *History of Philadelphia, 1609–1884*, 3 vols. (Philadelphia: L. H. Everts and Co., 1884), 3: 2040–41.

7. "The Story of a Busy Life," *NYT*, June 28, 1894; Charles Austen Bates, *American Journalism from the Practical Side* (New York: Holmes Publishing Co., 1897) 42, 46; *The Encyclopedia of Greater Philadelphia*, s.v. "Printing and Publishing" (by James J. Wyatt), http://philadelphiaencyclopedia.org/ (accessed Mar. 6, 2017).

8. "Success of the *Philadelphia Record*," *NYT*, June 5, 1894.

9. Bates, *American Journalism*, 46–47.

10. Julius Chambers, *News Hunting on Three Continents* (New York: Mitchell Kennerley, 1921), 16.

11. See Haller's *Medical Protestants*, ch. 6; see also Haller's *History of American Homeopathy*, 173, 204, 26.

12. *Philadelphia Record*, Mar. 1, 1880, editorial quoted in Charles H. Lothrop, *Medical and Surgical Directory of the State of Iowa for 1880 and 1881* (Clinton, Iowa: Allen Steam Printing and Binding, 1880), 83.

13. "The Diploma Swindle," *AJP* (Apr. 1880): 235; "Attack upon the Philadelphia University," *PhInq*, June 15, 1880, 3; "Dean Miller Arraigned for Forgery," *PhInq*, Aug. 4, 1880, 2; "Local Briefs," *PhInq*, Mar. 17, 1881, 3.

14. "Report of the Attorney General," *Commonwealth of Pennsylvania, 1880–81*, 2.

15. "Doctor Buchanan Again in Trouble," *PhInq*, Jan. 7, 1880, 3; "Police Intelligence," *PhInq*, Jan. 14, 1880, 3; "Philadelphia Pickings," *Harrisburg Patriot*, Jan. 8, 1880, 1; "The Chester Mystery," *PhT*, Jan. 7, 1880, 4.

16. "Bogus Medical Colleges," *Chicago Medical Times* 12, no. 2 (May 1880): 95–96; "Bogus Diplomas," *Michigan Medical News* 3, no. 12 (June 25, 1880): 181; "Bogus Diplomas—the American University Again," *PhInq*, Mar. 31, 1880, 2.

17. *Report of the Commissioner of Education for the Year 1880* (Washington, D.C.: GPO, 1882), 161; "Bogus Diplomas—the American University Again," *PhInq*, Mar. 31, 1880, 2.

18. "A Dejected Dean," *PhInq*, June 11, 1880, 2; "The National Disgrace," *PhRec*, June 10, 1880, 1; "Report of the Commissioner of Education," *Executive*

Documents of the House of Representatives for the Third Session of the Forty-Sixth Congress, 1880–1881, vol. 11 (Washington, D.C.: GPO, 1881), 164.

19. Abrahams, *Extinct Medical Schools,* 441.

20. "National Disgrace," *PhRec,* June 10, 1880, 3.

21. Ibid.

22. "Soft Hearted Brothers," *PhRec,* Apr. 22, 1880, 1; "Ingraham on the Rack," *PhRec,* May 6, 1880, 1.

23. "Doctor Goerssen," *PhRec,* Apr. 14, 1880, 1

24. "Miscellaneous," *PhInq,* Apr. 6, 1880, 3; Report of the Commissioner of Education," *Executive Documents of the House of Representatives,* 161; Lothrop, *Medical and Surgical Directory of the State of Iowa,* 78.

25. "Bogus Diplomas—the American University Again," *PhInq,* Mar. 31, 1880, 2.

26. "Buchanan," *DetFrP,* Sept. 11, 1880, 1.

27. Unless otherwise indicated, the account of John Buchanan's arrest and the search of the EMC is drawn from the following sources: "Suppressing a Crying Evil," *WR,* June 12, 1880, 1; "A Dejected Dean," *PhInq,* June 11, 1880, 2; "Bogus Medical Diplomas," *NYT,* June 10, 1880; "The National Disgrace," *PhRec,* June 10, 1880, 1; and "The Diploma Mill," *PhRec,* June 12, 1880, 1.

28. Appendix F4, *Journal of the Legislative Council of New South Wales, 2nd Session 1887* (Sydney: Charles Potter, Government Printer, 1887), 93. Evidence taken by the New South Wales Legislative Council on a medical practice law, included testimony and documentation from a witness (Andrew Houison), on attempts to join the physician registry using fraudulent documents. Included were long extracts from the article in the July 17, 1880, *Philadelphia Record* reviewing the materials seized in the June 1880 raid on the EMC.

29. Ibid., 95.

30. Ibid., 93.

31. "Bogus Doctors," *New Haven (Conn.) Register,* July 19, 1880, 1; "Buchanan and his Bogus Diplomas," *CMG* 44, no. 12 (Dec. 1880): 364; "Philadelphia Diploma Shops," *CMG* 44, no. 8 (Aug. 1880): 261.

32. "A Dejected Dean," *PhInq,* June 11, 1880, 2.

33. See advertisements in *Augusta (Ga.) Chronicle,* Feb. 9, 1872; *Weekly Louisianan,* June 13, 1874, 3.

34. Appendix F4, *Legislative Council of New South Wales,* 93–96.

35. "A Dejected Dean," *PhInq,* June 11, 1880, 2.

36. Unless otherwise indicated, sources for John Buchanan's ordeal in obtaining bail are drawn from "Buchanan at Liberty," *PhRec,* June 19, 1880, 1; "A Dejected Dean," *PhInq,* June 11, 1880, 2; "Bogus Medical Diplomas," *NYT,* June 10, 1880; "Criminals and Their Deeds," *NYT,* June 11, 1880; "Pine Street College," *PhInq,* June 17, 1880, 2.

37. "Suppressing a Crying Evil," *WR,* June 12, 1880, 1.

38. "Moving on the Colleges," *PhRec,* June 15, 1880, 1.

39. Appendix F4, *Legislative Council of New South Wales*, 93.

40. "Arrest of a Pine Street College Professor," *PhInq*, July 7, 1880, 2; "The Case of Professor Kenroth," *PhInq*, July 8, 1880, 3; U.S. Census Bureau, *1880 Federal Census*, Philadelphia, Pennsylvania, Supervisor District 1, ED 102, 5.

41. See "A Notary's Arrest," *PhRec*, July 13, 1880, 1, and July 14, 1880, 4.

42. Ibid.

43. Unless otherwise indicated, the account of this additional evidence-gathering by Norris and the *Record* is taken from "Buchanan's Audacity," *PhRec*, Aug. 5, 1880, 1.

8. THE "DEATH" OF JOHN BUCHANAN

1. "Buchanan's Fatal Leap," *PhRec*, Aug. 18, 1880, 2.

2. "Old Bogus," *PhInq*, Mar. 25, 1881, 8.

3. Abrahams, *Extinct Medical Schools*, 302; "Mysterious Disappearance of Philadelphia Physician," *PhInq*, June 23, 1870, 2.

4. "Report of the Select Committee of the Senate, appointed to investigate . . . the alleged corrupt issuing of medical diplomas . . . ," *Session of 1872*, 1267–68.

5. See the *Philadelphia Inquirer* for the following articles: "The Barker Case," July 28, 1875, 2; "The Harbison-Gordon Case," Mar. 30, 1876, 2; "Central Station," June 9, 1876, 3; "The Irvin Murder," May 9, 1879, 3; and "Dr. Harbison and the Irvin Tragedy," July 3, 1879, 2. See the *Philadelphia Times* for these articles: "The Mystery Unsolved," July 28, 1875, 4; and "Harbison's Hospital," Apr. 27, 1876, 3.

6. "Buchanan Drowns Himself," *NYT*, Aug. 18, 1880, 1.

7. "Again Arrested: Ladner Brothers Brought Back to City," *PhInq*, Sept. 13, 1884, 2.

8. "Death or Fraud?" *PhInq*, Aug. 18, 1880, 2; "Bogus Buchanan," *PET*, Sept. 13, 1880, 1.

9. "Buchanan—The Rumpus," *PhInq*, Aug. 20, 1880, 2; "Death or Fraud?" *PhInq*, 2.

10. "Buchanan—The Rumpus," *PhInq*, Aug. 20, 1880, 2.

11. "The Swimming Match," *NYT*, July 22, 1875; see also, "An Extraordinary Swim," *PhInq*, Aug. 6, 1876, 3; and "Breasting the Waves," *PhInq*, Aug. 14, 1877, 2.

12. "A Fifty Dollar Job," *PhRec*, Aug. 19, 1880, 1; "Dr. Buchanan's Alleged Suicide," *NYT*, Aug. 21, 1880, 1; "Buchanan—The Rumpus," *PhInq*, Aug. 20, 1880, 2.

13. "Buchanan—The Rumpus," *PhInq*, Aug. 20, 1880, 2.

14. Chapman may have approached others soliciting an impersonator. Albert Urian gave an affidavit to that effect before a notary and the *Record*'s John Norris. Chapman responded with a perjury charge against Urian that was ultimately dismissed. See "Old Bogus," *PhInq*, Mar. 25, 1881, 8; "Dr. Buchanan and His Abuses," *PhInq*, Aug. 26, 1880, 2.

15. "Buchanan—The Rumpus," *PhInq*, Aug. 20, 1880, 2.

16. "United States District Court," *PhInq*, Aug. 17, 1880, 2.

17. "Buchanan—The Rumpus," *PhInq*, Aug. 20, 1880, 2.

18. "Old Bogus," *PhInq*, Mar. 25, 1881, 8.

19. "Buchanan's Fatal Leap," *PhRec*, Aug. 18, 1880, 1; "A Doctor Disappears," *Cincinnati Daily Gazette*, Aug. 18, 1880, 4.

20. "Dragging the Delaware," *New York Truth*, Aug. 18, 1880, 1.

21. Ibid.

22. "Death or Fraud?" *PhInq*, Aug. 18, 1880, 2; "Buchanan's Fatal Leap," *PhRec*, Aug. 18, 1880, 2.

23. Thomas Coyle, *Everybody a Swimmer* (Chester, Pa: Melville and Haas, 1884), 7.

24. "Suicide of Dr. Buchanan," *PhRec*, Aug. 17, 1880, 1.

25. "Buchanan—The Rumpus," *PhInq*, Aug. 20, 1880, 2.

26. "Buchanan's Fatal Leap," *PhRec*, Aug. 18, 1880, 1.

27. "Alleged Suicide," *PhInq*, Aug. 21, 1880, 2.

28. The *Philadelphia Record* and the *Detroit Free Press* had the inside track on covering the Buchanan story but the *Philadelphia Press* had a well-informed source in Jennings. His statements on Buchanan's whereabouts and many other facts of the case were remarkably accurate and predated the *Record* and *Free Press* stories. Yet Jennings's efforts to capture Buchanan failed, while the efforts of Norris and the *Record* gathered steam. See "Buchanan Alive," *NYH*, Aug. 21, 1880, 2; and "Buchanan in Detroit," *NYH*, Aug. 22, 1880, 6.

29. "Was Buchanan in Wilmington?" *PhRec*, Aug. 24, 1880, 1.

30. "Dr. Buchanan's Whereabouts," *PhInq*, Aug. 23, 1880, 2; "Buchanan," *PhT*, Aug. 20, 1880, 4.

31. Buchanan's attitude is surmised based on his remarks to a Philadelphia bartender, who identified the doctor as a regular patron who offered unguarded comments when he stopped by for his usual milk punch, shortly after the announcement of the mail fraud charges. See "Buchanan in Canada," *PhRec*, Aug. 25, 1880, 1.

32. It is unclear precisely when Buchanan slipped out of Philadelphia. The *Detroit Free Press* placed Buchanan in Detroit by August 10 or earlier for a meeting at the office of Dr. Henry S. Thomas (at 146 Michigan Avenue) to discuss prospects for a medical school. This conflicts with Philadelphia press reports, citing unnamed sources, which asserted that Buchanan had been inquiring about ferry schedules and tides several days before August 17. Moreover, a statement in the *Free Press* account that Dr. William Paine, the former dean of Philadelphia University, had met with Buchanan as a party to these talks was not repeated either in subsequent *Free Press* editions or in any other periodical. The *Free Press* account, therefore, was probably incorrect.

33. "Busy Buchanan," *DetFrP,* Aug. 24, 1880, 8.

34. Ibid. The encounter with Buchanan is reconstructed from this article.

35. Ibid.

36. "Caged Again," *PhRec,* Sept. 13, 1880, 1.

37. Henry S. Thomas and John J. Siggins, eds., "Detroit University Faculty Roster," *JPM* 1, no. 1 (July 1882): title page.

38. Wilder, *History of Medicine,* 735; "Bogus Buchanan," *PET,* Sept. 13, 1880, 1.

39. The *Philadelphia Record* identified the man as Mooney. It is unclear which name is correct.

40. "Dr. Buchanan," *DetFrP,* Sept. 10, 1880, 1.

41. Ibid.

42. "Hunted Down," *PhInq,* Sept. 11, 1880, 8.

43. "Bogus Buchanan," *PET,* Sept. 13, 1880, 1.

44. "Buchanan and His Abuses," *PhInq,* Aug. 26, 1880, 2.

45. "Buchanan," *DetFrP,* Sept. 11, 1880, 1.

46. Stephanie Hoover, *Philadelphia Spiritualism and the Curious Case of Katie King* (Charleston, S.C.: History Press, 2013), 24, 40.

47. The description of Buchanan's spiritualist evening is drawn from "Caged Again," *PhRec,* Sept. 13, 1880, 1; "Bogus Buchanan," *PET,* Sept. 13, 1880, 1; "Buchanan," *DetFrP,* Sept. 11, 1880, 1; and "Hunted Down," *PhInq,* Sept. 11, 1880, 8.

48. "Caged Again," *PhRec,* Sept. 13, 1880, 1.

49. "Bogus Buchanan," *PET,* Sept. 13, 1880, 8.

50. "Caged Again," *PhRec,* Sept. 13, 1880, 1.

51. Unless indicated otherwise, the account of Norris's tracking and capture of John Buchanan is derived from the contemporary newspaper accounts. See "Bogus Buchanan," *PET,* Sept. 13, 1880, 1; "Buchanan," *DetFrP,* Sept. 11, 1880, 1; and "Hunted Down," *PhInq,* Sept. 11, 1880, 8.

52. "Caged Again," *PhRec,* Sept. 13, 1880, 1.

53. *Dictionary of American Biography,* s.v. "Palmer, Henry Wilbur."

54. "Report of the Attorney General for 1879 and 1880," *Reports of the Heads of Departments of the Commonwealth of Pennsylvania* (Harrisburg: Lane S. Hart, State Printer, 1881), 3–4.

55. "Buchanan Capture," *PhRec,* Sept. 11, 1880, 1.

9. TRIAL AND IMPRISONMENT

1. Unless otherwise indicated, the account of Buchanan's extradition hearing and return to Philadelphia is taken from "Buchanan," *DetFrP,* Sept. 11, 1880, 1.

2. "Bogus Buchanan," *PET,* Sept. 13, 1880, 1.

3. Ibid.; "Captured at Last," *PhInq,* Oct. 23, 1880, 2.

4. The interview sequence with the *Herald* reporter is drawn from "Bogus Buchanan," *PET*, Sept. 13, 1880, 1.

5. Abrahams, *Extinct Medical Schools*, 452.

6. "Caged Again," *PhRec*, Sept. 13, 1880, 1.

7. "Diploma Buchanan," *NYH*, Sept. 14, 1880, 4; "The Pine Streeter," *PhInq*, Sept. 14, 1880, 3.

8. "Pine Streeter," *PhInq*, Sept. 14, 1880, 3; "United States District Court," *PhInq*, Nov. 16, 1880, 2.

9. "Pine Streeter," *PhInq*, Sept. 14, 1880, 3; "Buchanan's Bail Forfeited," *PhInq*, Sept. 15, 1880, 2; "Captured at Last," *PhInq*, Oct. 23, 1880, 2.

10. "The Buchanan Conspiracy Trial," *PhInq*, Nov. 23, 1880, 2; "Blind Goddess," *PhInq*, Nov. 25, 1880, 2.

11. Ibid.

12. The song title may be unfamiliar, but the tune would be recognizable to many from Walt Disney's *Dumbo*. The reworked lyrics for *Bogus Dr. John* probably featured a more upbeat tempo to reflect its bawdier subject matter.

13. "Bogus Dr. John," Air: "Baby Mine" ([Philadelphia]: A. W. Auner, ca. 1880–81), imprint held by the American Antiquarian Society, Boston, Mass. See the appendix for the entire song.

14. The description of Buchanan's trial on mail fraud charges is drawn from "Dr. Buchanan's Acquittal," *PhInq*, Dec. 1, 1880, 2; "Acquitted on a Technicality," *PhRec*, Dec. 1, 1880, 1; and "Editorial," *PhRec*, Dec. 1, 1880, 2.

15. The description and quotations from Buchanan's sentencing are drawn from "United States District Court-Sentence Imposed on Buchanan," *PhInq*, Dec. 7, 1880, 12.

16. "Dr. Buchanan in the Penitentiary," *PhInq*, Feb. 7, 1881, 3; "Admission and Discharge Book, 1875–1888," Roll #442, Justice Population Records, Eastern State Penitentiary, RG-15, Records of the Department of Justice, Pennsylvania State Archives, Harrisburg, Pa.

17. "History of Eastern State," Eastern State Penitentiary (website), https://www.easternstate.org/research/history-eastern-state (accessed Feb. 23, 2017).

18. Paul Kahan, *Eastern State Penitentiary: A History* (Charleston, S.C.: History Press, 2008), 16–20.

19. *Dictionary of American Biography*, s.v. "Haviland, John."

20. See chapter 3 of Norman Johnston's *Eastern State Penitentiary: Crucible of Good Intentions* (Philadelphia, Pa.: Philadelphia Museum of Art, 2004).

21. Alexis de Tocqueville and Gustave de Beaumont, *On the Penitentiary System in the United States and its Application in France*, trans. Francis Lieber (Philadelphia, Pa.: Carey, Lea and Blanchard, 1833), 74.

22. This and the description of the prison population derive from a sampling

based on the pages of prison records in which John Buchanan was listed. See "Discharge Descriptive Docket, 1873–1890," Oct. 6, 1881; "Reception Descriptive Book, 1879–1884," Feb. 5, 1881; and "Commutation Book, 1865–1883," Feb. 5, 1881, all in Justice Population Records, Eastern State Penitentiary, RG-15, Records of the Department of Justice, Pennsylvania State Archives, Harrisburg, Pa.

23. "Buchanan in Canada," *PhRec*, Aug. 25, 1880, 1.

24. *Eighteenth Annual Report of the Inspectors of the Eastern State Penitentiary of Pennsylvania* (Philadelphia: Ed. Barrington and Geo. D. Haswell, 1847), 11.

25. "Insane Convicts at Eastern Penitentiary," *PhInq*, Feb. 15, 1881, 2.

26. Kahan, *Eastern State Penitentiary*, 9, 29, 31, 44.

27. "An End of Two Buchanan Colleges," *PhInq*, Oct. 1, 1880, 3; "The Two Bogus Colleges Finally Wiped Out," *MSR* 43, no. 15 (Oct. 9, 1880): 329.

28. John Buchanan's confession is drawn from "60,000 Bogus Diplomas," *PhRec*, Mar. 25, 1881, 1; "Old Bogus," *PhInq*, Mar. 25, 1881, 8; "Confession," *Cleveland Leader*, Mar. 25, 1881, 1; "Bogus Sheepskins," *WR*, Mar. 25, 1881, 1; and "Buchanan the Diplomatist as a Confessor," *BMSJ* 104, no. 14 (Apr. 7, 1881): 331.

29. "Bogus Diplomas," *PhT*, June 20, 1876, 4.

30. "Itemized," *PhInq*, Mar. 31, 1881, 3.

31. Details of Buchanan's sentencing hearing are drawn from "Dr. Buchanan Detained for Sentencing," *PhInq*, Oct. 7, 1881, 2; and "Again Sentenced," *PhInq*, Oct. 11, 1881, 2.

10. OLD TRICKS AND A NEW CAREER

1. "Eclectic Medical Society," *Montpelier Argus and Patriot*, June 7, 1882, 1.

2. "Physicians: The Law for their Registration," *PhInq*, Aug. 5, 1881, 3.

3. See "The Doctors' Register," *PhInq*, Mar. 21, 1882, 2; and *PhInq*, June 17, 1882, 2.

4. Samuel B. Hoppin, *The Physicians' Protective Register* (Philadelphia, Pa.: Physicians' Protective Register Co., 1881), 6.

5. "Ready for Business," *PhInq*, Nov. 23, 1882, 2.

6. Hoppin, *Physicians' Protective Register*, 6.

7. "Dr. Buchanan: Arrested on a Capias," *PhInq*, June 12, 1883, 8; "New Jersey Matters," *PhRec*, June 12, 1883, 4.

8. "Broken-Down Buchanan," *Philadelphia Times*, reprinted in *DetFrP*, Nov. 6, 1883, 3; "News Topics," *Baltimore American and Commercial Advertiser*, June 13, 1883, 2.

9. Unless otherwise indicated, Buchanan's discussion of the state of medicine is taken from his *Family Physician and Domestic Practice of Medicine* (Philadelphia, Pa.: R. Russell, 1884), 17–19.

10. See Ludmerer, *Learning to Heal*, 27; Rothstein, *American Physicians*, 285; Dan-

iel Drake, "Selection and Preparatory Education of Pupils," in *Medical America in the Nineteenth Century*, ed. Gert H. Brieger (Baltimore, Md.: Johns Hopkins Univ. Press, 1972), 13; and Andrew Boardman, "An Essay on the Means of Improving Medical Education and Elevating Moral Character," in Brieger, *Medical America*, 25, 34.

11. See "Buchananism," *EMJ* 40, no. 8 (Aug. 1880): 389; and "The Bogus Diploma Traffic," *EMJ* 41, no. 5 (May 1881): 243.

12. "The Bold Buchanan," *PhRec*, Jan. 21, 1885, 1.

13. "All Sorts," *PhInq*, Jan. 19, 1885, 2; Buchanan's Trial," *PhInq*, Mar. 10, 1885, 3.

14. "Bold Buchanan," *PhRec*, Jan. 21, 1885, 1; "All Sorts," *PhInq*, Jan. 19, 1885, 2.

15. See "In the Toils Again," *PhInq*, Jan. 21, 1885, 2; "Public Tribunals," *PhInq*, Feb. 7, 1885, 3; "Law and Equity," *PhInq*, Mar. 3, 1885, 2; and "Buchanan's Ordeal," *PhRec*, Mar. 10, 1885, 1.

16. Trial details and quotes are drawn from "Buchanan's Trial," *PhInq*, Mar. 10, 1885, 3; "Buchanan's Ordeal," *PhRec*, Mar. 10, 1885, 1; "Tribunals," *PhInq*, Mar. 11, 1885, 3; "Buchanan Convicted," *PhRec*, Mar. 11, 1885, 4; and "Money Down," *SF Bul*, Mar. 16, 1885, 3.

17. "Local Summary," *PhInq*, Sept. 15, 1885, 3.

18. "Buchanan's Trial," *PhInq*, Mar. 10, 1885, 3; "Public Tribunals," *PhInq*, Feb. 7, 1885, 3.

19. "Minor Paragraphs: Ohio University," *New York Medical Journal* 43 (Apr. 3, 1886): 386.

20. Ibid. See also *Annual Catalog of the Ohio University, 1885* (Athens, Ohio: Athens Journal, 1885).

21. The 1900 federal census listed John and Rebecca Buchanan as father and daughter. See U.S. Census Bureau, 1900 Federal Census, New York, New York, Borough of Manhattan, ED 861, Sheet 5. "R. R. Russell" was listed as the publisher for two of Buchanan's books, *The Family Physician and Domestic Practice of Medicine* (1884) and *An Encyclopedia of the Practice of Medicine Based on Bacteriology* (1890). For information on Buchanan's death and his preceding years' business arrangements with Russell, see the following *PhRec* articles: "Veiled Woman Lavish with Cash," Jan. 10, 1908, 3; "Faints in Court at Name Sister," Jan. 11, 1908, 3; and "Buchanan Tangle up to the Court," Jan. 12, 1908, 3.

22. Janik, *Marketplace of the Marvelous*, 184–88.

23. Ibid., 190, 192, 199.

24. Author has in his possession an 1891 copy of *The Germicide* bearing the print stamp of an Indianapolis, Indiana, druggist, George W. Sloane.

25. Janik, *Marketplace of the Marvelous*, 204–7.

26. J. M. Toner, "Statistical Sketch of the Medical Profession in the United States," *Indiana Journal of Medicine* 4 (1873): 4–5.

27. The figure given for eclectic physicians as a percentage of all physicians in Philadelphia is derived from the author's review of all Philadelphia physicians

as listed in the *Medical and Surgical Directory of the United States* (New York: R. L. Polk and Co., 1886), 789–828.

28. Stephen Petrina, "Medical Liberty: Drugless Healers Confront Allopathic Doctors, 1910–1931," *Journal of the Medical Humanities* 29 (Dec. 2008): 213.

29. See "Buchananism," *EMJ* 40, no. 8 (Aug. 1880): 389; and "Not Our Joseph R. Buchanan," *EMJ* 40, no. 1 (Jan. 1880): 52.

30. George E. Potter, "Status of Eclectic Medicine: Pennsylvania," *Transactions of the National Eclectic Medical Association . . . for the Years 1886–87 . . .*" 14 (Orange, N.J.: Chronicle Book Printing Office, 1887), 85, 93.

31. Henry B. Piper, "Annual Address Before the National Eclectic Medical Association at Atlanta, Georgia, June 16, 1886," *Transactions of the National Eclectic Medical Association . . . for the Years 1886–87 . . .* , 52; "The Bogus Diploma Traffic," *EMJ* 41, no. 5 (May 1881): 243.

32. "Letter from Philadelphia: The Diploma Traffic," *BMSJ* 103, no. 3 (July 15, 1880): 65–66; "Medical Legislation," *CMG* 44, no. 10 (Oct. 1880): 325.

33. "A Buchanan Diploma Mill in California," *Pacific Medical and Surgical Journal* 23, no. 5 (Oct. 1880): 218–220, quotation on 219.

34. See "Buchanan's Disciples," *The Medical Standard* 6, no. 5 (Nov. 1889): 154; "At a Recent Meeting," *The Medical Standard* 6, no. 6 (Dec. 1889): 183–84.

35. "Letter from Philadelphia: The Diploma Traffic," *BMSJ* 103, no. 3 (July 15, 1880): 65; "Bogus Diploma Business," *Hahnemannian Monthly*, new series 2, no. 9 (Sept. 1880): 574.

36. See "Enforcing the Medical Practice Act in New York," *JAMA* 26, no. 12 (Mar. 21, 1896): 592; "Irregular Practitioners in Germany," *Ninth Annual Report of the State Board of Health and Vital Statistics of the Commonwealth of Pennsylvania* (Harrisburg, Pa.: Clarence Busch, state printer, 1894), 627–31.

37. "Diploma Vendors, Skunks," *EMJ* 41, no. 12 (Dec. 1881): 575–76; Appendix F4, *Legislative Council of New South Wales*, 89–90.

38. Historical matter from AMA Council on Medical Education, *Medical Colleges of the United States*, 8.

39. "Another Diploma Mill," *BMSJ* 107 (Dec. 7, 1882): 545–46; "A Typical Anti-Vaccinationist," *JAMA* 23, no. 2 (July 14, 1894): 83–84; Martin Kaufman, "American Medical Diploma Mills," *Medical Faculty Bulletin*, Tulane University 26 (1967): 56.

40. Historical matter from AMA Council on Medical Education, *Medical Colleges of the United States*, 12, 16.

41. "The Bogus Diploma Business in Boston," *MSR* 43, no. 16 (Oct. 16, 1880): 352; "Buchanan the Diplomatist as Confessor," *BMSJ* 104 (Apr. 7, 1881): 33; Appendix F4, *Legislative Council of New South Wales*, 96.

42. Illinois State Board of Health, *Conspectus of the Medical Colleges of America* (Springfield: H. W. Rokker, 1884), 79.

43. Kaufman, "American Medical Diploma Mills," 56.

44. Haller, *Kindly Medicine*, 74; "Philadelphia Diploma Shops," *CMG* 44, no. 8 (Aug. 1880): 262.

45. See historical matter from AMA Council on Medical Education, *Medical Colleges of the United States*, 6–17.

46. See the story series appearing on the front page of the *St. Louis Star*, from Oct. 15 through Oct. 25, 1923.

47. See "Laws Regulating the Practice of Medicine—State Boards of Health" and "Medicine and Special Legislation," *EMJ* 40, no. 1 (Jan. 1880): 48–49, and *EMJ* 40, no. 2 (Feb. 1880): 58.

48. Reginald Fitz, "Legislative Control of Medical Practice," *BMSJ* 131 (July 5, 1894): 1.

49. "State Boards," *EMJ* 40, no. 9 (Sept. 1880): 406. See also Mohr, *Licensed to Practice*, chs. 6–7, for the post-*Dent* push for medical legislation and a depiction of "hard-line Regularism" (p. 55) at the expense of irregulars during the early days of the West Virginia Board of Health.

50. Ludmerer, *Learning to Heal*, 234.

51. Johnson and Chaudhry, *Medical Licensing and Discipline*, 87–88.

52. Nathan Colwell, "Improvements in Medical Education in Sixteen Years," *Fed Bull* (Aug. 1920): 200; "Medical Education in the United States," *JAMA* 73, no. 7 (Aug. 16, 1919): 499–533, esp. 517.

53. Johnson and Chaudhry, *Medical Licensing and Discipline*, 36; Starr, *Social Transformation*, 115.

54. Illinois State Board of Health, *Conspectus of Medical Colleges*, xxiv–xxv.

55. Ibid., xxv–xxvi.

Epilogue

1. Buchanan's children prevailed in the courts. The judge labeled Russell's testimony as "conflicting" and filled with unsubstantiated facts. See *Buchanan et al. v. Buchanan*, *Atlantic Reporter*, 68 A. (St. Paul, Minn.: West Publishing Co., 1908), 780–84.

2. Unless otherwise indicated, the sources for descriptions of Buchanan's death and estate trial are drawn from "Say Doctor's Clerk Took His Estate," *PhInq*, Jan. 10, 1908, 3; "Sister Was Not Buchanan's Child," *PhInq*, Jan. 11, 1908, 2; "Reba Hurff Buchanan Faints in Court," *Bridgeton (N.J.) Evening News*, Jan. 11, 1908, 2; "Veiled Woman Lavish with Cash," *PhRec*, Jan. 10, 1908, 3; "Faints in Court at Name Sister," *PhRec*, Jan. 11, 1908, 3; and "Buchanan Tangle up to the Court," *PhRec*, Jan. 12, 1908, 3.

3. "Died: Buchanan," *PhInq*, Feb. 28, 1873, 4.

4. "Denounces Sister in Court," *NYT*, Jan. 11, 1908, 9.

5. "Decides Against Miss Hurff," *New York Sun*, Jan. 22, 1908, 4.

6. "Died: Sites," *PhInq*, Oct. 31, 1878, 5.

7. "Necrology," *JAMA* (Nov. 28, 1896): 1169.

8. "Obituaries: Marshall Calkins, M.D.," *BMSJ* (Dec. 14, 1922): 906.

9. See William Paine Papers, box 32, folder 905, Eclectic Medical College Records, 1845–1942; Collection No. 3, Series X. Lloyd Library and Museum, Cincinnati, Ohio; "Dr. Paine Arrested," *PhInq*, Mar. 13, 1892, 5; "The Peabody Hotel," *PhInq*, July 21, 1892, 6.

10. "Surprise to Dr. Bowlsby," *Brooklyn Daily Eagle*, Mar. 4, 1901, 5; "Obituary—Dr. William H. Bowlsby," *Brooklyn Daily Eagle*, Aug. 28, 1901, 3; "Is It a Clue?" *NYTrib*, Oct. 26, 1871, 12.

11. "Rosenzweig," *NYH*, Feb. 23, 1873, 7; "Jacob Rosenzweig," *New York Evening Post*, Nov. 13, 1873, 3; "Pages of Foolscap," *Auburn Daily Bulletin*, Nov. 18, 1873, 4.

12. See "Dr. Buchanan's Son on Trial," *PhInq*, Mar. 30, 1883, 8; "Grand Jury Work," *PhInq*, July 9, 1890, 5; "A Business Venture: 'Dr.' George Buchanan Unsuccessfully Tries the Shoe Trade," *PhInq*, July 27, 1890, 6; "Dr. Buchanan Acquitted," *PhInq*, Apr. 7, 1891, 7.

13. "Dentist Held for Court," *PhT*, Nov. 26, 1885, 3; "Whipped," *PhT*, May 5, 1886, 3; "Police Intelligence," *PhInq*, Mar. 2, 1883, 3; "Dr. Chapman to Pay $5 Per Week," *PhInq*, July 11, 1883, 2; "New Jersey News Notes," *PhInq*, May 22, 1902, 3; "Dentist Will Make a Fight," *PhRec*, Apr. 24, 1902,3; *Beecher's Manual and Dental Directory of the United States* (New York: Beecher and Co., 1884), 118; *Boyd's Business Directory of Philadelphia City* (Philadelphia, Pa.: C. E. Howe Co., 1900), 150.

14. "John Norris Dies in His 58th Year," *NYT*, Mar. 22, 1914.

15. "Palmer, Henry Wilbur (1839–1913)," Biographical Directory of the United States Congress (website), http://bioguide.congress.gov/scripts/biodisplay.pl?index=P000040.

16. "Gendell Takes Meredith's Place," *PhInq*, Dec. 27, 1906, 2; "City Solicitor Gendell Yields to Long Illness," *PhInq*, Nov. 14, 1910, 1.

17. "The Story of a Busy Life," *NYT*, June 28, 1894; "William M. Singerly Dead," *NYT*, Feb. 28, 1898, 7; *Dictionary of American Biography*, s.v. "Singerly, William M."

18. "Resignation of Dr. Rauch," *BMSJ* 125, no. 3 (July 16, 1891): 68; "Dr. John H. Rauch," *JAMA* 51 (Dec. 12, 1908): 2074–75; John Moses, *Illinois: Historical and Statistical* (Chicago: Fergus Printing Co., 1892), 1037–38.

Index

Page numbers in italics refer to illustrations.

Buchanan and Company, 228–31
Bureau of Education (U.S. Interior Department), 142
Butler, Samuel Worcester, 90
Butler (U.S. District Court judge), 153, 165, 197–204
Buzzell, James M., 34, 55

California, medical licensing in, 122
Calkins, Marshall, 31–32, 34, 37, 55, 243
calomel, 17–18, 20, 23
Campbell, J. P., 85
Canon of Medicine (Avicenna), 4
Catto, Octavius, 87
Centennial Practice of Medicine, The (Buchanan), 46, 47
Central Medical College of New York, 28
Chapman, Martin V.: bail for Buchanan by, 153; and Buchanan's "suicide," xxv, 162, 165, 170; on EMC faculty, 111; extradition and escape by, 190–97; later legal troubles of, 220, 245; in Michigan and Canada, 172, 176–88; trial and sentencing of, 197–98, 204
Chase, Thomas G., 29–31
Chatfield, Charles, 67
Chatham Planet, 175–76
"Cherry Hill," 206. *See also* Eastern State Penitentiary
cholera epidemic (1848–1849), 19–22, 24
Christian Recorder, 84
Cincinnati Medical Gazette, 150
Civil War: and medical licensing laws, 115–16; and medical school enrollment, 41, 56–57; postwar political structure of Philadelphia, 81
Clark, William, 53
Cleary, Daniel, 153
Cochran, James, 37, 71, 152
College Courant, 67–73
College of Medicine of Maryland, 61
Comstock Law (1873), 106
Conklin, Walter, 75
Connecticut: diploma mills in, 234; and medical regulation in antebellum era, 22
consultation clause (American Medical Association), 25
Cook, William H., 234
Cooke, Thomas: and early eclecticism, 10–11; EMC departure by, 55; EMC early operations, 29–30, 32, 34, 35;

EMC founding by, 17–18, 26–29
Court of Quarter Sessions (Philadelphia), 196–97, 215
Coyle, Thomas, 163–65
Craik, James, 18
Cregar, Phillip A., 147, 156–57
Croswell, Charles, 184, 191
Culpeper, Nicholas, 7
Curtis, Alva, 10, 11, 14–15, 234

Darling, H. E. (Buchanan), 175
Davies, Idris, 92, 94–95
Davis, Jonathan, 85, 96
Davis, Nathan, 221
Dawson, George Austin (Norris), 144, 148, 156, 191–93, 200
Dawson, Henry (Norris), 144–45, 191–92
"Death of Marie Roget, The" (Poe), 75
DeBeust, Robert H., 76–77
degree of merit, Buchanan's definition of, 93
Dent v. West Virginia, 235
de Tocqueville, Alexis, 207
Detroit Eclectic Medical College, 148, 175, 190
Detroit Free Press: on Buchanan's whereabouts, 171–74; pursuit of Buchanan by, 181–89
Detroit University for Rational Medicine and Surgery, 175
Dick, Elisha, 18
Dickens, Charles, 204–5
Diller, David, 152
diploma sales: African American students sought by EMC, 53–55; *Allen v. Buchanan*, 100–103, 108, 139; "Buchanan diplomas," 232–33; Buchanan's arrest (1880, Michigan), 181–88; Buchanan's arrest (1880, Philadelphia), 148–59; Buchanan's arrest (1885), 224–27; Buchanan's Detroit eclectic school plans, 148, 175, 190, 214; Buchanan's purchase of blank diplomas, 107; Buchanan's *Record* interview about, 210–15; Buchanan's sales following legal challenges of 1872, 108–11; and business model of nineteenth-century colleges, 61–62; early newspaper accounts of, 67–74; estimated number of diplomas sold, 149, 212, 233; and faculty turnover at EMC, 55, 153; and financial

materia medica and Buchanan's writing, 47; and orthodox medical profession's criticism of, 62–63, 231–32; and
orthodox medical profession's scan-
dals, 17–22; regulation in antebellum
era, 22–25; rise of eclectic medicine,
10–16; size of industry, 118, 231
*Eclectic Practice of Medicine and Surgery,
The* (Buchanan), 46, 47
Eden Methodist Church (Philadelphia),
139
Edinburgh University (Missouri and Chi-
cago), 233
Educational Committee of the State Leg-
islature, 212
Edwards, Davis, xxv
Elliot, William, 86–88, 96
EMC. *See* Eclectic Medical College
(EMC) of Pennsylvania
*Encyclopedia of the Practice of Medicine
Based on Bacteriology, An* (Buchanan),
46, 47
*Epitome of the Eclectic Practice of Medicine,
The* (Paine), 34
European Anatomical, Pathological and
Ethnological Museum (Philadelphia),
70
Evans, George O., 98
Everts, William, 142
Everybody a Swimmer (Coyle), 168
"Evil of the Age, The" (*New York Times*),
75–76
examining boards, inception of, 237–38.
See also medical licensing laws

Fairchild (Buchanan), 172
Fairman, George, 90
*Family Physician and Domestic Practice of
Medicine, The* (Buchanan), 46, 47,
220–24
Fanning, John William (Norris), 144–46,
148, 156, 191–94, 200
Female Medical College of Pennsylva-
nia, 52
Fitler, Joseph, 80, 81, 86, 103
Fitzpatrick, John (Buchanan's son-in-
law), 157–59
Fitzpatrick, John (decoy), 158
Fitzpatrick, W. L., 245
Fletcher, W. J., 157, 159
Fondey, John, 32, 34, 35, 49, 55, 103

Foster, J. (Buchanan), 178
Foster, Walter H. ("W. H. Foster," "Fos-
ter"), 161, 214
Four Years at Yale (Chatfield), 67
Fox, Daniel, 83, 87
Franklin, Benjamin, 205
Franklin Medical College, 27
Fulmer, John J., 156

Galen, 4–5
Gamble, William, xxii
Geary, John W., 98
Gendell, J. Howard, 131, 134, 183, 247
Germany: Buchanan on diploma sales in,
213; White on diploma sales to, xxiv–
xxv, 142, 145–48, 156
Germicide, The, 229, 229–30
Gibbons, John, 149, 153, 197
Givin, Samuel, 149, 167–68
Glasgow College, 45, 212, 219
Godman, John, 5
Goodrich, J. T., 54
Gove, Mary, 8
Graham, Sylvester, 8
Gram, Hans Burch, 8
Great Britain, Buchanan on diploma sales
in, 213
Green, Job, 181

Hack, J. W. H., 85
Hahnemann, Samuel, 8–9
Hahnemannian Monthly, 81
Hahnemann Medical College (Philadel-
phia), 124
Hall, John, 85
Hamilton, W. R. (journalist), xxii, xxvi
Hamilton, William (engraver), 225
Hanmore, Howard, 97
Harbison, William C., 96, 161–62, 214
Harrison, William Henry, 17–18, 21–22
Harvard Medical School, 22, 32, 126,
221–22
Haviland, John, 206
head draping practice, of prisoners,
204–5
Hearst, William Randolph, 246
Hering, Constantine, 8
History of Medicine, The (Wilder), 29
*History of the American Eclectic Practice of
Medicine* (Paine), 35
Holland, Joseph B., 34

Philadelphia Press: on diploma sales, 67–68, 73–74, 82, 97; Norris's career at, 135
Philadelphia Public Ledger, 135, 136
Philadelphia Record, 131–59; on Buchanan family discord, 220, 242; Buchanan interview by, 210–15; on Buchanan's arrest (1885), 225; and Buchanan's extradition to Pennsylvania, 189–97; and Buchanan's mail fraud indictment, xxiv, xxv; and Buchanan's medical training, 45; and Buchanan's obscenity charge, 105–6; on Buchanan's "suicide," xxii–xxvii, 167, 168; and Buchanan's trials (1880), 197–204; on Buchanan's use of bribery, 100, 105; editorial by, 203–4; and EMC arrests, 152–59; on EMC closure, 128; and EMC sting operation, 142–51; location of, 148; Pennsylvania attorney general's meeting with, 131–34, *133;* Philadelphia University exposed by, 134–42; and pursuit of Buchanan in Michigan, 168, 181–88; Singerley's ownership of, 131–38, *133, 137,* 181–82, 247. *See also* Norris, John
Philadelphia School of Anatomy, 37
Philadelphia Times, 135, 141–42
Philadelphia University: and American College of Medicine, 34, 39; charter revoked, 141; Illinois State Board of Health on, 127–28; inception of, 39–41; Paine's rivalry with Buchanan, 37–41, *38,* 79, 211; Pennsylvania state legislature inquiry of, 90, 97–99; *Philadelphia Record*'s exposure of, 132, 134–42; as Philadelphia University of Medicine and Surgery, *13,* 39, *39, 40;* and physician registry, 218–19
phrenology, 8
physicians: population of (nineteenth century), 118, 231; professionalization trend of medical field, 115 (*see also* medical licensing laws); quacks (term origin), 122. *See also* eclectic medicine history; medical education; medical licensing laws; orthodox medicine (allopathy); *individual names of medical schools*
Physicians' Protective Register, 219
Physio-Eclectic Medical College (Cincinnati), 234

Physiological and Therapeutic Uses of Our New Remedies, The (Buchanan), 46, 47
Physio-Medical College (Cincinnati), 234
Physio-Medicals, 10, 14
Pinel, Philippe, 5
Poe, Edgar Allan, 75
Polk, Charles G., 152, 192
Polk, James, 18
Potter, Stephen H., 29–30, 34, 35, 55
Potter, Thomas, 43
Practical Treatise on Midwifery and Diseases of Women and Children, A (Buchanan), 46, 145
Practical Treatise on the Diseases of Children (Buchanan), *43,* 46
prostitution: Buchanan on legalization of, 50; Buchanan's alleged brothel plans, 195
pseudo-homeopaths, 14
public health concerns. *See* medical licensing laws
Puck, "The Philadelphia Physician Factory" (cartoon), *143*
Pulitzer, Joseph, 246
Pure Food and Drug Act (1906), 230–31
purgatives, 6–7, 9, 17–18, 20, 24, 47

quacks, term origin for, 122

Rand, Howard, 90–92, 94–95
Randall, William M., 90
Rauch, John, 122–28, *123,* 247
Rauch, William, xxii
Recherches sur les Effets de la Saignee (Louis), 19–20
Reed, Joseph, 67–68, 97
Reformed Medical College of Georgia, 28
Reformed Medical College of New York, 11
Registration Act (1869), 82
Reinhardt Brothers, 229
Reuter (federal deputy marshall), 149
Revels, Hiram, 85
Revels, Willis Richardson (W. R.), 85–86, *86*
Rhode Island, and regulation in antebellum era, 22
Robinson, Professor (Mumey), 176
Rogers, Mary, 75
Rogers, Robert E., 89–91
Roney, W. C., 175